Indigenous Cultures and Mental Health Counselling

North America's Indigenous population is a vulnerable group, with specific psychological and healing needs that are not widely met in the mental health care system. Indigenous peoples face certain historical, cultural-linguistic, and socioeconomic barriers to mental health care access that government, health care organizations, and social agencies must work to overcome. This volume examines ways Indigenous healing practices can complement Western psychological service to meet the needs of Indigenous peoples through traditional cultural concepts. Bringing together leading experts in the fields of Aboriginal mental health and psychology, it provides data and models of Indigenous cultural practices in psychology that are successful with Indigenous peoples. It considers Indigenous epistemologies in applied psychology and research methodology and informs government policy on mental health services for these populations.

Suzanne L. Stewart (Yellowknife Dene First Nation) is a psychologist and Associate Professor of Indigenous healing in Clinical and Counselling Psychology at the Ontario Institute for Studies in Education, University of Toronto, Canada.

Roy Moodley is Associate Professor of Clinical and Counselling psychology in the Department of Applied Psychology and Human Development at the Ontario Institute for Studies in Education, University of Toronto, Canada.

Ashley Hyatt is a doctoral student of Clinical and Counselling Psychology at the Ontario Institute for Studies in Education, University of Toronto, Canada.

Explorations in Mental Health Series

For a full list of titles in this series, please visit www.routledge.com

Books in this series:

Psychological Approaches to Understanding and Treating Auditory Hallucinations
From theory to therapy
Edited by Mark Hayward, Clara Strauss and Simon McCarthy-Jones

Primitive Expression and Dance Therapy
When dancing heals
France Schott-Billmann

A Theory-Based Approach to Art Therapy
Implications for teaching, research and practice
Ephrat Huss

The Interactive World of Severe Mental Illness
Case Studies from the U.S. Mental Health System
Diana J. Semmelhack, Larry Ende, Arthur Freeman, and Clive Hazell with Colleen L. Barron and Garry L. Treft

Therapeutic Assessment and Intervention in Childcare Legal Proceedings
Engaging families in successful rehabilitation
Mike Davies

Trauma, Survival and Resilience in War Zones
The psychological impact of war in Sierra Leone and beyond
David A. Winter, Rachel Brown, Stephanie Goins and Clare Mason

Cultural Foundations and Interventions in Latino/a Mental Health
History, Theory, and within Group Differences
Hector Y. Adames & Nayeli Y. Chavez-Dueñas

Indigenous Cultures and Mental Health Counselling
Four Directions for Integration With Counselling Psychology
Edited by Suzanne L. Stewart, Roy Moodley, and Ashley Hyatt

Indigenous Cultures and Mental Health Counselling

Four Directions for Integration With Counselling Psychology

Edited by Suzanne L. Stewart, Roy Moodley, and Ashley Hyatt

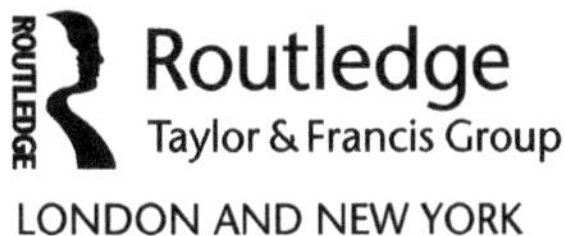

LONDON AND NEW YORK

First published 2017 by Routledge

2 Park Square, Milton Park, Abingdon, Oxfordshire OX14 4RN
52 Vanderbilt Avenue, New York, NY 10017

Routledge is an imprint of the Taylor & Francis Group, an informa business

First issued in paperback 2018

Library of Congress Cataloguing-in-Publication Data
Names: Stewart, Suzanne L., editor. | Moodley, Roy, editor. | Hyatt, Ashley, editor.
Title: Indigenous cultures and mental health counselling : four directions for integration with counselling psychology / edited by Suzanne L. Stewart, Roy Moodley, and Ashley Hyatt.
Description: New York : Routledge, [2016] | Series: Explorations in mental health series ; 16
Identifiers: LCCN 2016013995 | ISBN 9781138928992 (hardback) | ISBN 9781315681467 (ebk)
Subjects: LCSH: Indians of North America—Mental health. | Indians of North America—Mental health services. | Indians of North America—Counseling of. | Community mental health services—North America. | Ethnopsychology—North America.
Classification: LCC RC451.5.I5 I64 2016 | DDC 362.2/208997—dc23
LC record available at https://lccn.loc.gov/2016013995

ISBN: 978-1-138-92899-2 (hbk)
ISBN: 978-0-367-19615-8 (pbk)

Typeset in Sabon
by Apex CoVantage, LLC

Contents

Foreword

Indigenous Healing Past and Present: Exploding Persistent Binaries

As a clinically trained, community engaged, and culturally attuned research psychologist, I explore the significance of "mental health" policies, practices, and institutions for community life in Native North America. On one hand, in the long wake of European settler colonization, Indigenous communities still reel from state-sponsored programs of subjugation that have fostered epidemic levels of debilitating distress. In the current historical moment, such distress is officially managed—when it is officially managed at all—through the technologies of the psy-disciplines as deployed in clinical settings under the rubric of "health care." In consequence, psychology and psychotherapy have achieved substantial inroads within Native community life, almost always as a result of external government support and sponsorship. On the other hand, in response to these palpable legacies of colonial subjugation, Native peoples have embarked on agentic projects of community renewal and self-determination. These efforts typically involve contemporary commitments to Indigenous cultural reclamation and revitalization, including the rediscovery and deployment of ancestral therapeutic traditions in service to individual and collective healing. As a result, Native spirituality and ritual practice have emerged as powerful and compelling alternatives for redressing community dysfunction, reconstituting collective identity, and resisting the hegemonic ideologies of surrounding settler societies.

Thus, *both* professional clinical and "traditional" spiritual approaches to therapeutic intervention for "mental health" problems are available in most Native communities and to most Native-identified individuals today. Some Indigenous persons in distress avail themselves of both kinds of therapies (as well as additional complementary and alternative health practices), while others avail themselves of neither kind, preferring instead to rely on personal fortitude and hardiness to guard their minds from intrusion by untrusted professionals and to protect their personal autonomy from external constraint. Perhaps more than ever before—owing to long histories of encounter, exchange, subjugation, and assimilation—we are witnessing the collapse of familiar and influential oppositions long used to characterize Native and Euro-North Americans: civilized versus savage, modern versus traditional, Western versus Indigenous, and so forth. For, as cultural psychologist Richard Shweder (1994) has observed, "In a postmodern world, your ancestry is less important than your travel plans" (p. 15). In short, cultural essentialism is out and cultural "hybridism" is in. Such is the broad global context for efforts dedicated to "Indigenizing mental health." As one fascinating and important expression of this commitment, this significant and substantial book undertakes a process of illuminating the indigenous paradigm in the theory and practice of counselling and psychotherapy.

Toward similar ends, one alternative I pursue with my Indigenous community partners is the appraisal of certain "traditional" healing practices with regard to their suitability for inclusion within established health clinics that serve American Indians. It seems impossible to undertake such work, however, without abutting questions such as the following: *What is American Indian traditional healing? Who is an authentic Native traditional healer?* These potentially contentious queries betray an even more fundamental set of concerns in Native North America surrounding privileged access to Indigenous tradition per se. In this regard, as a provocation to intellectual engagement, I sometimes ask American Indian audiences in the United States to nominate the individuals they consider to be the most renowned Native American healers of, not the 19th century, but rather the 20th century. I myself propose two names: the Lakota holy man Black Elk (*Hehaka Sapa*, 1863–1950), who famously "spoke" through the American poet John Neihardt in 1932 (DeMallie, 1984), and the Cherokee/Choctaw televangelist Granville Oral Roberts (1918–2009), who rose from obscurity in rural Oklahoma to preside over a multimillion-dollar healing ministry (Herrell, 1985). The fun in pairing these two individuals is the surprise inclusion of Oral Roberts, who most do not think of as Native American,[1] and Christian faith healing, which most do not think of as a spiritual tradition worthy of therapeutic credence.

One irony, of course, is that even Black Elk was an extremely devout Christian for the majority of his adult life—he converted to Roman Catholicism around age forty, repenting from his Indigenous ceremonial practices and bringing hundreds of other Indians into the church during his subsequent life as a catechist and missionary. A second irony is that a small but visible minority of Indigenous people in tribal communities throughout North America today continue to actively practice Oral Roberts–style (i.e., "charismatic," "seed faith," or "word of faith") Christian healing. We might wonder, then, at what point does Indigenous participation in such practices render them Indigenous healing traditions. Again, in response to such thorny questions, we are invited to consider issues of cultural authenticity and historical continuity with the ancestral past. Importantly, such considerations are not limited to cross-sectional religious comparisons within any given Indigenous community but also pertain to intergenerational dynamics within particular Native families. I offer as illustration an example from my own extended family that has lived as part of the Gros Ventre tribal community for generations on the Fort Belknap Reservation in North Central Montana. In the summer of 1994, as part of a project associated with my studies at school, I interviewed my own grandmother, Mrs. Bertha (Gone) Snow (1918–2016), in an effort to understand Gros Ventre cultural identity in Gros Ventre terms.

Among the many things I learned from this conversation was her own (ambivalent) convictions about Gros Ventre healing tradition. For most of my lifetime, my late grandmother was the matriarch of the Gone family, the firstborn of Frederick P. and Mary (John) Gone. During her long life, she spanned a remarkably shifting reservation social world, including interactions with monolingual Gros Ventre–speaking grandparents who lived the celebrated life of the equestrian buffalo hunt, bilingual parents who were converts to Roman Catholicism and who believed that the future prospects of the Gros Ventre people depended on forsaking Gros Ventre traditions to better compete in a White-dominated world, and children and grandchildren who sought to return to the Gros Ventre tradition in the wake of the Red Power movement of the 1970s. With specific reference to Gros Ventre traditions, then, Grandma Bertha was exposed to these interactions to the degree that they featured in early 20th-century reservation life. She herself witnessed an old-time Gros Ventre "sucking" doctor, Spotted Bird, treat her ailing infant sister when Grandma was a small girl (as recounted in Gone, 2010). But most of her views on traditional matters resulted from the authoritative descriptions and interpretations offered to her by her father, Fred Gone (1886–1967). Interestingly, as a consequence of these experiences, Grandma expressed considerable respect for the power of early reservation-era Gros Ventre medicine men.

For example, Grandma told me the following story about one of our famed medicine men named Stiffarm during our conversation in 1994. Note that her father, who later recounted the story to his eldest daughter, directly witnessed the event, which she then told to me, partly in her father's voice, using quoted speech in keeping with Gros Ventre narrative tradition:

> They called [Old Man] Stiffarm to come and doctor [this woman]. And there's certain songs they sing. Four times they sing . . . to call this medicine, to get it to going. And my grandma and grandpa was there. And my dad was there, and he was singing. And, here, he said, "Stiffarm had a ferret pelt, about that big, about that long. Round one. Then he went and put it over there by the door, and this woman was laying over there." And [Stiffarm would] back away from [that ferret pelt while blowing a bone whistle], just like he was coaxing it with that whistle . . . He was blowing it, and he'd back up towards that woman. Pretty soon this [ferret pelt] moved, come this way. And [Stiffarm would] come after it again, and he'd blow his whistle. And [that ferret] would go [that way].

Clearly, in order for the lifeless pelt of this ferret to move in this way, sacred power was involved. Such animating power was a core feature of Northern Plains Indian religious understanding and was arguably the central attribute of historical Indigenous healing practices.

As if the ritual animation of the ferret pelt was not amazing enough, what happened next, according to Grandma, was truly astonishing:

> About the fourth time [Stiffarm] did that, [this ferret] just . . . lit right in there, just buried his head in this woman's stomach. And he pulled something out. "It looked like a tumor," [my dad] said, "about that big around. He showed it to us. He put it in our hands." In the meantime, he had them make a fire outside. And dad said, "There was veins. It looked like a tumor with veins all over it," he said. "You could see the veins. It felt like a piece of liver, but it had a membrane over it, like a gland. It looked like a big gland," he said. "He showed it to us. He put it in my hand . . . It was bloody," he said. Then, here, this ferret was laying alongside of her. It was a hide again. Just a dried hide. But they'd seen it attack her and go in. And so they took [that tumor] out, and they put it in that fire, and it burnt up. Now that's what you call a medicine man!

Thus not only did Grandma credit old man Stiffarm with remarkable doctoring power, but she also passed along her regard by narrating this account in the context of kinship relations spanning four generations (see also, Gone, 1999; Gone, Miller, & Rappaport, 1999). Most importantly, she told this story to underscore a specific, important point for younger generations of Gros Ventres.

That point, in sum, was that bona fide Gros Ventre "ways" are gone. In other words, for Grandma, there was no historical continuity of authentic Gros Ventre sacred tradition, including Gros Ventre healing tradition. Instead, she asserted, "that power is gone":

> My kids, you know, they depend on what I tell them. I just tell them what I think I know, what I got from my grandfolks, and my dad. They told me that there was no such thing [as exercising power] anymore. It's gone. All those that had that power is gone. And I don't think there's a living soul today that can go up there on [that mountaintop to fast and pray for a vision] and get power.

In fact, a major function of the Stiffarm narrative for Grandma was that modern claims to authentic healing power require strong supporting evidence: "You got to prove that power. You got to prove it beyond a doubt. My dad had proof of power of a medicine man right in his hand." And so, her clear message for younger generations of her family (and perhaps for younger tribal members more generally) underscored the end of authenticity and the discontinuity of sacred (healing) tradition on the Fort Belknap Reservation sometime during the early part of the 20th century, when all the "old-timers" (of her grandparents generation) had passed on. And yet today, even at Fort Belknap and against all odds, sacred tradition has once more been renewed.

More specifically, as the contributors to this book make so plainly evident, an important component of such cultural and spiritual renewal is the reclamation or revitalization of Indigenous healing traditions. These contemporary healing traditions find clear lines of continuity with the past even as they have been reconfigured for modern modes of living in Indigenous communities. They are less likely today to entail dramatically visible workings of power; indeed, even the language of sacred "power" has been displaced by its New Age counterpart: "energy." They are less likely today to be deployed for restorative healing (i.e., curing discrete sicknesses) and more likely to be adopted for transformative healing (i.e., reorienting vulnerable selves) in Indigenous lives (Waldram, 2013). They are more likely today to presume or instill a robust psychological-mindedness in keeping with globalized "therapy culture" (Furedi, 2004). Finally, they are not uncommonly used in integration with or as adjunctive to biomedicine, as well as in concert with a wide range of other designated "complementary and alternative" health discourses and practices (Gone, 2011). And why not, given that Indigenous people today exist in so many respects as both modern and "Western"? In sum, many contemporary Indigenous healing traditions throughout North America are now ideally suited for integration with counselling and psychotherapy in the mental health domain.

As a consequence, this volume is a wonderful introduction and thorough orientation to the role that traditional healing might play in addressing the "mental health" concerns of Indigenous communities at the outset of a new millennium. We are fortunate to benefit from its many insights.

Joseph P. Gone
University of Michigan

Note

1. The case of Oral Roberts is actually controversial and illustrates the sensitive ethnoracial politics of American Indian identity in the USA. Roberts routinely claimed Cherokee ancestry through his mother, Claudius Priscilla (Irwin) Roberts. This acknowledgement provides one criterion by which American Indian ethnoracial identity might be attributed: self-identification. Interestingly, census entries for Roberts's family recorded during his Oklahoma youth show that all members of his immediate circle—including his mother—were listed as "White" for U.S. census purposes. This designation provides another criterion by which American Indian ethnoracial identity might be attributed: government ascription. In 1963, Roberts was selected as "American Indian of the Year" by the organizers of the Oklahoma American Indian Exposition, an annual Native-run powwow and fair. He is still listed on their roster of honorees as "Choctaw." This appreciation provides a third criterion by which American Indian ethnoracial identity might

be attributed: recognition within the Native community. Finally, Wikipedia—apparently on the basis of other unsubstantiated Internet sources—asserts that Roberts was a "card-carrying member" of the Choctaw Nation of Oklahoma. Intrigued by the possibility that Roberts or his mother may have been enrolled tribal members, I contacted a colleague at the Cherokee Nation of Oklahoma in 2011 to see whether they maintain any record of Roberts or his ancestors on their tribal rolls—they reportedly do not. I also contacted the enrollment office of the Choctaw Nation of Oklahoma, but they invoked privacy rules prohibiting the release of any information about Roberts's status with the tribe. Irrespective of the outcome, this possibility provides a fourth criterion by which American Indian ethnoracial identity might be attributed: tribal enrollment (or citizenship).

References

DeMallie, R. J. (Ed.) (1984). *The sixth grandfather: Black Elk's teachings given to John G. Neihardt*. Lincoln, NE: University of Nebraska Press.

Furedi, F. (2004). *Therapy culture: Cultivating vulnerability in an uncertain age*. London: Routledge.

Gone, J. P. (1999). "We were through as Keepers of it": The "Missing Pipe Narrative" and Gros Ventre cultural identity. *Ethos, 27*(4), 415–440.

Gone, J. P. (2010). Psychotherapy and traditional healing for American Indians: Exploring the prospects for therapeutic integration. *The Counseling Psychologist, 38*(2), 166–235.

Gone, J. P. (2011). The red road to wellness: Cultural reclamation in a Native First Nations community treatment center. *American Journal of Community Psychology, 47*(1–2), 187–202.

Gone, J. P., Miller, P. J., & Rappaport, J. (1999). Conceptual self as normatively oriented: The suitability of past personal narrative for the study of cultural identity. *Culture & Psychology, 5*(4), 371–398.

Herrell, Jr., D. E. (1985). *Oral Roberts: An American life*. Bloomington, IN: Indiana University Press.

Shweder, R. A. (1994). Fundamentalism for highbrows: The aims of education address at the University of Chicago. *Academe, 80*(6), 13–21.

Waldram, J. B. (2013). Transformative and restorative processes: Revisiting the question of efficacy in indigenous healing. *Medical Anthropology, 32*(3), 191–207.

Preface

Although the growth of multicultural counselling and psychotherapy has been increasing since the 1960s, there has been very little research and publication on Indigenous healing practices (see Duran, 2006; Gone, 2010; McCormick, 2005; Poonwassie & Charter, 2005; Stewart, 2008). As Gone (2010) states, "Despite routine celebrations of indigenous healing practices within the multicultural counseling literature, almost no substantive description and explication of specific forms of traditional healing and associated therapeutic paradigms have been published" (p. 226). The traditional knowledge that gave rise to these practices and the ways in which psychology theory building can be advanced through the inclusion of Indigenous healing methods is still to be explored in a systematic and creative way. Indeed, there are several courageous attempts to infuse culture into counselling psychology (see Arthur & Collins, 2005; Pedersen & Lonner, 2015; Vontress, 2010), but with a breadth of areas and issues to be focused on, there was very little room left for Indigenous healing practices to get the quality of discussion it deserves.

However, there is wide spread acknowledgement and acceptance within the multicultural counselling and psychotherapy movement that there is tremendous potential for clinical practice if Indigenous healing methods are explored and systemically discussed in the mainstream mental health disciplines (McCormick, 2005; Stewart, 2008). The need to engage with First Nations and other Indigenous healers and healing is paramount since mainstream counselling psychology is in a crisis, having exhausted its repetitive therapeutic approaches, and is now in need of newer models and methods to add to its repertoire of healing. While Indigenous healing traditions date back to thousands of years, they could also be seen as therapeutic ways for the future, where the rich knowledges of the distant past are frameworks within which future discomforts and psychological distress could be addressed, such as stress and environment changes, innovations in human relational practices, and the use of sacred ceremonies in the search for truth and reconciliation. Moreover, the imperative for the use of Indigenous healing traditions is political, particularly for North American Indigenous communities. Through the ruthlessness of colonialism, Indigenous healing was delegitimized, prohibited, and forbidden. The focus on Indigenous research and theory building in psychology will provide Indigenous and non-Indigenous scholars with capabilities to reclaim wisdoms of the past, recontextualize traditional knowledges in the land of its origin, and establish a form of critical resistance towards the colonial project (much of which still remains intact today). Psychology's engagement with Indigenous healing practices will clearly address the larger questions of human rights and cultural rights, the issue of equity and diversity related to culturally relevant mental health services for Indigenous clients, and many more. The critical issue for any form of engagement with Indigenous healers and healing methods by Western psychology is not solely about integration, however noble this pursuit is and will always be, but the fundamental issue is the question of rights and freedom of Indigenous communities to practice and receive their own traditions of healing in a context within which they are able to make choices about their health and quality of life.

While the political and ideological frame constructs the motivation to engage with Indigenous and traditional healing, Gone (2010) offers a timely reminder of the ideological dilemma and complexity within which any pursuit of Indigenous healing is engaged with in the face of modernity. Joseph Gone succinctly puts forth the argument that

> Native people who are choosing to engage in community-based projects of cultural reclamation and revitalization without succumbing to a postmodern nostalgia for some pristine and untainted "authentic" premodern indigenous tradition by which all subsequent modifications and adaptations are found wanting in comparison. Processes of cultural change are endemic in the human condition, and despite much Native grief in the face of sudden and pervasive colonial disruptions, exiling indigenous peoples to the conceptual state of eternal premodernity will not serve Native interests in an increasingly globalized world.
>
> (p. 215)

Clearly, any engagement with Indigenous healing tradition is a sociocultural and political act(ion). If integration, which is loosely defined in the social sciences as bringing together peoples of different ethnicities into unrestricted and equal associations, is applied to Indigenous healing traditions, the problems of such a process tend to surface. Given the colonial legacy in North America, it seems unlikely that integration is possible or desirable at the current stage in the process and perhaps not until the complex question of land rights, reparations, and restitutions are addressed adequately. For equality to be experienced by Indigenous peoples, Western psychology may need to start with these questions rather then look for ways in which Indigenous healing traditions can be appropriated for its utility to prompt a Western healing science that is fast becoming outdated and culturally irrelevant in a multicultural and multiracial society.

Moving in the direction of integration, Duran (2006) in *Healing the Soul Wound*, introduced the concept of hybridism, which is defined as the bringing together of the best of two worldviews, Indigenous and Western, into the practice of counselling psychology. In the spirit of hybridism, all the chapters in this book are constructed through a post-structuralist framework, which sets the tone for integration by using an Indigenous paradigm of knowledges: the Indigenous four sacred directions are used as the thematic sections formatted to enter a realm of creativity, healing, and wellness. The four directions were chosen by us to honor Indigenous knowledge systems as the central concept within which local, traditional, and Indigenous meanings can be resymbolized so that the principles and values of Indigeneity can be shared and not reconfigured within Western psychology and counselling. It is our understanding, through cultural teachings and experiences, that all healing for all people begins with the spiritual, as put forth by the four directions, thus the first section of the book is the easterly direction, often known by many Indigenous peoples to represent the spirit.

The spiritual aspect of healing work is just one aspect of the Indigenizing psychology movement. Indigenizing psychology thus becomes an imperative, not only for Indigenous clients and practitioners but also for all users of psychology. With this objective and value in mind, the various chapters in this book present a range of theoretical and empirical accounts of the dilemmas and issues facing both students and professionals in the mental health fields and how these may be remediated in counselling psychology, graduate mental health education, and academic research. In exploring these dynamics, the chapters in this book contribute to an understanding of the nature of current shifts in professional psychological practice, particularly in relation to knowledge transfer, integration of Western and Indigenous healing and pedagogies, cross-cultural collaborations, Indigenous research methodologies, traditional prevention and control of specific disorders, and clinical and ethical accountability. Ultimately, the chapters in this book strive to contribute to a broader discussion about Indigenizing mental health within the global traditional healing movement.

Global Traditional Healing Movements

The Indigenizing psychology movement began in the late 1970s across the globe in several non-Western countries as a response to colonialism and nationalism that arose after independence (see Hwang, 2005 for discussion). It was not until the 1990s that the growth of traditional healing was seen across the globe, in part because of the excellent research in alternative and complementary healing practices in mainstream medicine. Also, the rise could be attributed to the need to transform Western models of health and mental health care due to Western psychology's failures and limitations to address diaspora immigrant's needs (Gielen, Fish, & Draguns, 2004; Moodley & West, 2005). These early explorations centred on a strong critique of Western psychology for its Eurocentric obsession with the psychology of behaviour, illness, and healing (Moodley & Stewart, 2011) and recommended that psychology needs to develop in local context, solving local problems since "the meaning of illness for an individual is grounded in . . . the network of meanings an illness has in a particular culture" (Good & Good, 1982, p. 148). This recommendation strongly suggested that a solely Western approach to solving mental health problems is not the way forward in the evolution of health and mental health care.

While these early beginnings originated through the rise of post-independence nationalism and a postcolonial critique of Western health and mental health theories, there was also a recognition that Western healing strategies were not appropriate since Western counselling, psychology, and psychotherapy are seen to be problematic as healing tools as they are constructed by the same cultural system that causes the racism, oppression, and illness in the first place. This mismatch fuels a liberal humanistic discourse of the global village mentality, which advocates for a universal psychology and health care that positions and values Western healing practices as central to human behaviour and health care. This form of cultural imperialism generates a tokenism towards culturally relevant and locally grounded theories of illness and wellness, further reducing any agency for Indigenous healing traditions research and practice.

Clearly, the failures of the use of Western psychological healing methods on non-Western clients, many of whom were not attending therapy because they saw it as foreign, or they terminated therapy due to culturally incompetent practices, resulted in a major shift in research related to traditional and Indigenous healing. Traditional healers and healing are a part of the health care system in China, India, Brazil, and, more recently, South Africa (see for example, Moodley, Gielen, & Wu, 2013). These services were initiated long before by the healers themselves, such as the Latin American Curanderos, the Hougans from Haiti, the Hakims from Pakistan, and Vaidyas and Shamans from India. While the need for local and culturally relevant healing practices required the use of traditional healing methods, these practices themselves were transformed, modified, or reconstituted to suit current contexts and health care needs (Moodley & Stewart, 2011). Indigenous healing practices are beginning to be accepted in large metropolitan cities such as New York, Toronto, and London, UK. According to Dein and Sembhi (2001), first- and second-generation immigrants practice traditional healing alongside conventional medicine to make up for the shortcomings of Western healthcare practices. Generally, immigrant communities seem to incorporate a form of medical pluralism using cultural and traditional healing practices as one of many sources of healing for their health and mental health needs. For example, Ataudo (1985) indicated that for 80 percent of the African population, traditional methods are synonymous with primary health care. Traditional healing methods were brought to North America during the time of slavery and have been transforming to suit current needs. For example, practices such as Black Magic and Voodoo have been a response to slavery and racism (see Chireau, 2003; Sutherland, Moodley, & Chevannes, 2014). While Maat, a modernized and transformed version of healing practices with its foundations in Africa, helps clients with racial discrimination and cultural marginalization (Graham, 2005). In Canada and the United States, these practices appear to be complementing existing Indigenous practices such as storytelling, sacred ceremonies, Medicine Wheel, the Pimaatisiwin circle (see Poonwassie & Charter, 2005), and sweat lodges (Smith, 2005). What is critical to note is that the rise of Indigenous healing practices in North America, on the other hand, constructs itself through a very different process: through a politics of resistance to current colonial social, political, and cultural frameworks, as well as racism and the systematic disavowal, disruption, and fragmentation of Indigenous cultures and its peoples.

Colonialism, Trauma, and Healing

Canadian and U.S. Indigenous peoples have experienced multiple historical colonial aggression and assaults. Both education and mental health as systems were used as tools of oppression for Indigenous peoples through Indian residential school. Residential schools were an extensive school system set up by the federal government and administered by churches from the early 1920s to the mid-1990s. The goal of residential schools was, according to the Indian Act, "To kill the Indian in the child," and was based on the premise that Indigenous cultures were inferior to White Christian ones. Many Canadian Indigenous children were forcibly removed, often by the Indian agent or the police, from their families and communities and shipped to the schools, where they were kept for months and years. Many children experienced sexual abuse and corporal punishment for speaking their language, and they were instilled with beliefs that being Indian was bad. For generations, parents and families were left with communities devoid of children. Most children were not educated academically but instead taught domestic and hard labour. Many children died from neglect and illness and many died trying to run away or by suicide. The identities of hundreds of dead students remain unknown. The health, social, and economic outcomes of this history continue to impact all Indigenous peoples today. Meanwhile, as residential schools spanned across Canada, federal policies were enacted to outlaw Indigenous healing practices. Indigenous traditional healers were jailed or sometimes killed, and Christianity and Western medicine were made available to Indigenous communities. Western medicine came mostly via doctors and nurses who were flown into Indigenous communities once or twice a month. In pre-1970s urban areas, many clinics servicing White Canadians refused to service Indigenous Canadians based on race and Indian status. Thus Indigenous peoples were left without their own healing practices to sustain them through intergenerational traumas and with inadequate Western services and beliefs as replacements. Currently, both education and mental health care continue to be sites of systemic and personal oppression for Indigenous peoples because Indigenous identities and knowledges continue to be disallowed and disrespected in most mental health practices, pedagogies, curriculum from preschool to postsecondary, and in most professional disciplines.

It is not easy or simple to define Indigenous traditional healing since it is rooted in Indigenous oral traditions of passing knowledge of healing and medicine from one generation to the next. According to Robbins and Dewar (2011), direct experience with healers and traditional healing is critical in understanding the nature of the healing practices, which is also influenced by the various Indigenous languages and cultures. Furthermore, they argue that in a respective Indigenous language, healing ideas and concepts may not be directly translatable into English or across other Indigenous languages and cultures. They suggest that, in Canada, the Métis language (Michif) constructs Métis health in a particular way that offers a particular worldview of how a Métis person sees himself or herself in relationship to the earth. Robbins and Dewar (2011) also argue that the term "traditional healing" is a British colonial concept disliked by many Indigenous groups, and it is a term that scholars have introduced to Indigenous peoples in English-speaking parts of the world, emphasizing that most Indigenous healing practitioners would have referenced a complex set of healing practices and beliefs as simply medicine.

Indeed, the current ways in which Indigenous healing for health and mental health are understood and practiced are also deeply ingrained in the colonial historical context of racism and oppression and also current ways in which microaggression plays out in society. From this perspective, Indigenous healing in health and mental health can be considered a social construct, rather than just a biological or technical process, due to the cognitive imperialism of Western psychology. Accepting this possibility and realization of the relationship of the social, economic, and the political in the lives of Indigenous peoples and their ways of healing can be seen as a radical divergence from the precepts of classical psychology. The divergence then surfaces the many ways in which Indigenous healing traditions cannot be integrated into classical psychological interventions. Besides the varied and extensive methods used in Indigenous healing, at the root is the epistemological difference that makes the possibility of integration an uneasy one, but a desirable pursuit within modernity. Ultimately, Indigenization of Western psychology is critical for both Indigenous and non- Indigenous peoples. Stewart (2008) writes that healing from colonialism is a major health issue, and grounding healing in an Indigenous paradigm of health and well-being could help many non-Natives in Canadian society. Since Western mental health systems have oppressed and harmed Indigenous peoples throughout history, reclaiming and reasserting the value of Indigenous healing traditions is paramount to offer psyche strength, emotional well-being, and physical wellness to all peoples who have been failed by the deficit and disease models of Western health and mental health practices.

One point of convergence for Indigenous and Western mental health is in the relational model where the relationship between the client and the healer is the basis for healing. The intimacy and intersubjective alliance, for example, is a process that is viewed as sacred in Indigenous healing and is now a major focus within the Western model of psychotherapy. Indeed, "most forms of traditional healing assume that therapeutic knowledge and practice are essentially dependent on relationships with more powerful others who compassionately share gifts of healing in exchange for respectful offerings and ritual observances" (Gone, 2010, p. 206). Acknowledging that the relationship is the basis of the healing will eventually lead to the reimagining of wellness for Indigenous peoples of North America. To conclude, in Gone's (2007) words: "Together, we must collaboratively re-imagine Native American wellness in local terms, along with the community based partnerships and programs ideally suited to its recovery and circulation" (p. 299).

How the Book is Organized

The aim of this edited compilation text is to critically analyze Indigenous traditional healing practices in relation to mental health in Western counselling and psychotherapy. In connecting with current debates concerning counselling and psychotherapy, the analysis of Indigenous healing practices may provide a critical point of departure for highlighting challenges and transformations within the field of psychology. Invited contributors represent leading and well-known practitioners, researchers, and educators within the multidisciplinary field of Indigenous mental health from disciplines of psychology, psychiatry, traditional Indigenous healing, nursing, and social work. Many of these contributors are Indigenous and represent diverse Original Peoples identities from across Turtle Island (North America). Some of the contributors are non-Indigenous; they are the trailblazers who invited the Indigenous paradigm into Western disciplines and provided a place of respect and reciprocity at the centre of Western edifices of knowledge. Contributors authored chapters on topics such as Indigenous healers and healing, cultural healing practices, the integration of traditional and Western mental health practices, professional training and education, Indigenous research methodology, and ethics. These contributions are in the form of empirical research, theoretical arguments and critiques, and professional reflections and narratives. Positioning current psychological practice within the context of historical and current colonialism is also a theme of the book.

The first section of the book, Part One: "East: Indigenous Spirituality in Western Psychology," represents the birth and celebration of integration of spirituality into Western psychological practice. In this section, chapters highlight how Indigenous conceptions and practices of spirituality can be a foundation in psychology and what it means to gain enlightenment and illumination from the ethereal and sacred place of Indigenous spirituality within Western psychological contexts.

Chapter One: "Reclaiming Grassroots Traditional Indigenous Healing Ways and Practices Within Urban Indigenous Community Contexts" by Barbara Waterfall, Dan Smoke, and Marylou Smoke. Prior to our colonization, traditional Indigenous healing practices were carried out organically through grassroots kinship systems of relationship. We can contextualize these systems of relationship as the kinship mutual-aid approach to helping (Waterfall, 2008). Indigenous peoples historically possessed profound knowledge(s), acquired over countless generations, about living in harmony and balance, counselling, holistic health, medicine, and healing (Baikie, 2009; Coyhis & White, 2006). The training of Indigenous healers and the practices of Indigenous healing modalities were organized through extended family ties. In spite of colonial impositions, Indigenous healing ways and practices, nonetheless, remain resilient today and can be clearly observed through current grassroots healing practices. This chapter explores two Indigenous healing initiatives that exist within Indigenous grassroots community contexts. Given that we currently reside in urban areas, these case studies reflect our work within Indigenous urban community contexts. The two case examples refer to Dan and Mary Lou Smoke's involvement as organizers and members of an Indigenous grassroots addictions recovery healing circle and Barbara Waterfall's and Mary Lou Smoke's work with the organization of Indigenous women's drumming and singing circles. The framework that informs our discussion about traditional urban healing ways and practices employs Indigenous cultural resiliency and postcolonial psychology theories within an overarching feminist anticolonial prism (cf. Waterfall, 2008). This chapter begins with a brief explication of this discursive framework for practice. We follow this discourse with a discussion of salient Indigenous cosmological understandings about the context and the basic premises of Indigenous healing practices. In so doing, the traditional organization of the grassroots approach for helping and healing will be clarified. The chapter will then give a brief portrayal of the social context that we currently work in within our healing practices. Finally, we will speak to two case examples of Indigenous approaches to healing and wellness that are located within grassroots urban Indigenous community contexts. These two case examples speak to the cultural resiliency of the Indigenous kinship approach to healing and helping, as well as to the affirmation that Indigenous grassroots cultural practices are legitimate forms of Indigenous intervention, treatment, and therapy.

Chapter Two: "A Laughing Matter: Native American Humour as an Indigenous Healing Tradition and Way of Life" by Michael Tlanusta Garrett, J. T. Garrett, Gloria K. King, Tarrell Awe Agahe Portman, Edil Torres-Rivera, Dale Brotherton, and Lisa Grayshield. In order to best work with Native clients, it is critical to have an accurate understanding of the essence of the people and a working knowledge of cultural communication styles. As humour is an integral piece to both of the aforementioned areas, it is important to understand the spiritual tradition of Native humour, as it exists in many forms. As such, Native American humour is explored as an essential healing element in Indigenous cultures, not only as a communication style but also as a spiritual tradition and way of life. The chapter includes a discussion describing the current literature on the use of humour in the helping professions and description of various forms and communication styles of Native humour as spiritual tradition. Finally, implications for awareness and possible use of Native humour in the therapeutic process with Native clients is offered by examining the use of humour as a metaphor for healing and to help clients become more integrated and more spontaneous in their relationships, to help clients learn helpful coping strategies, to spontaneously and creatively facilitate development of the helping relationship and understanding of client issues, and provide important insight into possible resources and/or courses of action that could be helpful in working through particular issues.

Chapter Three: "Gifts of the Seven Winds Alcohol and Drug Prevention Model for American Indians" by Rockey Robbins, E. Allen Eason, Stephen Colmant, Derek Burks, and Brenda McDaniel. Gifts of the Seven Winds is a culturally grounded Cherokee drug and alcohol group prevention program for Cherokee adolescents and their parents. The intervention is designed to increase interpersonal connection between adolescents and parents, facilitate participants' utilization of tribal healing and storytelling traditions, enhance psychological immunity to drug and alcohol misuse, and build leadership capacities. Seven Winds emphases were generated collaboratively with tribal community members. The curriculum focuses on community rather than individual healing, holistic wellness rather than cognitive education, stories rather than problem solving, and strengths rather than on problems and deficits. All phases of implementation, from participant and facilitator recruitment to the purification ceremony to the concluding honoring feast, as well as group activities (including process questions) and accompanying projects are described in detail.

Chapter Four: "Traditional Spiritual Healing" by Wendy Hill. Throughout the years working as a traditional healer in different communities, Wendy Hill has gained valuable insight into the spiritual power that individuals have, which she shares in this chapter. Many people have been given limited resources to understand themselves. Part of Hill's work as a healer is to help people understand themselves as spiritual people, which is one aspect of healing. If people do not believe that they have control and power within themselves, then how can they feel responsible for their healing? Illness, pain, and emotional trauma are all linked in a traditional healing and spiritual perspective. The healing that is necessary for any individual to feel better is unique and based in on that individual's unique needs; there is no universal approach to a person's healing. If a person is shy or unwilling to admit the events that have led to the emotional, mental, or physical problems that he or she has, then the spirit cannot be healed. The knowledge and awareness of what an individual needs to bring the healing into his or her life can only come from a higher power. A healer is the person responsible for giving the support to this process, whether it is through words or bringing the spirits into the space of the person to allow that experience to happen.

The second section of the book, Part Two: "South: Innovative Integration in Psychological Practice," represents the emotional aspects of human nature, the self, and the world for many Indigenous cultures. This section has chapters that identify how psychological practice puts the notion of trust at the forefront: trust within the therapeutic alliance and trust within the discipline of psychology to move out of its comfort zone to invite Indigenous healing into the structured Western world where erstwhile practices of cognitive imperialism and oppression harmed Indigenous and non-Indigenous clients and patients.

Chapter Five: "Indigenous North American Psychological Healing Ways and the Placement of Integration and Decolonization" by Glen McCabe. Indigenous North Americans, referring to the Métis, First Nations, and Inuit in Canada and American Indians and Alaska Natives in the United States, have been seeking help from traditional healers and Elders for as long as anyone in their communities can remember (Angel, 2002; Peat, 2005). They reside in different countries and in different political jurisdictions within these countries, but tend to experience the same social, emotional, and mental health issues and also seek similar resources for help in efforts to deal with their problems. Currently, Indigenous North Americans are seeking help from traditional helpers and from mainstream counsellors at unprecedented rates. At the same time, Indigenous North Americans still experience high rates of mental health complaints (Cockerham, 2000). Also, they experience higher than normal rates of violent and accidental deaths, family breakdown, and criminal incarceration (French, 1997). Added to this is a substantial interest among non-Indigenous people in the healing practices of Indigenous healers and Elders. Many of the people who use traditional healer services claim that they feel helped by the interventions they experience. In addition to this, Indigenous people are pursuing the services of mainstream mental health practitioners at a significant rate, while honouring their traditional beliefs and methods (Mehl-Madrona, 1997; Peat, 2005). Many also claim to feel helped. These phenomena have given rise to increased attention from researchers and clinical practitioners both inside and outside the Indigenous community. Much of the attention has been focused on the kind of techniques used by traditional Indigenous helpers and on the similarities and differences that they bear when compared to mainstream interventions. In this chapter, Glen McCabe outlines the nature of a model of psychotherapy that is used by Indigenous North Americans that was the central focus of a qualitative research project McCabe undertook about a decade ago. Glen McCabe's research is an integrated model made up of methods used in both the mainstream and Indigenous communities and grounded in the same theoretical understanding associated with these techniques. Since the model described here is composed of conditions that are also highly prized in many mainstream therapies, you could with some justification assume that there is a culturally hybridized therapy, or integrated model, if you like, that might be emerging and evolving from the interaction between these two communities. As one will hopefully see by the end of this chapter there is some truth in this assumption, but perhaps it is a somewhat limited truth.

Chapter Six: "Counselling Indigenous Peoples in Canada" by Suzanne L. Stewart and Anne Marshall. Indigenous peoples represent approximately 4 percent of Canada's total population (Statistics Canada, 2009). Over 50 percent of the Indigenous population is under the age of twenty-four and 40 percent are under the age of sixteen. Thus the population is growing with a high concentration of youth. Since the 1970s, there has been a large migration of Indigenous peoples from rural areas and First Nation reserves to cities. Currently, over 600,000 self-identified Indigenous people live in cities—54 percent of the total Aboriginal population—and the numbers are expected to grow according to demographic trends. The Indigenous population is becoming increasingly urban; in 2006, 54 percent lived in an urban centre, an increase from 50 percent in 1996. From 2001 to 2006, the Indigenous population in Canada increased by 196,475; over this period, the Indigenous population grew by 20.1 percent, a rate five times that of the non-Indigenous population. Mental health is a vital aspect of overall health for Canadian Indigenous peoples. However, Indigenous cultural understandings of mental health and healing are distinctly different from understandings that have prevailed in most North American mental health provider settings, including counselling contexts. Counsellor training in Canada and the United States is based almost exclusively on a Western paradigm of health that differs from an Indigenous worldview (Gone, 2004). These differences in paradigmatic worldviews can form a barrier to effectively helping Native peoples who seek counselling services from formally trained counsellors, including those who may be trained in cross-cultural or multicultural approaches. Further, Duran (2006) suggests that counselling Indigenous individuals from a non-Indigenous perspective (i.e., Western perspective) is a form of continued oppression and colonization, as it does not legitimize the Indigenous cultural view of mental health and healing. "A postcolonial paradigm would accept knowledge from differing cosmologies as valid in their own right, without their having to adhere to a separate cultural body for legitimacy" (Duran & Duran, 1995, p. 6). Some counselling educators, researchers, and practitioners are increasingly recognizing the inseparability of cultural foundations and mental health needs and are attempting to devote more effort to explore traditional cultural conceptions of mental health and healing. For example, Indigenous mental health and healing training, education, and practice have been incorporated into many postsecondary-training programs across the country (cf. Stewart, 2009). In order to address more culturally relevant knowledge regarding mental health and healing, this chapter presents a brief history of Indigenous peoples and its implications for mental health and healing, an overview of key issues for Indigenous clients, and two models of Indigenous counselling.

Chapter Seven: "Lessons From Clinical Practice: Some of the Ways in Which Canadian Mental Health Professionals Practice Integration" by Olga Oulanova and Roy Moodley. Traditional healing continues to play an important role in the lives of Canadian Aboriginal communities, and it has been suggested that competent mental healthcare services need to integrate this helping approach. The authors interviewed Canadian mental health professionals who use both Western psychological interventions and Aboriginal traditional practices, with the aim of divulging what such integration looks like in clinical practice. By means of three case illustrations, this chapter will discuss the following aspects of integration: traditional healing medicines inside the therapy room, naturalistic healing outside the therapy room, and holistic counselling. Implications for mental healthcare delivery within Aboriginal communities are addressed.

The third section of the book, Part Three: "West: Trauma and Contemporary Indigenous Healing," brings together chapters that discuss the themes of introspection and insights, ideas grounded in the body, or physical aspect of trauma in psychology.

Chapter Eight: "Injury Where Blood Does Not Flow" by Eduardo Duran and Judith Firehammer. This chapter introduces the reader to a different way of experiencing a different cultural life-world. The discussion reviews and compares Western and traditional Native ways of interpreting trauma. Internalized oppression, a symptom of historical trauma, is explored through the historical "Indian agents' " psychology and how this impacts present communities through workplace dynamics. Clinical implications of treating Native veterans are dealt with in juxtaposition with best Western clinical practices because the authors believe that this issue opens critical discourse into the origins of historical trauma and paves the way to a liberation narrative.

Chapter Nine: In "Historical Perspectives on Indigenous Healing" by Allison Reeves and Suzanne L. Stewart. The authors review commonalities among Indigenous healing practices in Canada and highlight how these approaches diverge theoretically and practically from Western approaches to mental health care provision. This discussion is contextualized within an understanding of how settler arrival and colonial imperialism impacted Indigenous health and well-being, and it offers a resilience-based perspective on the value of incorporating Indigenous healing practices into mental health care provision.

Chapter Ten: "Colonial Trauma and Political Pathways to Healing" by Terry Mitchell. This chapter discusses the unacceptable burden of psycho-social-physical-health inequalities borne by Indigenous peoples, which are identified as a signifier of social injustice with political pathways to resolution. Historical and contemporary forms of colonial violence and related colonial trauma are social issues that settler societies need to increase awareness of, sensitivity to, and accountability for. Mitchell provides an overview of the social constructs of Indigeneity, colonialism, and colonial trauma. These constructs provide a foundation for the introduction of six political pathways to advancing social justice as a mental health strategy for promoting the health and wellness of Aboriginal peoples in Canada within a larger framework of reconciliation.

The fourth and final section of the book, Part Four: "North: Healing Through Western and Indigenous Knowledges," identifies themes of the mental aspect of people and psychological practice. At an abstract level, these chapters are about logic, wisdom, and thinking; concretely, these chapters hold discussions and guidelines for ethics, teaching, and shifts in paradigm. There is a theme in this section that change only happens when it is supported. In bringing together empirical evidence and the clinical and professional experience of leading experts, this section provides support to mental health practitioners, researchers, and educators who are interested in multiple ways of knowing and in reconciling the oppressive colonial history of mental health on Indigenous peoples and all peoples who have been failed by Western mental health interventions.

Chapter Eleven: "Cultures in Collision: 'Higher' Education and the Clash Between Indigenous and Non-Indigenous 'Ways of Knowing' " by Michael Chandler. The author explores the "worldviews" and "epistemic practices" common to many Indigenous learners and looks at how these distinct "ways of knowing" can shape the ongoing educational prospects of Canada's contemporary First Nations, Métis, and Inuit students. Although such culturally driven "beliefs about belief" contribute to many of the academic missteps that stymie Indigenous learners on every rung of the usual educational ladder, special attention will be focused here on the common difficulties faced by those who, against odds, have succeeded in gaining admission to institutions of "higher" learning. The broad thesis explored here is that, rather than being counted as fair commentary on the competencies of individual students, the whole panoply of academic difficulties encountered by Indigenous learners is better understood as the aftermath of a drive-by shooting—a collective wound inflicted in the course of that ongoing cultural war still being waged against those whose "ways of knowing" are foreign to, and regularly at odds with, what Rorty (1987, p. 57) has called the dominant "Judeo-Graeco-Roman-Christian-Renaissance-Enlightenment-Romanticist framework to" of understanding, that over centuries has dominated mainstream Eurocentric educational practice. Any serious attempt to defend the possible merits of this thesis—the idea that the educational inequities suffered by Indigenous learners are part and parcel of an across-the-board effort to discount the very possibility of bona fide Indigenous ways of knowing—requires persuading the reader of at least three things. The first of these arguments is easily, if painfully, won and only requires rehearsing that familiar litany of defamatory statistics regularly used to demonstrate that, in comparison to their culturally mainstream counterparts, Indigenous learners often prove to be academic underachievers, frequently leave school at a tender age, and are sorely underrepresented among those who graduate from high school, or succeed at various levels of postsecondary training. If there are any remaining surprises in these well-rehearsed educational woes, it is, perhaps, that something like half of those Indigenous students who do make it all the way to some institution of "higher" learning regularly end up leaving empty handed, without the "degree" that they and their communities had so much hoped for (DeGagné, 2002). In short, the common plight of far too many Indigenous learners is a recurrent story of lost opportunities and failed prospects—failures that, if anything, increase in volume and volubility in the ideologically driven world of postsecondary education. The second and more expansive of the arguments takes the form of a synopsis of those emerging lines meant to persuade you that Indigenous persons, in Canada and around the world, actually do subscribe to distinctive ways of knowing or folk epistemologies that set them apart from, and put them at a serious educational disadvantage relative to, their non-Indigenous counterparts. In concluding this chapter, an attempt will be made to "connect the dots" by arguing that responsibility for many of the educational shortfalls that defeat some Indigenous learners, can be legitimately laid at the door of all those who insist that anything short of a full, root-and-branch conversion to classic Eurocentric beliefs about belief is equivalent to a stubborn refusal to take advantage of what bona fide Westernized knowledge is widely imagined to be. The chapter ends with a gesture in the direction of the sort of research program that would seem to be required if existing claims about Indigenous ways of knowing are to be taken with new seriousness by the usual guardians of Western scientific respectability

Chapter Twelve: "An Ally in Northern Community Health: Respectful Engagement in Healing Relationships," by Linda O'Neill. Throughout history, all cultures have developed explanations for abnormal or unhealthy behaviours and culture-specific methods, referred to as Indigenous methods, for dealing with resulting problems. Culture-specific conceptualizations, emic in source, exist for a variety of psychological problems. Western practitioners will often have very different perceptions of what "good" mental health looks like, as well as what constitutes effective intervention strategies. Western-based practitioners need to be able to validate the client's cultural conception of mental health problems because this conception of mental illness affects help-seeking action, the expectations of treatment outcome, and the manifestation of symptoms. A major factor in developing a culturally congruent manner in the helping profession is the cultural awareness of the practitioner and the development of cultural competence. This chapter provides lessons learned and wisdom gained from a quarter century of cross-cultural engagement and work as a helping practitioner in a northern community. The developmental process of becoming an ally with Aboriginal clients and community members includes an ongoing critique of dominant theories of helping practice, advocacy for changes in mental health policy to address healthcare inequalities, and in-depth reflection on cultural heritage and influences. To become an ally, culture had to be understood and presented as a phenomenon far greater than tradition, but rather as moral visions that guide us to what is good and right and healthy. The role of a true ally is considered in this chapter to be someone who works for cultural growth and expansion of resources with acknowledgement of the possibility that no single cultural system holds comprehensive resources for coping, resilience, and healing. The goal in this chapter is to help other practitioners reflect on ways to become allies and bridge the gaps between their various cultures' beliefs on mental health and healing and those of their clients.

Chapter Thirteen: "*A'tola'nw*: Indigenous-Centred Learning in a Counselling Graduate Program" by Anne Marshall, Larry Emerson, Lorna Williams, Asma Antoine, Colleen MacDougall, and Ruby Peterson. This chapter discusses Aboriginal learners "training" to be counsellors and helpers who will eventually return to their communities. However, the Western academy is difficult to negotiate and navigate if deep Indigenous-centred decolonized learning must happen. As learners, the authors found new space to learn, think, and feel, that are in fact free from oppression and colonial control. Traditional leaders tell us the answers lie within. Yet there are few maps to follow with little time and few opportunities for the type of deep learning we desire. Simultaneously engaging Western and Indigenous learning is not easy. Things can get traumatic. We know and don't know our cultures and languages. We are of mixed ancestry. We have inherited unresolved residential school trauma whether we know it or not. We understand and don't understand community, kinship, and place. We are connected and disconnected. We feel both joy and pain. We are humanized and dehumanized. We sense beauty and contradictions among ourselves. But we are here to learn. We have hopes and aspirations for healthy communities and nations. We understand what the Western academy wants from us. However, there are obstacles out there. We must be vigilant and courageous learners or we will be immobilized and discouraged and among ourselves will wind up reproducing the very same conditions that have disrupted our communities. How do we learn? How do we know what to know? How can we as a learning community successfully understand ourselves, assess our situation without harsh judgment, and restore and regenerate our capacity to articulate our own solutions using principles of traditional knowledge and cultural self-determination as a guide for healing, decolonization, transformation, and mobilization? We must do this while remembering to remember the promise to our communities, families, and ourselves.

Chapter Fourteen: "A Partnership With the People: Skilful Navigation of Culture and Ethics" by Melinda A. García, Gayle S. Morse, Joseph E. Trimble, Denise M. Casillas, Beth Boyd, and Jeff King. In recent years, there has been a striking increase in mental health research conducted among Indigenous and other ethnic groups. At the same time, there has been an increase in efforts to develop robust methods that respect the integrity of the community as well as the scientific validity of the research. This has been in response to the concerns that arose in many ethnocultural communities from their experiences with researchers and teams who misinterpreted data from the community's point of view and who shared community data inappropriately. For some researchers, these challenges to the prior ways of conducting research are only beginning to be actively acknowledged at any level, including the methodological, procedural, and conceptual levels. Responsible and robust research with ethnocultural communities requires a relationship with the community that is based on mutual respect as defined by the community and is based on community-sourced ethics. Indeed, many ethnocultural communities have developed their own community-based research review committees to ensure ethical researcher community relationships. This chapter reviews the history of how research has been conducted in ethnocultural communities with the use of culturally inappropriate designs, methodology, and interpretation. It then describes how research can be both scientific and healing for communities when it is conducted with integrity and transparency, in addition to being executed in a manner recognized by the community as ethical. When a researcher enters into a partnership with a community, the resulting research methodology will be solidly grounded in respecting the ethics and integrity of the community.

References

Angel, M. (2002). *Historical Perspectives on the Ojibwa Midewiwin: Preserving the Sacred*. Winnipeg: The University of Manitoba Press.

Arthur, N., & Collins, S. (2005). *Culture-infused counselling: Celebrating the Canadian mosaic*. Calgary: Counselling Concepts.

Ataudo, E. S. (1985). Traditional medicine and biopsychosocial fulfillment in African health. *Social Science in Medicine, 21*, 1345–1347.

Baikie, G. (2009). Indigenous-centered social work: Theorizing a social work way of being. In R. Sinclair, M. A., Hart, & G. Bruyere, G. (Eds.), *Wicihitowin: Aboriginal Social Work in Canada* (pp. 42–61). Halifax: Fernwood Publishing.

Chireau, Y. P. (2003). *Black Magic: Religion and the African American conjuring tradition*. Berkeley, CA: University of California Press.

Cockerham, W. C. (2000). *Sociology of mental disorder*, 5th ed. Upper Saddle River, New Jersey: Prentice Hall.

Coyhis, D. L. & White, W. L. (2006). *Alcohol problems in Native America: The untold story of resistance and recovery—"The truth about the lie."* Colorado Springs: White Bison Inc.

DeGagné, Michael D. (2002). *Interaction without integration: The experience of successful First Nations Students in Canadian post-secondary education*. (Doctoral dissertation). Department of Educational Administration, Michigan State University, East Lansing, MI.

Dein, S., & Sembhi, S. (2001). The use of traditional healing in South Asian psychiatric patients in the UK: Interaction between professional and folk psychiatries. *Transcultural Psychiatry, 38*, 243–257.

Duran, E. (2006). *Healing the soul wound: Counseling with American Indians and other Native peoples*. New York: Teachers College Press.

Duran, E., & Duran, B. (1995). *Native American postcolonial psychology*. Albany, NY: State University of New York.

French L. A. (1997). A review of US/Indian policy: A unique chapter in U.S. history. *Free Inquiry in Creative Sociology, 25*(2), 169–177.

Gielen, U. P., Fish, J. M., & Draguns, J. G. (2004). *Handbook of culture, therapy and healing*. Mahwah, NJ: Lawrence Erlbaum.

Gone, J. P. (2004). Mental health services for Native Americans in the 21st century United States. *Professional Psychology: Research and Practice,* 35(1), 10–18.

Gone, J. P. (2007). "We never was happy living like a Whiteman": Mental health disparities and the postcolonial predicament in American Indian communities. *American Journal of Community Psychology, 40*(3–4), 290–300.

Gone, J. P. (2010). Psychotherapy and traditional healing for American Indians: Exploring the prospects for therapeutic integration. *The Counseling Psychologist, 38*(2), 166–235.

Good, M.-J. D. (1982). Towards a meaning-centred analysis of popular illness categories: 'Fright-illness' and 'heat distress' in Iran. In A. J. Marsella & G. M. White (Eds.), *Cultural conceptions of mental health and therapy* (pp. 141–66). Dordrecht: Reidel.

Graham, M. (2005). Maat: An African centered paradigm for psychological and spiritual healing. In R. Moodley & W. West (Eds.), *Integrating traditional healing practices into counseling and psychotherapy* (pp. 210–20). Thousand Oaks, CA: Sage Publications.

Hwang, K.-K. (2005). A philosophical reflection on the epistemology and methodology of indigenous psychologies. *Asian Journal of Social Psychology, 8*(1), 5–17.

McCormick, R. (2005). The healing path: What can counsellors learn from Aboriginal people about how to heal? In R. Moodley, & W. West (Eds.), *Integrating traditional healing practices into counseling and psychotherapy* (pp. 293–304). Thousand Oaks, CA: Sage.

Mehl-Madrona, L. (1997). *Coyote medicine: Lessons from Native American healing*. New York: Fireside.

Moodley, R. (2011) The Toronto Traditional Healers Project: An introduction. *International Journal of Health Promotion and Education, 49*(3), 74–8.

Moodley, R., Gielen, U. P., & Wu, R. (2013). *Handbook of counseling and psychotherapy in an international context*. New York: Routledge.

Moodley, R., & Stewart, S. L. (2011). Special issue: Integrating traditional healing practices into health promotion and education. *International Journal of Health Promotion and Education, 49*(3), 69–136.

Moodley, R., & West, W. (2005). *Integrating traditional healing practices into counseling and psychotherapy*. Thousand Oaks, CA: Sage.

Peat, F. D. (2005). *Blackfoot physics: A journey into the Native American universe*. Boston, MA: Weiser Books.

Pedersen, P. B., & Lonner, W. B. (2015). *Counseling across cultures*, 7th ed. Thousand Oaks, CA: Sage.

Poonwassie, A., & Charter, A. (2005). Aboriginal worldview of healing: Inclusion, blending, and bridging. In R. Moodley, & W. West (Eds.), *Integrating traditional healing practices into counseling and psychotherapy* (pp. 15–25). Thousand Oaks, CA: Sage.

Rorty, A. O. (1987). Persons as rhetorical categories. *Social Research, 54*(1), 55–72.

Robbins, J. A., & Dewar, J. (2011). Traditional indigenous approaches to healing and the modern welfare of traditional knowledge, spirituality and lands: A critical reflection on practices and policies taken from the Canadian indigenous. *The International Indigenous Policy Journal*, 2(4), Retrieved from: http://ir.lib.uwo.ca/iipj/vol2/iss4/2 doi: 10.18584/iipj.2011.2.4.2.

Smith, D. P. (2005). The sweat lodge as psychotherapy. In R. Moodley & W. West (Eds.). *Integrating traditional healing practices into counseling and psychotherapy* (pp. 196–209). Thousand Oaks, CA: Sage Publications.

Statistics Canada. (2009). Aboriginal peoples in Canada in 2006: Inuit, Métis and First Nations, 2006 Census. Statistics Canada, Ottawa.

Stewart, S. L. (2008). Promoting indigenous mental health: Cultural perspectives on healing from Native counsellors in Canada. *International Journal of Health Promotion and Education, 46*(2), 49–56.

Stewart, S. (2009). *Indigenous graduate student stories on success and challenges of postsecondary education.* Research Report submitted to Centre for Studies in Post Secondary Education, OISE, University of Toronto.

Sutherland, P., Moodley, R., & Chevannes, B. (2014). *Caribbean healing traditions: Implications for health and mental health.* New York: Routledge.

Vontress, C. E. (2010). Culture and counseling: A personal retrospective. In R. Moodley, & R. Walcott (Eds.), *Counseling across and beyond cultures* (pp. 19–42). Toronto: Toronto University Press.

Waterfall, B. (2008) *Decolonizing Anishnabec social work education: An Anishnabe spiritually-infused reflexive study* (Unpublished doctoral thesis). Toronto: Ontario Institute for Studies in Education of the University of Toronto.

Part 1

East

Indigenous Spirituality in Western Psychology

1 Reclaiming Grassroots Traditional Indigenous Healing Ways and Practices Within Urban Indigenous Community Contexts

Barbara Waterfall with Dan Smoke and Mary Lou Smoke

Prior to our colonization, traditional Indigenous healing practices were carried out organically through grassroots kinship systems of relationship. We can contextualize these systems of relationship as the kinship mutual-aid approach to helping (Waterfall, 2008). Indigenous peoples historically possessed profound knowledges, acquired over countless generations, about living in harmony and balance, counselling, holistic health, medicine, and healing (Baikie, 2009; Coyhis & White, 2006). The training of Indigenous healers and the practices of Indigenous healing modalities were organized through extended family ties. In spite of colonizing impositions, Indigenous healing ways and practices, nonetheless, remain resilient today and can be clearly observed through current grassroots healing practices.

This chapter will speak to two Indigenous healing initiatives that exist within Indigenous grassroots community contexts.[1] Given that we currently reside in Urban centres, these case studies reflect our work within Indigenous urban community contexts. The two case examples refer to Dan and Mary Lou Smoke's involvement as organizers and members of an Indigenous grassroots addictions recovery healing circle, and Barbara Waterfall's and Mary Lou Smoke's work with the organization of Indigenous women's drumming and singing circles.

The framework that informs our discussion about traditional urban healing ways and practices employs Indigenous cultural resiliency and postcolonial psychology theories, within an overarching feminist anticolonial prism (cf. Waterfall, 2008). This chapter begins with a brief explication of this discursive framework for practice. We follow this discourse with a discussion of salient Indigenous cosmological understandings about the context and basic premises of Indigenous healing practices. In so doing, the traditional organization of the grassroots approach for helping and healing will be clarified. The chapter will then give a brief portrayal of the social context that we currently work in within our healing practices. Finally, we will speak to two case examples of Indigenous approaches to healing and wellness that are located within grassroots urban Indigenous community contexts. These two case examples speak to the cultural resiliency of the Indigenous kinship approach to healing and helping and to the affirmation that Indigenous grassroots cultural practices are legitimate forms of Indigenous intervention, treatment, and therapy.

Discursive Framework

Dei (2000) contends that the employment of a "discursive" rather than a "theoretical" approach opens up space for the inclusion of ever-changing social realities and questions, as well as for the infusion of multiple Indigenous theoretical practices and perspectives. Influenced by Dei's work, the framework that informs this discussion is an overarching feminist anticolonial discursive prism (Dei & Asgharzadeh, 2001; Waterfall, 2008) with infused salient Indigenous cultural resiliency (Dumont, Hopkins, Dell, & Menzies, 2014; Heavy Runner & Morris, 1997) and postcolonial psychology perspectives (Archibald, 2006; Wesley-Esquimaux & Smolewski, 2004). A detailed delineation of this framework appears in Waterfall (2008).

A feminist anticolonial stance has been previously defined as the absence of colonial imposition, as the agency to govern our own lives, and as the practice of such agency based upon our ancestors', women-centred principles of life-giving and nurturance (Wane & Waterfall, 2005). Informed by feminist anticolonial discourse, our entry point for work within Indigenous communities begins by centering the traditional mutual-aid paradigm and traditional healing ways and practices, particularly those that are grassroots initiatives. While it is recognized that there are many understandings about what the term "grassroots" refers to, we define the domain of grassroots activity as that which stems from outside of and independent from the government funding sector.

For purposes of further augmenting the role and importance of the traditional grassroots paradigm, Indigenous cultural resiliency theory is also employed within this discursive framework. Indigenous cultural resiliency theorizing stems from Indigenous grassroots perspectives and presents as a positive and proactive traditionalist stance. Informing practice, this theory presents as a proclamation of the present-day resiliency of traditional Indigenous ways and systems of practice (Heavy Runner & Morris, 1997). Connected to cultural resiliency theorizing is discourse pertaining to the legitimacy of Indigenous cultural practices as intervention, treatment, and therapy. With respect to the addictions recovery literature, this discourse is referred to as culture as treatment (Coyhis & White, 2006; Dumont et al., 2014).

Given that the two grassroots healing initiatives discussed in this chapter have been created in direct response to the Indigenous peoples' personal and intergenerational responses to colonialism, we infuse within our discursive prism postcolonial psychology theorizing. We acknowledge that the current social problems that exist within Indigenous communities, such as poverty, homelessness, addictions/substance abuse, and violence are the direct consequences of historic and ongoing colonial impositions (Archibald, 2006;

Wesley-Esquimaux & Smolewski, 2004). We also conceptualize that the overall impacts of colonialism have created the psychological issues of unresolved historic grief and intergenerational post-traumatic stress and trauma (Wesley-Esquimaux & Smolewski, 2004; Whitebeck, Xiaojin, Hoyt, & Adams, 2004).

The Relationships Between North American Indigenous Cosmologies, the Social Organization of Traditional Indigenous Societies, and Indigenous Healing Practices

Within pre-colonial existences, Indigenous societies were matrifocal and, in some Nations, there was matriarchal governance (Anderson, 2000). In all Nations, women were highly respected, having central and pivotal roles in all aspects of family and community life, inclusive of economic, social, political, and spiritual/cultural activities (Anderson, 2000; Mihesuah, 2003). This understanding is supported by our recorded libraries, or pictographic drawings, as well as by our Elders' oral teachings (Thunderbird, 2011). Women possessed personal and collective freedoms and powers in these societies, such as the freedom to enter and end intimate relationships of their own choosing, as well as decision-making powers (Anderson, 2000). With respect to the matriarchal, Hau de no sau nee people considered women to be owners of all property (Maracle, 2003). Anderson (2000) contends that women's centred positioning did not mean that men were excluded, nor were there struggles or competitiveness between genders. Anderson (2000) described that within many Indigenous societies, men's and women's positioning was one where each gender had complimentary roles.

Many Nations contextualized human beings' relationship with the natural ecology as existing within a circular cosmological understanding. This circular cosmology has often been referred to as the Sacred Hoop, or the Medicine Wheel (Nabigon, 2006). Life within the Medicine Wheel understanding is conceptualized as being made up of four distinct areas corresponding to the four cardinal directions of east, south, west, and north; the four seasons of the year of spring, summer, autumn, and winter; the four stages of life from birth, youth, adulthood, and Elder hood, and the four components of self as emotional, mental, physical, and spiritual (White Bison, Inc., 2002).

Traditionally, there is a belief in a Creator of Life, understood to have both female and male traits, as well as a universal creative life force/intelligence within the universe. It is also understood that the Creator of Life exists within all life forms, inclusive of the four elements of the earth, water, air, and fire, as well as rocks, trees, plants, animals, birds, and fish, as examples. Within traditional Indigenous thought, there is a deep respect and reverence for plants and historically, medicinal plants were never used excessively nor abused (Coyhis & White, 2006). As an example, alcohol can be understood to be a medicine derived from plant life. While a few North American Indigenous

Nations used alcohol prior to European contact, this substance was never consumed in excessive or abusive ways (Coyhis & White, 2006).

Indigenous peoples commonly understood and understand today that the Creator of Life resides within the heart of every human being. Nabigon, an Oji-Cree Elder's (2006) depiction of an "inner spiritual fire" supports this standpoint. This fire is deemed the source of our personal power, healing, and renewal, as well as our will or self-determination. From a traditional healing stance, it is understood that the true healer is ultimately the person seeking healing. While overt measures can and are used by traditional healers, such as performing healing ceremonies or directing the person to the use of a healing plant medicine, the underlying objective of any Indigenous healing practice is to assist persons in connecting to and utilizing the majestic power of the Creator, or inner fire, for their own healing (Antone, Miller, & Myers, 1986). As natural conductors of this inner power, human beings are understood to possess innate ways to heal themselves from any form of disharmony or disease, such as talking, crying, or laughing (Nabigon, 2006).

Indigenous methodologies were thus developed to assist people with healing themselves of any form of distress and maintaining harmony, such as employing healing or drumming and singing circles. Pertinent to this discussion is the understanding that the sacred items employed by Indigenous people, such as ceremonial pipes, rattles, and drums are imbued with a specific spirit and possess interconnecting, restorative, and healing qualities. Goudreau, Weber-Pillwax, Cote-Meeks, Madill, & Wilson (2008) assert that the practice of drumming, as an example, was historically an important aspect of Indigenous cultures. Amadahy (2003) argues that Indigenous drum music assisted Indigenous peoples with maintaining an essential peace and unity.

There exists within traditional Indigenous cultures a deep respect for all of life (Nabigon, 2006). It is also believed that human beings' relationship with all that exists within our universe is one of a "universal system of kinship ties." Prior to colonialism, our societies were organized along tightly knit extended family lines. Traditional societies were organized to promote peaceful and balanced relations. Traditional ethics, systems, ceremonial practices, and everyday social relations were organized to ensure and maintain a spirit of respectful coexistence with all of creation. For many Indigenous nations, governance and decision making were structured around kinship systems that fostered a consensual paradigm. The purpose of our structures and internal processes were to promote peace and unity among our peoples (Alfred, 2005). From this foundational perspective, it can be understood that all people within a family, community, and nation were responsible for the health and well-being of the people. It is this ethic of being responsible for the people and for future generations that constitutes the axiological foundation from which Indigenous knowledges, systems, and methods of practice originate. Alfred (2005) contends that "reciprocity and mutual obligation were the foundations of (traditional) human interactions and of relationships with other elements in creation" (p. 84). Relating this understanding to Indigenous healing and helping methods, we can contextualize that great Indigenous power can be derived by gathering together and supporting each other collectively. The employment of healing drumming and singing circles were used, and many Nations made use of circular ceremonial practices, such as the sweat lodge, full moon ceremonies, and the sun dance (Anderson, 2000; Hart, 2002; White Bison, Inc., 2002).

Informed by the understanding of "natural law,"[2] traditional life revolved around a preventative medicine. When issues of unrest or unbalance were noticed, it was argued that these issues were immediately attended to (The Truth and Reconciliation Commission of Canada, [TRC], 2015). While it has been noted that in some circumstances abuse of women did exist, there were social structures in place to ensure that this issue was addressed, and there were severe consequences for anyone committing such an offense (Anderson, 2000). Important to this discussion is the understanding that the present-day, government-funded helping systems that are part of Indigenous peoples present-day experiences, did not exist within our pre-colonial history. We did not have soup kitchens, welfare lines, children's aid societies, battered women's shelters, addictions treatment centers, or hospitals for psychiatric patients, as examples.

The Current Context of Our Healing Practices

All of the Indigenous people we work with within our healing practices have been impacted in some form by historic and ongoing colonizing forces. It is not within the scope of this chapter to speak to the specifics of how colonialism has been organized or the effects it has had on Indigenous peoples lives. As has been reported by the TRC (2015),

> for over a century, the central goals of Canada's Aboriginal policy were to eliminate Aboriginal governments, ignore Aboriginal rights, terminate the Treaties, and, through a process of assimilation, cause Aboriginal peoples to cease to exist as distinct legal, social, religious, and racial entities in Canada. The establishment and operation of residential schools were a central element in this policy, which can best be described as "cultural genocide."
>
> (p. 1)

So too have Indigenous feminist scholars portrayed how the combined forces of church and state have actively suppressed Indigenous women's traditional economic, political, social, and cultural/spiritual powers (Anderson, 2000; Mihesuah, 2003).

It is noteworthy that colonialism is not only that which encompasses our past, but rather is ongoing and reformulating, continuing to impact upon the lives of Indigenous peoples today (Alfred, 2005; Dei & Asgharzadeh, 2001). Alfred (2005) has also argued that the government-funded sector can serve as a force for ongoing reformulating colonizing impositions. A very important understanding about Indigenous peoples relationship to colonization is that in many respects, Indigenous peoples have not been passive victims of oppression. Rather, Indigenous peoples, since early contact, have been actively resisting colonizing impositions and influences, as well as finding creative culturally based responses to combat that oppression[3] (Coyhis & White, 2006).

In our healing practices within our urban communities, we work with women, men, children, and youth from diverse Nations and diverse economic backgrounds. Some of the adults we work with are well educated by Western standards and earn high incomes. Some are teachers, counsellors, administrators, cultural resource people, and/or are serving in leadership roles in our communities. At the other end of the spectrum are people who are newly released from corrections facilities. Also, some are getting away from street life, or are currently living in poverty—subsisting on income assistance. Some are also currently living in, or have recently lived in, abusive conditions. Most of the people we work with have been emotionally, physically, sexually, or spiritually abused at some time in their lives. Many are in recovery from substance abuse, addictions, and/or are dealing with emotional or mental health issues. Some struggle with anger, rage, anxiety, depression, identity confusion, low self-esteem, and post-traumatic stress syndrome. Others have been able to overcome these and other issues, and they offer a breadth of support to our communities through the revitalization of traditional kinship systems of support.

As healers within our communities, we have been most impressed with our people's will and determination to live balanced, healthy, and productive lives. Many of the people that we serve are able to gain balance and wellness by returning to the traditional cultural teachings, practices, and traditional ways of life practiced by our ancestors. Our healing practices have been predicated on the principle that connection to and involvement with Indigenous cultural practices is a legitimate context for intervention, treatment, and healing. Much of our work within our communities has involved supporting persons recovering from substance abuse and addictions; supporting women, children, and youth who have been in abusive family relationships; assisting people to release painful emotions that have been associated with living within a colonized existence; and creating grassroots, culturally rooted, and kinship-based circles of support, healing, and mutual aid. To that end, Mary Lou and Dan have been involved with the creation and maintenance of a culture-based support circle for persons recovering from addictions. Recognizing that Indigenous women's power and authority has been the target of colonizing processes, we also strategically prioritize assisting Indigenous women to reclaim their power and traditional roles within their families and communities. To facilitate this objective, Barbara and Mary Lou have spent extensive time committed to creating and nurturing Indigenous women's drumming and singing circles.

The following will describe two case examples of our grassroots efforts in our communities.

The Resilience of the Traditional Kinship Systems of Helping Within Urban Indigenous Contexts: Two Case Examples

The Fire Starter, Medicine Wheel Circle

Mary Lou and Dan Smoke became involved in the work of organizing a culturally rooted approach within their urban community for Indigenous persons desiring to recover from substance abuse and addiction. While there were many Alcoholics Anonymous meetings available to attend in the city, there was not a specific space for Indigenous people to gather in an Indigenous-centred manner. Indigenous community members were intrigued by the Indigenous-centred recovery movement of White Bison, Inc. (2002) in the United States, which has been predicated on the premise that the resurgence and practice of Indigenous cultures serves as the locus of addictions treatment (Coyhis & White, 2006).

Employing the recovery paradigm of Alcoholics Anonymous through the usage of the twelve steps, White Bison, Inc. (2002) created a unique culture-based approach that employs the Medicine Wheel as its overarching metaphor and methodology for recovery. To that end, the original twelve steps of Alcoholics Anonymous have been reworded to resonate with Indigenous peoples' understandings and experiences. Making use of the Medicine Wheel metaphor, the recovery process is contextualized as beginning in the eastern direction—a place of new beginnings—and involves a process of moving around the wheel through the directions of east, south, west, and north. Congruent with this conceptualization, the recovery journey is understood to encompass four crucial processes of recognizing that the person has a problem with alcohol or drug abuse or addiction, acknowledging that the person must be committed to recovery and that great effort is required to obtain recovery, forgiving oneself and others for the harms and hurts acquired through the person's life's journey, and changing and thereby stopping the negative behaviours that are associated with drinking and using chemical substances. This approach to recovery also focuses on wellness and addresses the issues that are the root causes of substance abuse and addiction.

Dan and Mary Lou, along with others in their community, decided to start an Indigenous recovery circle meeting that was based upon the White Bison, Inc. (2002) model. In February of 1997, the first circle meeting was held, and this circle has been referred to as the "Medicine Wheel Fire Starters Circle." It is noteworthy that the term "Fire Starters Circle," and the association of the work to create an Indigenous-centred Twelve Step approach as a "Fire Starters Circle" is a term now commonly employed by White Bison, Inc. (Coyhis & White, 2006, p. 182). There are now many Fire Starters Circles in various parts of Canada and the United States. With respect to the Medicine Wheel Fire Starters Circle, this meeting is held one evening every week,[4] and currently they have over thirty members. This circle also now has long-term recovery success stories. Each week, at least twenty members come to these circles, and they also have many visitors from other Indigenous communities and from other Twelve Step meetings.

Visiting this circle, one can easily see the resilience of the traditional kinship and mutual-aid approach to helping. While not necessarily biologically related, in this urban context, members of the circle become supportive kin, or extended family, to each other. This support is offered both within and outside of the circle meetings to facilitate members being able to work through the recovery process. It is also important to note that all voices are valued within the circle, and there is a great deal of diversity reflected in the social location of its members. As indicated earlier, people come from all different walks of life, be they persons who are newly out of prison, who are getting out of street life, who left abusive relationships, who are on income assistance, or who come from higher income brackets. None of these social conditions bear any relevance given the Indigenous truism that "within the circle, we all are of equal height." Moving beyond rhetoric, one can see this occurring in practice. Women and men share an egalitarian space, with decision making occurring through consensual decision-making processes. Indeed, the facilitation of the circle is shared among members with stable recovery.

Their weekly circle process begins with the facilitator of the circle lighting sage and passing around sage as a medicine for purification. This ritual referred to as "smudging", facilitates the ability to connect inwardly, thereby enabling participants to speak their truth. A popular Indigenous prayer is recited. Currently, their process also includes a member of the circle reading from the Coyhis (2007) book, *Meditations with Native American Elders: The Four Seasons*. This provides a context for Indigenous Elders teachings and a focus for discussion. As well, members of the circle are asked if they have any topics to speak about. Congruent with Indigenous sharing circles, the process then involves passing an eagle feather around the circle, and participants are given an opportunity to share. As has been recorded about this methodology, "we take the eagle feather and it goes all the way around the Circle so everyone's had a turn to talk" (Coyhis & White, 2006, p. 142).

Unlike Alcoholics Anonymous meetings, this circle is not restricted to a specific time limit. Participants are welcome and encouraged to share for as long as is desired or required. Through the process of sharing, many participants feel safe to release pent up feelings of hurt, sadness, or frustration by discharging tears. These circles are predicated on a common traditional Indigenous understanding that there is great merit and healing when focused on the activity of listening (Nabigon, 2006). As Nabigon (2006) contends, "the first step towards healing is to listen to the dark side" within our being. He further asserts that, "listening helps us to make the appropriate changes from negative to positive behaviour" (p. 72). This Indigenous premise is very overt in the Medicine Wheel Fire Starters Circle, as participants spend more time listening to others than they do speaking. Another dissimilarity to Alcoholics Anonymous is that within this circle, membership is not restricted to persons who are dealing with alcohol issues. Rather, the circle accepts persons with diverse issues, including persons who are attempting to recover from drug abuse or addiction, compulsive overeating, or emotional or mental health issues.

Indigenous Women's Drumming and Singing Circles

The act of drumming and singing is an important strategy for Indigenous resistance and self-determination. Within today's context, the picking up of drumming and singing has profound consequences for Indigenous women. Goudreau et al. (2008) attest to the health-promoting impacts of Indigenous women's hand drumming and singing. Some of these impacts are described by Goudreau et al. (2008) as finding one's voice and empowerment, the building of healthy identities, connection to culture and traditions, expressing feelings and providing comfort, relaxation and disease prevention, positive thinking and confidence, family bonding, sharing and listening, a sense of belonging, and building social support networks. Amadahy (2003) supports the aforementioned standing impacts of drumming and singing and also reports that this practice can be an important tool for maintaining sobriety.

Waterfall's (2005) work has also asserted that Indigenous hand drumming and singing is a legitimate Indigenous-centred therapeutic tradition and a useful practice for mental health and well-being. She also asserts that the Indigenous drum itself can be a healer, as well as a teacher. As it reminds us of the heartbeat that we felt when we were in the wombs of our mothers, the drumbeat connects us to the heartbeat of Mother Earth (Goudreau et al., 2008). The resonance of the drumbeat connects us to earth-based energies of nurturance and sustenance, as well as to our own inner will, or personal fire of self-determination. When we hear the drum beat, we are reminded of our original kinship connections with the world around us. The significance of "picking of the drum" for Indigenous women is that it moves us beyond remembering how things used to be to reasserting that history in our present-day context. So too when playing in unison with other drummers, the rhythm of the drumbeat also teaches us how to work cohesively together for the collective good. Thus the act of drumming is a powerful tool for Indigenous self-determination.

Congruent with a grassroots approach, Mary Lou and Barbara, in different urban settings, facilitate hand drumming and singing circles in their homes. It is noteworthy that diversity is most welcome in these circles, and as such, women come from different economic backgrounds as well as from different Indigenous Nations. Young girls have also been welcomed to join these circles, thereby encouraging these youth to be involved in healthy and productive activities. Similar to the Medicine Wheel Fire Starters Circle, the process of gathering together to drum begins with the lighting of medicines, such as sage, and the offering of a prayer. The burning medicine is passed around the circle, giving circle members an opportunity to clear away any type of negative emotion that they may be carrying. The process often then involves giving circle members an opportunity to share around the circle about how they are feeling, or to speak to the events that have occurred prior to our last meeting. Usually a sacred item is passed around the circle, such as an eagle feather or a stone, to facilitate focused sharing and respectful listening among circle members. The opportunity to share at the beginning of the circle gives members an opportunity to get to know each other personally, to connect with each other at an emotional level, and to develop trust and rapport.

Healing does occur within these circles, and one of the main objectives of these circles is to assist women in connecting with their personal and collective power. This is accomplished by teaching women traditional protocols about the care of their drums, how to conduct themselves in drumming circles, as well as how to specifically drum and sing Indigenous songs. It is noteworthy that Indigenous songs often begin with a lead line sung individually by a member of the circle. At the onset of women joining the circle, Mary Lou and Barbara as song keepers lead all of the songs. However, when women have gained a momentum with the basics of drumming and singing, they are encouraged to take turns sharing the lead with the songs. Usually, Indigenous women are very shy to do this at first, given the historic experiences of colonialism that have strategically silenced their voices. With nurturance and encouragement, however, women do take turns singing the leads of songs. As has been noted about other Indigenous women's drum circles, "no one is considered a failure; drumming is something that almost anyone can do, and one's singing is never criticized" (Goudreau et al., 2008, p. 78). Mary Lou and Barbara have also observed that when women begin singing, especially when taking on the responsibility of leads, they usually respond with awe and surprise when hearing their own voices. We contend that the presence of this phenomenon indicates the extent to which colonizing processes suppressed and silenced Indigenous women's voices.

It is noteworthy that being around the vibration of drumming, combined with the singing of Indigenous songs, can facilitate the bringing up of emotional pains and trauma (Goudreau et al., 2008). It is thus not uncommon for time to be given throughout a circle gathering for the sharing and discharging of deep emotional pain. Through the context of sharing deep emotions, circle members develop strong emotional and spiritual bonds. Similar to the Medicine Wheel Fire Starters Circle, members may not be blood related, yet they learn to treat each other as extended family, or kin. Indeed, deep bonds of Indigenous sisterhood are formed. The resilience of the kinship-based, mutual-aid paradigm becomes predominant within these circles. As an example, it is not uncommon for circle members to assist each other outside of drumming and singing sessions with childcare, procuring and preparing of food, and transportation to important appointments or functions, as well as emotional and spiritual support.

The impacts of Indigenous women drumming and singing have many ripple effects within their families and communities. One outcome has been the revitalization of Indigenous women's traditional-centred roles. We have observed favourable responses from our communities to our women's drumming and singing groups. This has been indicated by our often being invited to drum and sing at community gatherings, such as traditional feasts, socials, funerals, powwows, and other events.

Conclusion

We have presented the perspective that Indigenous societies prior to our colonization were ones that promoted harmony, peace, health, and well-being. Organized through kinship systems of relationship, the locus of Indigenous strategies for helping and healing were ones that focused on people connecting their own personal and collective power. Contextualized as the inner flame, Indigenous ways of healing and helping promoted Indigenous self-determined agency. As Indigenous peoples, we possess the knowledge and the capability to address our current life's challenges. Yet Indigenous peoples' ability to do this has been constrained by historic and ongoing colonizing processes (Alfred, 2005). Related to this understanding is the perspective that much of the social issues and challenges that Indigenous peoples experience today are in direct response to historic and ongoing forms of colonialism.

Dei and Asgharzadeh (2001) have asserted an effective Indigenous intervention must offer a social and political correction. We contend that the two case studies delineated in this chapter are important contributions to Indigenous mental health discourse, as they offer a prescriptive strategy away from ongoing forms of colonization. Designed to strategically address two critical impacts of colonialism—substance abuse and the disruption of women's power and authority within Indigenous societies—our case studies have spoken to an urban Indigenous addictions recovery circle and urban Indigenous women's drumming and singing circles. Informed by a feminist anticolonial discursive framework, these examples reflect grassroots, Indigenous self-determined initiatives that have been free to develop in accordance with our ancestors' ways of practice and organically outside of the parameters of the government-funded sector. We contend that these two cases speak to the legitimacy, efficacy, and utility of Indigenous culturally rooted, kinship-based, mutual-aid approaches to healing and helping.

Notes

1. Motivated by a respect for Indigenous protocol, we do not speak to specifics about Indigenous sacred ceremonial healing practices. That is, knowledges about Indigenous sacred ceremonies remain within the realm of our oral traditions, and

we do not have permission to share this information in written form. Giving these parameters around the sharing of traditional Indigenous healing practices, we will speak about two examples of generic grassroots healing activities that take place in the public domain.

2. Natural law is a system of law whose principles are rooted in nature and the reasoning of the "good" human mind (Confederated Native Court, 1997).
3. An example of this aforementioned resistance has been Indigenous peoples responses to the European introduction of alcohol into Indigenous systems. The historical accounts portray Indigenous peoples' initial response to the introduction of alcohol in many Nations was one of outright rejection (Coyhis & White, 2006). Coyhis and White's (2006) research also reveals that if alcohol was consumed in the early contact period, a great deal of personal restraint was used. The documented history reveals that the introduction of alcohol into Indigenous systems and the encouragement of Indigenous people becoming intoxicated was a deliberate strategy used by Europeans to exploit Indigenous peoples during treaty and trade negotiations (Hawkins & Blume, 2002). Yet, in spite of these acts of exploitation, Indigenous peoples as early as the 1750s developed culturally rooted strategies to attend to the rise of this new social issue. One such example was the Seneca prophet, Handsome Lake, who, while in an alcoholic coma, received visions of how to lie with and respect alcohol. Recovering from his comma, he became a spiritual leader for his people and reasserted culture-based teachings while encouraging his people to completely abstain from alcohol consumption (Coyhis & White, 2006).
4. In recognition for their service and success with respect to the Wellbriety recovery movement, the Medicine Wheel Fire Starters Circle was given an award of recognition by White Bison, Inc. (Coyhis & White, 2006).

References

Alfred, T. (2005). *Wasase: Indigenous pathways to action and freedom.* Toronto: Broadview Press.

Amadahy, Z. (2003). The healing power of women's voices. In. K. Anderson, & B. Lawrence (Eds.), *Strong women stories: Native vision and community survival* (pp. 144–155). Toronto: Sumach Press.

Anderson, K. (2000). *A recognition of being: Reconstructing Native womanhood.* Toronto: Sumuch Press.

Antone, R., Miller, D., & Myers, B. (1986). *The power within people: A community organizing perspective.* Deseronto: Peace Tree Technologies.

Archibald, L. (2006). *Decolonizing and healing: Indigenous experiences in the United States, New Zealand, Australia and Greenland.* Ottawa: Aboriginal Healing Foundation.

Baikie, G. (2009). Indigenous-centered social work: Theorizing a social work way of being. In R. Sinclair, M. A. Hart, & G. Bruyere (Eds.), *Wicihitowin: Aboriginal social work in Canada* (pp. 42–61). Halifax: Fernwood Publishing.

Confederated Native Court. (1997). *Confederated Native court judgement and reason.* Retrieved from http://sisis.nativeweb.org/sov/confjudg.html

Coyhis, D. L. (2007). *Meditations with Native American elders: The four seasons.* Colorado Springs: Coyhis Publishing.

Coyhis, D. L., & White, W. L. (2006). *Alcohol problems in Native America: The untold story of resistance and recovery—"The truth about the lie."* Colorado Springs: White Bison Inc.

Dei, G. J. S. (2000). Towards an anti-racist discursive framework. In G. J. S. Dei, & A. Calliste. (Eds.), *Power, knowledge and anti-racism education: A critical reader* (pp. 23–40). Halifax: Fernwood.

Dei, G. J. S., & Asgharzadeh, A. (2001). The power of social theory: The anti-colonial discursive framework. *Journal of Educational Thought, 35*(3), 297–323.

Dumont, J., Hopkins, C., Dell, C., & Menzies, P. (2014, February). *Culture as intervention in addictions treatment: Appreciating evidence within indigenous knowledge*. Presentation given at the Chiefs of Ontario Health Forum, Intercontinental Hotel: Toronto. Retrieved from http://health.chiefs-of-ontario.org/sites/default/files/news_files/Culture%20as%20Intervention%20in%20Addictions%20Carol%20Hopkins.pdf

Goudreau, G., Weber-Pillwax, C., Cote-Meeks, S., Madill, H., & Wilson, S. (2008). Hand drumming: Health promoting experiences of Aboriginal women form a northern Ontario urban community. *Journal of Aboriginal Health, 4*(1), 72–83.

Hart, M. A. (2002). *Seeking mino-pimatisiwin: An Aboriginal approach to helping.* Halifax: Fernwood.

Hawkins, E. H., & Blume, A. W. (2002). Loss of sacredness: Historical contexts of health policies for indigenous people in the United States. In P. D. Mail, S. Heurtin-Roberts, S. E. Martin, & J. Howard (Eds.), *Alcohol use among American Indians: Multiple perspectives on a complex problem* (NIAAA Research Monograph No. 37, pp. 25–46). Bethesda, MD: National Institutes of Health, National Institute on Alcohol Abuse and Alcoholism.

Heavy Runner, I., & Morris, J. S. (1997). Traditional Native culture and resilience. *Research Practice, 5*(1). Minneapolis: University of Minnesota. *Center for Applied Research & Educational Improvement, College of Education and Human Development.* Retrieved from http://www.coled.umn.edu/carei/Reports/Rpractice/Spring97/traditional.htm

Maracle, S. (2003). The eagle has landed: Native women, leadership and community development. In K. Anderson, & B. Lawrence (Eds.), *Strong women stories: Native vision and community survival* (pp. 70–80). Toronto: Sumach Press.

Mihesuah, D. A. (2003). *Indigenous American women: Decolonization, empowerment, activism.* Lincoln: University of Nebraska Press.

Nabigon, H. (2006). *The hollow tree: Fighting addiction with traditional Native healing.* Montreal and Kingston: McGill-Queen's University Press.

Thunderbird, S. (2011). *Indigenous women's rights.* Retrieved from http://www.shannonthunderbird.com/Indigenous_women_rights.htm

The Truth and Reconciliation Commission of Canada. (2015). *Honouring the truth, reconciling for the future: Summary of the final report of the Truth and Reconciliation Commission of Canada.* (Executive Summary) Retrieved from website www.trc.ca/websites/ . . . /File/ . . . /Exec_Summary_2015_05_31_web_o.pdf

Wane, N. N., & Waterfall, B. (2005). Hoops of spirituality in science & technology. In P. Tripp, & L. Muzzin (Eds.), *Teaching as activism: Equity meetings environmentalism* (pp. 47–63). Montreal and Kingston: McGill-Queen's University Press.

Waterfall, B. (2005). *Anishnabec hand drumming as Native-centered social work practice.* Presentation given at the Annual spirituality and social work conference, London, Ontario, Kings University College.

Waterfall, B. (2008). *Decolonizing anishnabec social work education: An anishnabe spiritually-infused reflexive study* (Unpublished doctoral thesis). Toronto: Ontario Institute for Studies in Education of the University of Toronto, Toronto.

Wesley-Esquimaux, C. C., & Smolewski, M. (2004). *Historic trauma and Aboriginal healing*. Ottawa: Aboriginal Healing Foundation.

White Bison, Inc. (2002). *The red road to wellbriety in the Native American way*. Colorado Springs: White Bison Incorporated.

Whitebeck, B. L., Xiaojin, C., Hoyt, D. R., & Adams, G. W. (2004). Discrimination, historical losses and enculturation: Culturally specific risk and resiliency factors for alcohol abuse among American Indians. *Journal of Studies in Alcohol, 65*(4), 409–418.

2 A Laughing Matter

Native American Humour as an Indigenous Healing Tradition and Way of Life

Michael Tlanusta Garrett, J. T. Garrett, Gloria K. King, Tarrell Awe Agahe Portman, Edil Torres-Rivera, Dale Brotherton, and Lisa Grayshield

The Dogs Hold an Election

Once a long time ago, the dogs were trying to elect a president. So one of them got up in the big dog convention and said, "I nominate the bulldog for president. He's strong. He can fight."

"But he can't run," said another dog. "What good is a fighter who can't run? He won't catch anybody."

Then another dog got up and said, "I nominate the greyhound, because he sure can run."

But the other dogs cried, "Naw, he can run all right, but he can't fight. When he catches up with somebody, what happens then? He gets the hell beaten out of him, that's what! So all he's good for is running away."

Then an ugly little mutt jumped up and said, "I nominate that dog for president who smells good underneath his tail."

And immediately an equally ugly mutt jumped up and yelled, "I second the motion."

At once all the dogs started sniffing underneath each other's tails. A big chorus went up.

"Phew, he doesn't smell good under his tail."

"No, neither does this one."

"He's no presidential timber!"

"No, he's no good, either."

"This one sure isn't the people's choice."

"Wow, this ain't my candidate!"

When you go out for a walk, just watch the dogs. They're still sniffing underneath each other's tails. They're looking for a good leader, and they still haven't found him (Lame Deer, in Itzkowitz, 1995, pp. 59–60).

Chasing Your Tail

Contrary to the stereotypical belief that Natives are solemn, stoic figures poised against a backdrop of tepees, tomahawks, and headdresses, the fact is, most Native people love to laugh and always love a good story, as illustrated by the anecdote in the opening of this chapter (Garrett & Garrett, 1994). However, even something as simple as a joke or story can offer much more insight into a culture than may be apparent at first sight. Stories, anecdotes, witty one-liners, these are all examples of an expression of the spirit of Native people in a tradition that is unique to every tribal nation, but shares the same power across tribes.

Spirituality has been defined as "a way of being and experiencing that comes about through awareness of a transcendent dimension and that is characterized by certain identifiable values in regard to self, others, nature, life . . ." (Kelley, 1995, p. 4). Native humour as a spiritual tradition often goes unnoticed by Western culture as a powerful healing force in the lives of Native people, as it has been for ages. The fact that so many Native nations have survived the horror of countless acts of cultural genocide committed by Western culture and nations in the name of civilization serves as a testament, in part, to the resilience of Native humour having stood the test of time (Garrett & Pichette, 2000).

That Native people have been cast as uncommunicative, distant, or mysterious by Western culture says little about the true essence of an entire nation of many nations of Native people. It says more about a history of stereotyping Native people either as faithful sidekicks barely able to speak a complete sentence or as strangely mystical beings that seem to transcend the world of physical reality. It may be that both are true, or neither. Regardless, countries such as Canada and the United States continue to hold steadfast in their fascination of Native people, while rarely grasping the true essence of the many cultures of Native nations as they exist today. That spells disaster for helping professionals working with Native clients.

In order to best work with Native clients, it is critical to have an accurate understanding of the essence of the people and a working knowledge of cultural communication styles. As humour is an integral piece in both of the aforementioned areas, it is important to explore, with respect, further into the spiritual tradition of Native humour as it exists in many forms. The purpose of this chapter is to briefly discuss the current literature regarding the use of humour in the therapeutic process of helping and then explore Native humour as a spiritual tradition and way of life with implications for the practice of psychology.

Humour and Counselling Professions

No one knows for sure where the notion of counselling or psychology, as an intensely serious process of curing the mind and soul, originated, though most point to Freud. We could speculate on that point; however, we find ourselves in a day and age where people of all walks of life endure countless stressors, wherein there seems to be little about which to laugh. The topic of using humour in counselling is nothing new, but has received more attention recently in the professional literature.

The use of humour in the helping process has been associated with increasing trust, reducing stress, promoting holistic wellness, creating needed perspective, boosting physiological well-being, and allowing clients to take control over their lives (Maples et al., 2001). In particular, Rollo May (cited in Goldin & Bordan, 1999, p. 405) described the use of humour in the therapeutic process as a "healthy way of feeling a 'distance' between one's self and the problem, a way of standing off and looking at one's problem with perspective." Other authors have similarly described the effects of using humour in the therapeutic process in terms of the perspective it creates (Amada, 1993; Burkhead, Ebener, & Marini, 1996; Cousins, 1979; Goldin & Bordan, 1999; Herring, 1994). This perspective may indeed be either the way in which humour brings about much-needed oneness between seemingly opposite dimensions (e.g., subject and object) or much-needed distance (Eberhart, 1993).

One of the main advantages of using humour in the counselling process is that it allows the counsellor to seem more genuine and empathic. One of the main disadvantages of using humour in the counselling process inappropriately is that it can help clients avoid areas of conflict or may restrict their expression of emotion (Kush, 1997). Therefore, humour in the therapeutic process can have both desired and undesired consequences and seems to depend a great deal on how it is introduced by the helping professional and how it is used in the counselling process. However, many benefits of using humour in the counselling process have been described that include helping clients cope with stress; recover from illness; overcome adversity; achieve therapeutic goals; experience decreases in anxiety and discomfort; and overcome depression, grief, sorrow, disappointment, and loss (Amada, 1993; Burkhead et al., 1996; Cousins, 1979; Goldin & Bordan, 1999).

Amada (1993) also notes the important function that humour serves in helping persecuted groups deal with tragedy by giving them a means of "poking fun at their oppressors" (p. 161). An example of this can be found in the movie, *Smoke Signals*, when the main characters, who are both Native, sing a jubilant yet sarcastic version of John Wayne's "teeth," something they seem to improvise as a way of poking fun at the classic symbol of White heroism and rugged individualism, who often shows his bravery by "beating the Indians," sometimes almost single-handedly. Therefore, humour with ethnic minority clients may serve additional functions beyond some of the benefits typically noted in the literature. Though little has been written in the counselling literature specifically on Native humour as a cultural phenomenon, several authors have explored the value of using humour in working with Native clients (Garrett & Garrett, 1994; Herring, 1994; Herring & Meggert, 1994). For a better understanding of Native humour, it is necessary to explore the cultural nuances from a Native perspective.

Relating Through Narrative

For many Native people, the oral tradition of storytelling serves as an important educational method for conveying traditional values, beliefs, and expectations about life (Garrett, 1996a; Portman & Garrett, 2006). It is through stories that Native people learn, and it is through that kind of learning that they come to an understanding of themselves, the world around them, and their relationship to everything in that world. Listening to a person's story involves being given an opportunity to understand that person's life experience and perspective as he or she understands it. With any given story, the importance of relationship cannot be overlooked. This includes

> neither the "objective" (structure) nor the "subjective" (culture) but the relationship between them; neither past nor present, but the relationship between them; neither dominant memory nor commonplace understandings, but the relationship between them; neither the personal/individual nor large-scale changes, but the relationship between them.
> (Casey, 1993, p. 12)

Given these many relationships, the narrator must make decisions about framing the text concerning "the emphasis to be placed on particular elements, the way in which the elements are to be assembled for presentation, and the underlying set of assumptions . . ." (Casey, 1993, p. 25).

Framing, according to Casey (1993), depends upon the narrator's worldview, which is "inextricably bound up with its relationship to other worldviews (in a system of intertextuality)" (p. 26). The narrator has understandings and interpretations (how the story is told as well as what is told) within particular contexts that allows his or her development of self, understandings of others, and responses to existing social arrangements. The narrator communicates through language, defined as "the way in which human beings make meaning, as well as worldviews that have been socially constructed in that process" (Casey, 1993, p. 3). Essentially, this communication involves jointly constructed understandings of the world based on the assumption that the significance and meaning are developed not separately within the individual, but in coordination with other human beings in cultural context. As such, the narrative, in this way, also relates the narrator's worldview and culture as a perceptual lens through which the person views the world. Therefore, the focus of the narrative approach is on understanding meanings communicated through language by particular persons *in relation* to particular contexts. As one Native Elder put it, "in order to truly know your place in the Circle, you must recognize where you stand in relation to everything around you."

Lessons of the Eagle Feather: Rule of Opposites

Eagle feathers are considered sacred among Native Americans who make use of them for a variety of purposes, including ceremonial healing and purification. Eagle Medicine, though varying in meaning and practice across many tribal traditions, tends to represent a state of presence achieved through diligence, understanding, awareness, and a completion of "tests of initiation," such as the vision quest or other demanding life experiences. In some Nations/Tribes highly respected Elder status is associated with Eagle Medicine and the power of connectedness and truth. It is through experience and patience that this medicine is earned over a lifetime. There is an old anecdote that probably best illustrates the lessons of the eagle feather:

> Once while acting as a guide for a hunting expedition, an Indian had lost the way home. One of the men with him said, "You're lost, chief." The Indian guy replied, "I'm not lost, my tipi is lost."

The eagle feather, which represents duality, tells the story of life. It tells of the many dualities that exist in the Circle of Life, such as light and dark, male and female, substance and shadow, summer and winter, life and death, and peace and war (Garrett & Barret, 2003; Garrett & Myers, 1996). The eagle feather has both light and dark colours, dualities and opposites. Though one can make a choice to argue which of the colours is most beautiful or most valuable, the truth is that both colours come from the same feather, both are true, both are connected, and it takes both to fly (Garrett & Garrett, 1996; Garrett & Garrett, 2002). The colours are opposite, but they are part of the same truth. The importance of the feather does not lie in which colour is most beautiful, but in discovering the purpose of the feather. In other words, there is no such thing as keeping the mountains and getting rid of the valleys; they are one and the same, and they coexist because of one another. In this way, perhaps the essence of Native Americans and humour is the constant cultural seeking of balance and harmony through perspective and revealing what is true both in the simplest terms of what becomes apparent if you stop and see something for what it is and deeper truths that only reveal themselves through that constant seeking of perspective in the world; all of this involves a valuing of one's basic place in the world through humility and recognition of one's faults, caring for others, giving of oneself for the good of others, and being connected with others through openness and respect.

Native Americans and Humour

When asked, "What is the most important thing that White people still don't know about Native people; what are some of the big lies and cultural myths that still linger on?" Clyde Hall (Shoshone-Métis) replies:

> That Natives don't laugh. We laugh about everything, that's the way we survive. It's kind of a dry, insane sense of humour. It's better than crying—we do that, too. But anytime you laugh about something, it shatters it. Then it doesn't have any power over you.
>
> (In Thompson, 1994, p. 126)

Hall probably best captures both the essence and function of Native humour as a communication style and as a way of surviving in a sometimes difficult world. Humour, from a Native perspective, is as integral a part of life as eating. Ironically, context is an important feature of Native humour as a critical part of the culture, especially around mealtime. It is amazing to watch the transformation that occurs when people come together around food and really begin to open up. In Native country, mealtime is sometimes the worst time to try to eat because everyone (yourself included) is laughing so hard, cutting up, sharing sidesplitting stories, and teasing each other.

Native humour takes many different forms, including stories, anecdotes, teasing or razzing, songs, dance, art forms, cultural symbols, and so forth. Probably one of the most common forms that Native humour has taken traditionally is that of stories intended to both entertain and educate. Many tribal oral traditions emphasize important life lessons through the subtle humour expressed in the stories. So often it is an arrogant, manipulative, vain, clown-like figure of Rabbit, Possum, Coyote, Dog, Turtle, or Raven, among others (the character depends on the tribe, but is always the one who thinks he or she knows it all) that ends up learning a hard lesson in humility in the end, much to the amusement of others and maybe as a reminder to others (Garrett, 1998; Garrett & Garrett, 1996; Harjo, 1998; Herring, 1994). Consider, as an example, the hard lessons learned by Possum in the following Cherokee story (in Garrett, 1998, pp. 68–72) handed down from generations past.

Why the Possum's Tail Is Bare

A long time ago, when people could still understand the language of the animals, Ujetsdi, Possum, used to have a long, beautiful bushy tail. In fact, he had the longest, most beautiful, bushiest tail of all of the animals, and he knew it. He was so proud of his tail that he liked to brush it every day, and he sang about it all the time.

The animals, who hadn't had a good powwow in a while, decided that it was high time for a traditional "Donelawega," and they decided together in council that as part of the festivities, there would be a contest to see who had the most beautiful tail. Well, all of the animals knew who was going to win, but it was a good time to celebrate, eat well, offer prayers, see old friends, and make some new ones.

The council sent Tsi-s-du, Rabbit, as a messenger to bring news of the powwow to all of the animals in the different communities. Rabbit, who had had no tail since Bear had pulled it out, was very jealous of Possum and decided he was going to get Possum good.

So Rabbit eventually went to Possum's house and greeted him. He told him about the powwow that was to be held and about the contest. "Can I tell the council that you will be at the powwow then?" asked Rabbit inquisitively.

"Oh, I'd love to come," responded Possum, "but you'll have to make sure that I have a special seat up front so that all of the animals can see my long beautiful tail."

Rabbit chimed, "I am sure that the council wouldn't *think* of having you sit anywhere else, Possum. After all, it would be such an honor to have you sitting up front where everyone could see your tail. I'll even have someone come to brush and prepare it in a *proper* way since this is such a special event. After all, a tail that beautiful deserves a little special attention, and you want it to be done right."

Possum couldn't agree more and was very pleased, saying, "Oh, that would be just lovely. My tail is quite beautiful as it is, but I'm sure a little extra attention wouldn't hurt any."

So Rabbit went along his way and soon came upon Cricket, who was considered an expert hair cutter by all the animals. Cricket happened to owe Rabbit a favor, and it was time to pay up, so Rabbit told him just what to do and, once again, went about his business.

The next morning, Cricket went to Possum's house, saying that he had been sent by Rabbit to prepare Possum's tail for the powwow. So Possum, who had already been busy brushing his tail, stretched out on a big soft bed of moss and closed his eyes while Cricket went to work. Cricket brushed Possum's tail (while Possum reminded him how beautiful it was) and told him he would wrap a long strip of red cloth around and around it to keep it smooth until the powwow. But all the while, without Possum knowing it, Cricket was clipping the hair off of Possum's tail all the way down to the roots!

That night, Possum went to the ceremonial grounds where the powwow was being held. All of the animals were there. Each of the animals danced into the Circle around the Sacred Fire, one at a time and showed their tails to the admiring community. And there was Possum, sitting right up front in his special seat just as Rabbit had promised, waiting for his turn, which would be last. And patiently he waited, noticing how other animals' tails were no match for the beauty of his own. One by one, the animals moved into the Circle and then out once again. First Eagle, then Raccoon, then Bear, then Deer, and so on, until all of the animals had had their turn. And then it came time for Possum.

Possum loosened the red cloth tied around his tail and danced elegantly into the Circle, singing, "Behold my beautiful tail! See how long and beautiful it is! See the way it shines!" Then he wiggled his tail for all the animals to see.

All of the animals roared, and Possum continued dancing around the Circle, again singing, "Behold my beautiful tail! See how long and beautiful it is! See the way it sweeps the air!" And again he wiggled his tail for all the animals to see.

Once more, the animals roared in laughter, and in response, Possum resonated even louder than before. "Behold my beautiful tail! See how long and beautiful it is! See how fine the fur is!" And once again, he wiggled his tail for all the animals to see.

By now the animals were laughing so hard that Possum began to wonder why. As he looked around, everyone was laughing and pointing at his tail. Possum peered behind him and saw that, to his surprise, there was no hair on his tail—it was completely bald! Well, he was so shocked and embarrassed that without saying a word, he fell to the ground and played dead. And to this day, when taken by surprise, Possum does this. And to this day, Possum's tail is still bare. And so, it is good.

Learning From Possum

In Native humour, one can easily end up as the butt (or tail) of a joke. In the preceding story, not only is the subtle humour evident (by the way, this is one of the few stories where Rabbit doesn't end up on the short end of the stick), but the emphasis on community as an important spiritual tradition in the lives the Cherokee people is strong as well. Humility and a sense of generosity are cultural values that seem to pervade Native nations across the United States (Garrett, 1996b). Stories and anecdotes are but one means of reinforcing and reminding in-group members of the cultural values and unspoken rules by which they live. Native people live for laughter, which plays a very important role in the continued survival of the tribal community. After all, laughter relieves stress and creates an atmosphere of sharing and connectedness. As George Good Striker (Blackfoot) puts it, "Humor is the WD-40 of healing" (cited in Garrett, 1998, p. 137).

So where does the popular stereotype of Native American stoicism come from? As Phil Lane Sr. (Yankton Lakota) (cited in Schaef, 1995) says,

> Our white relatives say the Native is stoic. This is not necessarily true. We just wait to see the true person. Given time, he [or she] will show his [or her] true self, so we wait and time will provide the proof.
>
> (April 8, para. 1)

Indeed, silence and careful observation are important parts of Native self-discipline, reflection, and communication style (Garrett, 1996b; Garrett & Garrett, 1994); however, humour is just as important in bringing people together and reaffirming bonds of kinship. To see Native people "laughing hard, cutting up, teasing" with one another is a sign of the closeness between them and the "honouring of relation" that is occurring.

Non-Native people often view Native humour as being "dry" based on their observation of the obvious and the use of exaggeration. This style of humour, sometimes referred to by Native people as "teasing" or "razzing," is rather unique in its pragmatism of stating the somewhat obvious, but using perspective to show the humorous side of things. Moreover, the wit of Native one-line retorts are classic, and not uncommon. Whenever non-Native people have come up to me and said, "How," in a joking manner, I (primary author) have quickly responded to them by saying, "I don't know how, you tell me." Consider a few other examples of these Native one-liners:

- When questioned by an anthropologist on what Natives called America before the white man came, a Native simply said, "Ours" (Deloria, 1988, p. 166).
- A young Native was asked one day what a peace treaty was. He replied, "That's when the white man wants a piece of your land" (Deloria, 1988, p. 166).
- A Pueblo artist was quizzed one day on why Natives were the first ones on this continent. "We had reservations," was his reply (Deloria, 1988, p. 166).
- Question: Are you a full-blooded Native? Reply: No, I'm a pint low. I just came from the blood bank (Northrup, 1997, p. 2).
- Question: Do Natives have psychic powers? Reply: I knew you were going to ask me that. I just knew it (Northrup, 1997, p. 12).
- Question: Why is the white man in such a hurry to get to Mars? Reply: They think we have land there (Northrup, 1997, p. 13).
- Question: How do you say moose in Ojibwe? Reply: Mooz (Northrup, 1997, p. 66).
- Question: How do you say moccasin in Ojibwe? Reply: Makizin (Northrup, 1997, p. 66).
- Question: What does a [Native] Santa say? Reply: Ho, ho, ho-wah (Northrup, 1997, p. 68).
- Question: What is Native Summer? Reply: It's that warm spell between Native Spring and Native Fall (Northrup, 1997, p. 85).
- Question: If you're a Native, why is your skin so light? Reply: Melanin Deficit Disorder (Northrup, 1997, p. 87).
- Question: How do you insult [a Native]? Reply: Call him or her a Columbus lover (Northrup, 1997, p. 122).
- Question: What is the unemployment rate on the Rez? Reply: I don't know, that's not my job (Northrup, 1997, p. 215).
- Question: What's the difference between praying in church and praying at the casino? Reply: At the casino, you really mean it (Northrup, 1997, p. 221).
- Question: Why do you call it a Rez instead of a Reservation? Reply: Because the white man owns most of it (Northrup, 1997, p. 226).
- Question: What do you call a Walmart bag? Reply: A Native suitcase (M. T. Garrett, personal experience).
- Question: How do you say "dog" in Cherokee? Reply: di-o-gee (M. T. Garrett, personal experience).
- A Native woman of mixed ancestry was giving a talk once to an audience in which a heckler remarked to the speaker, "You don't look Native." And the speaker quickly retorted, "You don't look rude" (M. T. Garrett, personal experience).

As for the much-debated issue of whether or not sports teams should use Native mascots, Northrup (1997, p. 118), a member of the Anishaabe Nation, shares a conversation on the topic between he and a relative:

> My cousin, Rathide, suggested we go to a Saints' or Padres' game dressed as Catholics. What a great idea, I thought. Get thirty Shinnobs, put miters and vestments on them. They could carry rosaries, let people kiss their ring and wash their feet. Rathide also reminded me when the Catholics first came, they had the Bible and we had the land. Out of respect, we shut our eyes and got down on our knees to pray with them. When we got up, we had the Bible and they had the land. I decided not to dress as a Catholic . . .

Often, Native humour is cleverly used to dissipate tension, deal with potential conflict, or subtly communicate a serious message. Deloria (1988, p. 152) shares another example:

> One story concerns a very obnoxious missionary who delighted in scaring people with tales of hell, eternal fires, and everlasting damnation. This man was very unpopular and people went out of their way to avoid him. But he persisted to contrast heaven and hell as a carrot-and-stick technique of conversion. One Sunday after a particularly fearful description of hell he asked an old chief, the main holdout of the tribe against Christianity, where he wanted to go. The old chief asked the missionary where *he* was going. And the missionary replied that, of course, he as a missionary of the gospel was going to heaven. "Then I'll go to hell," the old chief said, intent on having peace in the world to come if not in this world.

Razzing, Native Style

What Is It?

Razzing is "a collective form of storytelling in which participants take some episode, humorous or not, from a present or past experience and relate it 'humorously' to the others in attendance" (Pratt, 1998, p. 57). The story used in razzing is often lengthy and typically embellished or changed by other participating people. Razzing is similar to "sounding" or "playing the dozens" of the African American oral tradition in which there is a skilled verbal duelling (i.e., participants direct verbal insults at one another) that occurs in the group context. Razzing is usually directed toward the divergent behaviour of an individual, group, or tribe. However, unlike sounding and playing the dozens, razzing is not directed toward family members, physical disabilities, or socioeconomic status (Pratt, 1998). As a matter of fact, one of the quickest ways to insult a Native person is to talk bad about his or her family.

What Is Its Purpose?

Traditionally, razzing or teasing, as it is sometimes called, has served a very important role in dealing with or reducing the likelihood of social conflicts, or making light of serious situations over which people have no control. It is not uncommon for Native people to use humour as a way of countering the ill effects of misfortune. As James Luna (Luisena/Diegueno) comments,

> In Native humor, you can make fun of anything and even at the worst times . . . but I think what I came to realize is that it's a way of easing the pain, that laughter is a good cure and that maybe if we didn't laugh so much, we would be depressed.
>
> (In Weintraub, Danto, & McErilley, 1996, p. 101)

We see the practical functions that Native humour serves, and we also see the powerful healing effect of perspective through a truly spiritual tradition in everyday interactions. Native humour is also used as a means of testing for anyone whose identity as a Native person is questionable or unknown (Pratt, 1998). As an intentional oral art form, the use of perspective through quick, witty remarks or the use of exaggeration in lengthy stories in the group's context is a prominent feature of Native humour, sometimes known as razzing, depending on geographic region and colloquialisms.

The Rules of Engagement

There are a couple of unspoken rules with regard to razzing, though these "rules" can be regional and thus differ slightly from tribe to tribe. Generally, razzing is restricted to participants of equal age status. However, there are exceptions, depending on the tribe, in which younger people may razz older people (depending on the topic), and older people may definitely razz younger people. It is generally understood across tribes that one does not disrespect an Elder, but again, this may vary from tribe to tribe. Second, it is not acceptable for those known as "candidate Natives" (anthropological term referring to people who can provide proof of tribal heritage, but have not been socialized in a Native environment) to razz other Native people (Pratt, 1998). When and if this occurs, it will usually be met with silence as a form of disapproval. Shunning of the offending person would be the extreme measure of social punishment for having broken any of the unspoken rules.

Shame Story

As mentioned earlier, razzing as a specific implementation of Native humour takes on various forms. One such form is the "shame story." In this form, one person becomes the object (like Possum) of the razz in which a past incident involving that person is meticulously recounted to those present who tend to join in with embellishments of their own. Each time the story is told, it can get more and more elaborate so that, it may indeed, barely resemble the original incident at all. Sometimes the object of the razz will self-select him or herself as the object of the razz and set him or herself up for it intentionally. As an example, I (primary author) remember a friend of mine, Joe Dudley (Yankton Lakota), saying in a Native peer group situation, "Well, I just got finished with my six-hour workout, and I'm not going to be able to go outside or *they'll* get me," implying that all the women would be after him. Another person responded, "Who, the flies?" whereupon the whole group burst out in laughter and joined in trying to contribute as many humorous remarks as they could. Another person said, "No, even the flies couldn't stand the smell of him right now!" Therefore, with razzing, Native people, among peers, will tease and leave themselves open to being teased, as it serves the purpose of keeping one humble and a part of the group. The creation and maintenance of relational connections is one of the main purposes of Native humour, as it has been for generations and in many forms.

Songs

Another implementation of razzing can occur through songs that are directed towards individuals or events. Probably one of the best-known examples of razzing through songs is the "forty-nines" originated by the Kiowa Nation of Oklahoma. The forty-nines, originally serving as celebration of past raiding parties, are generally held after a powwow. The topics of forty-nines are limitless, but still must conform to the rules described earlier. Other less formal styles of razzing can occur through song as people sitting around together spontaneously invent musical tributes to some humorous person, topic, or event, as evidenced in some classic Native films such as *Powwow Highway, Smoke Signals, Medicine River*, or *Thunderheart* to name a few.

An Overall Understanding of Native Americans and Humour

Native Americans understand all too well the importance of not taking yourself too seriously. This has served as one of the many useful coping methods for generations of Native people who have learned how to survive in the face of persecution, exploitation, and genocide. The thinking behind this is that people who are not open to teasing or cannot handle laughing at themselves probably cannot handle being part of the group if they are too wrapped up in themselves and their problems. The use of humour in Native tradition has contributed to the survival of many Native nations as a coping skill by restoring harmony and balance among Native people, serving as an everyday communication skill that preserves connections, and supporting the life-learning of younger generations as an oral tradition that shows people how to live or not live.

Overall, Native humour as a spiritual tradition takes various forms, gets played out in various ways, and serves a number of important purposes.

Among these purposes are the maintenance of Native culture, controlling social situations, teaching people how to live, creating unity, increasing social and political awareness, testing others' identity or cultural competency as Natives, and simply as a way of interacting and enjoying being together (Deloria, 1988; Pratt, 1998). With this in mind, it is important to translate knowledge and awareness of Native humour into practice in the counselling process through a culturally appropriate way that benefits the therapeutic process and demonstrates respect for Native clients.

Implications for Counselling

As a metaphor for counselling, healing ceremonies in many tribal traditions generally include some kind of informal sharing (e.g., sharing of a meal, sharing of stories) that invariably results in spontaneous use of humour. It just "flows" into the process, and things would not be the same without it. That may seem contrary to what many outsiders would expect who maintain a false image of "healing practices" (Native or otherwise) as a serious, intense, humourless processes of expelling pain and suffering. In Native tradition, one of the most powerful healing forces in existence is being able to be real and being able to laugh with family, friends, and strangers alike.

The use of humour in the counselling process does not have to take away from the seriousness of the counselling process or somehow dilute its effectiveness; in fact, it could enhance the process. One of the major goals of humour, according to the literature, should be to help clients become more integrated and more spontaneous in their relationships, as well as learning helpful coping strategies (Weaver & Wilson, 1997). In addition, humour in the counselling process can be used spontaneously and creatively to facilitate development of the therapeutic relationship, but never at the expense of the client's feelings. To be more specific, counselling professionals working with Native clients can encourage client sharing of funny stories or anecdotes that may say a lot about that client's identity and the issues with which he or she is dealing. In the process, these stories or anecdotes may also tell a lot about the client's family, clan, and tribe as important or unimportant determinants in how he or she sees him or herself. It also may open the doors to deeper trust in the therapeutic relationship. Moreover, it may provide some important insight into possible resources and/or courses of action that could be helpful in working through particular issues.

Although humour is found across cultural boundaries, the way in which it manifests concerning specific cultural meanings and style of communication varies. In addition, in the therapeutic relationship itself, the ability of counselling professionals and clients to use humour together as part of the therapeutic process is also affected by cultural differences between the two persons involved and by any power differentials resulting from those differences. Therefore, counsellors, as out-group members, must exercise caution, sensitivity, and tact when using humour in the helping process with clients of another ethnic group. The literature recommends that counselling professionals never use humour in a way that is denigrating to the client or communicates the message that he or she is not taking the client seriously (Goldin & Bordan, 1999; Maher, 1993). There is also a recommendation offered by Gladding (1995) that humour not be used when it a) avoids dealing with the client's feelings, b) is viewed by the client as irrelevant to his or her reason for being in the helping process, c) is experienced as a put-down, d) is used too frequently, or e) is inappropriately timed.

The implications for use of humour in the helping process also hold true for working with Native clients. Native humour serves as an important, culturally relevant coping mechanism and way of connecting. It can be a powerful tool in the helping process. It is important, however, to assess the client's level of acculturation to avoid making inaccurate assumptions about that person's cultural identity (see Garrett & Pichette, 2000 for further information).

Having a clear understanding of the client's cultural identity and level of acculturation, humour should only be used with Native clients when and if the client invites it, meaning that the client trusts the counsellor enough to connect on that level. What in one situation can be humorous between two people, in another situation, without the trust and sense of connection, can be interpreted as ridicule or "wearing a mask" (i.e., not being genuine). In addition, helping professionals using humour in the therapeutic process should be aware of the cultural restrictions (mentioned earlier in this article) around family, physical disability, and socioeconomic status, as well as requirements regarding age status and cultural identity (i.e., Native vs. non-Native persons).

All in all, both Native and non-Native helping professionals working with Native clients should exercise caution using humour in the therapeutic process, but definitely should not overlook it as a powerful therapeutic technique in itself. Native humour as a spiritual tradition serves the purpose of reaffirming and enhancing the sense of connectedness and resiliency experienced as being part of the family, clan, and tribe. To the extent that humour can serve that purpose in the therapeutic relationship, for assisting the counselling professional and client's work together, and for helping clients achieve their goals, all the better. Otherwise, we as helping professionals could just end up like dogs chasing our tails, or sniffing around the tails of other dogs.

References

Amada, G. (1993). The role of humor in a college mental health program. In W. F. Fry, & W. A. Salameh (Eds.), *Advances in humour and psychotherapy* (pp. 157–181). Sarasota, FL: Professional Resources.

Burkhead, E. J., Ebener, D. J., & Marini, I. (1996). Humor, coping, and adaptation to disability. *Journal of Applied Rehabilitation Counseling, 27*(4), 50–53.

Casey, K. (1993). *I answer with my life: Life histories of women teachers working for social change.* New York: Routledge.

Cousins, N. (1979). *Anatomy of an illness*. New York: Norton.

Deloria, Jr., V. (1988). *Custer died for your sins: An Native manifesto*. Norman, OK: University of Oklahoma Press.

Eberhart, E. (1993). Humor as a religious experience. In W. F. Fry, & W. A. Salameh (Eds.), *Advances in humour and psychotherapy* (pp. 97–119). Sarasota, FL: Professional Resources.

Garrett, J. T., & Garrett, M. T. (1994). The path of good medicine: Understanding and counseling Native Americans. *Journal of Multicultural Counseling and Development, 22*(3), 134–144.

Garrett, J. T., & Garrett, M. T. (1996). *Medicine of the Cherokee: The way of right relationship*. Santa Fe, NM: Bear & Company.

Garrett, M. T. (1996a). "Two people": An American Indian narrative of bicultural identity. *Journal of American Indian Education, 36*(1), 1–21.

Garrett, M. T. (1996b). Reflection by the riverside: The traditional education of Native American children. *Journal of Humanistic Education and Development, 35*(1), 12–28.

Garrett, M. T. (1998). *Walking on the wind: Cherokee teachings for harmony and balance*. Santa Fe, NM: Bear & Company.

Garrett, M. T., & Barret, R. L. (2003). Two-spirit: Counseling Native American sexual minority persons. *Journal of Multicultural Counseling and Development, 31*(2), 131–142.

Garrett, M. T., & Garrett, J. T. (2002). Ayeli: Centering technique based on Cherokee spiritual traditions. *Counseling and Values, 46*(2), 149–158.

Garrett, M. T., & Myers, J. E. (1996). The rule of opposites: A paradigm for counseling Native Americans. *Journal of Multicultural Counseling and Development, 24*(2), 89–104.

Garrett, M. T., & Pichette, E. F. (2000). Red as an apple: Native American acculturation and counseling with or without reservation. *Journal of Counseling and Development, 78*(1), 3–13.

Gladding, S. T. (1995). Humor in counseling: Using a natural resource. *Journal of Humanistic Education and Development, 34*(1), 3–12.

Goldin, E., & Bordan, T. (1999). The use of humor in counseling: The laughing cure. *Journal of Counseling and Development, 77*(4), 405–410.

Harjo, S. S. (1998, May). Without reservation. *Native peoples: The Arts and Lifeways, 11*, 50–55.

Herring, R. D. (1994). The clown or contrary figure as a counseling intervention strategy with Native American Native clients. *Journal of Multicultural Counseling and Development, 22*(3), 153–164.

Herring, R. D., & Meggert, S. S. (1994). The use of humor as a strategy with Native American children. *Elementary School Guidance & Counseling, 29*(1), 67–76.

Itzkowitz, M. (Ed.) (1995). *Concepts and cultures: A reader for writers*. Boston: Allyn & Bacon.

Kelley, E. W. (1995). *Spirituality and religion in counseling and psychotherapy: Diversity in theory and practice*. Alexandria, VA: American Counseling Association.

Kush, J. C. (1997). Relationship between humor appreciation and counsellor self-perception. *Counseling and Values, 42*(1), 22–29.

Maher, M. (1993). Humor in substance abuse treatment. In W. F. Fry, & W. A. Salameh (Eds.), *Advances in humor and psychotherapy* (pp. 85–96). Sarasota, FL: Professional Resources.

Maples, M. F., Dupey, P., Torres-Rivera, E., Phan, L. T., Vereen, L., & Garrett, M. T. (2001). Ethnic diversity and the use of humor in counseling: Appropriate or inappropriate? *Journal of Counseling and Development, 79*(1), 53–79.

Northrup, J. (1997). *The rez road follies: Canoes, casinos, computers, and birch bark baskets*. New York: Kodansha International.

Portman, T. A. A., & Garrett, M. T. (2006). Native American healing traditions. *International Journal for Disability, Development, and Education, 53*, 453–469.

Pratt, S. B. (1998). Ritualized uses of humor as a form of identification among American Natives. In D. V. Tanno, & A. Gonzalez (Eds.), *Communication and identity across cultures* (pp. 56–79). New York: Sage.

Schaef, A. W. (1995). *Native wisdom for white minds*. New York: Ballantine.

Thompson, M. (1994). *Gay soul: Finding the heart of gay spirit and nature*. San Francisco, CA: Harper San Francisco.

Weaver, S. T., & Wilson, C. N. (1997). Addiction helping professionals can benefit from appropriate humor in the work setting. *Journal of Employment Counseling, 34*(3), 108–114.

Weintraub, L., Danto, A., & McErilley, T. (1996). *Art on the edge and over: Searching for art's meaning in contemporary society 1970's-1990's*. Litchfield, CT: Art Insights.

3 Gifts of the Seven Winds Alcohol and Drug Prevention Model for American Indians

Rockey Robbins, E. Allen Eason, Stephen Colmant, Derek Burks, and Brenda McDaniel

The Gifts of the Seven Winds Drug and Alcohol Prevention Model is a culturally competent foundational substance use curriculum for Cherokee adolescents and their parents developed by psychologists, social workers, and Eastern Band Cherokees. The program philosophy is community-based, involving collaboration in both curriculum development and eventual implementation. The emergent curriculum makes use of stories, music, a sweat ceremony, traditional meals, and experiential exercises reflecting the historical and cultural context of Cherokee communities.

For American Indian youth, often living in a larger society whose values and customs are at odds with those in their American Indian communities, there is a struggle to hold an identity whose worth is acknowledged (Mitchell & O'Nell, 1998). LaFromboise and Rowe (1983) have suggested that many psychoeducational skills programs provided to American Indians have been culturally biased and do not acknowledge traditional American Indian perspectives. These programs have subsequently been unsuccessful because of resistance many American Indians may exhibit towards such forms of outside influences. Less prescriptive and more flexible social skills programs are needed. The Gifts of the Seven Winds Drug and Alcohol Preventions Model for Cherokee Families is not meant to be a step-by step guide for clinicians but a template for prevention efforts with American Indian groups.

The general goals of the program are to create an environment of trust and openness where personal reflections and group discussion foster evaluation of one's feelings, beliefs, and attitudes relating to Cherokee culture and drug and alcohol misuse. It specifically targets alcohol and other drug misuse as well as parent/child communication and bonding, while simultaneously focusing on tribal knowledges and rituals. Participants appropriate for this program include Cherokee adolescents and parents or similarly situated caregivers of high school juniors and seniors.

Alcohol and Drug Use Among American Indians

Underage drinking continues to be a widespread practice among American Indian adolescents. Novins, Beals, Moore, Spicer, and Manson (2004) monitored underage drinking throughout the 1990s until the present and argue that efforts to address the problem have failed. The National Epidemiological Survey on alcohol and related conditions (2006) reported that American Indian adolescents had the highest rate of alcohol treatment need among any other race at 14.1 percent, with Whites being second at 6.9 percent, as well as the highest illicit drug use treatment need at 11.8 percent with Whites being second at 5.8%.

Wallace et al. (2009) surveyed Native American students and found that 39 percent had tried more than just a few sips of alcohol by the end of the eighth grade and 72 percent by the end of the twelfth grade. Underage alcohol use threatens the development of young people with alterations in brain development and potential addiction. Early alcohol use is also associated with academic problems, delinquency, unprotected sexual activity, increased suicide and homicide, and car accidents (National Institute on Alcohol Abuse and Alcoholism, 2004/2005). In a comprehensive literature review, Hawkins, Cummins, and Marlatt (2004) found that American Indian youth tend to initiate substance use at a younger age, continue use after initial experimentation, and have higher rates of polysubstance use when compared with other racial groups. Substance initiation in Indian communities typically occurs between the ages of ten and thirteen years, with the onset for some as early as five or six years of age (Okwumabua & Duryea, 1987). Spear, Longshore, McCaffrey, and Ellickson (2005) reported that studies suggest early use in girls is at least as high as boys, if not higher.

Radin et al. (2006) reviewed literature on the role of peer influence and self-esteem in adolescent substance abuse. Their review showed that peer influence is more directly correlated with teen drug use than is self-esteem. However, the importance of both factors seems to vary substantially through the teenage years. Radin and colleagues conducted a ten-year prospective longitudinal study in a community sample of 224 urban American Indian adolescents and found that younger versus older teens were differentially influenced by their peers in terms of alcohol use. Furthermore, peer deviance was found to mediate the effects of self-worth on alcohol-related problems in earlier adolescence. However, as adolescents entered adulthood, self-esteem was found to be more directly related to alcohol problems.

Rodgers and Fleming (2004) examined personal-, family-, and community-level factors associated with alcohol use and abuse in a sample of 341 sixth through twelfth grade Native American students residing on a reservation. Results indicated that initiation of alcohol use at an earlier age was moderately related to alcohol abuse. The mean age of the sample was fourteen years, and the mean age of initiated alcohol use was eleven to twelve years. Adolescents who reported higher stress scores were more likely to use or abuse alcohol. Lower levels of parental monitoring and parental support were also risk factors. The presence of a nonparental adult who was willing to monitor youth behaviour was a significant protective factor and even stronger than parental monitoring or support on a reservation.

Garrett and Carroll (2000) have suggested that there are nine underlying reasons for substance dependence among Native Americans:

1) Historical factors: drinking patterns that developed during the 1880s with the introduction of alcohol into Native American tribes through boarding schools and relocation programs for the purpose of exploitation, discrimination, and assimilation and because of the disruption of traditional cultural and familial patterns that resulted from such programs.
2) Isolation: displacement from community and traditional roles, feeling cut-off from sources of belonging and communal meaningfulness.
3) Generational splits: lack of traditional function for Elders serving as role models/teachers for young people.
4) Sociodemographics: unemployment, inadequate housing, low educational levels, poverty-level incomes, and isolated living conditions.
5) Physiology: difficulties for many Native American people in physically absorbing sugars in an appropriate manner, which contributes to alcohol addiction.
6) Social facilitation: substance use as a facilitator of social cohesion and social interaction.
7) Peer pressure: not wanting to reject the sharing and generosity of one's peers when offered substances.
8) Coping mechanism: method of dealing with stress, boredom, powerlessness, sense of emptiness associated with acculturation and identity confusion.
9) Non-interference: avoidance behaviour of community members in maintaining cultural value of not imposing one's will on another and the lack of family/community sanctions against substance use.

American Indian Therapy Models for Alcohol Misuse

Therapists should be careful not to contribute to the ongoing colonialization process that American Indians endure daily by indiscriminately imposing models of treatment whose philosophical foundations are imbued with Western ideas (LaFromboise & Low, 1989). Many American Indian in-treatment facilities now successfully utilize sweats and talking circles as integral elements of their therapy (Gutierres & Todd, 1997).

Many programs are currently using the Red Road to Wellbriety curriculum (White Bison, 2002). This program offers American Indian interpretations of the Twelve Steps of Alcoholics Anonymous (AA). They use Medicine Wheel teachings to explain the goals of balance and harmony. They utilize the Talking Circle, where members discuss their problems and journeys to recovery with the aid of rituals and symbols, such as burning cedar, using eagle feathers, and discussing the colours and meanings of the four directions and traditional values. Each of the twelve steps is contextualized within the framework of traditional tribal values. The Recovery Medicine Wheel is another program for American Indians that works conjunctively with AA (Coggins, 1998). There are four areas within the wheel that correspond to the four realms of human existence: 1) physical realm (North), 2) introspective thought (West), 3) knowledge and enlightenment (East), and 4) spiritual realm (South). Each of these areas contains four steps, making sixteen steps toward recovery.

The efforts of the aforementioned programs to address drug and alcohol problems with American Indians deserve the highest praise. We are confident that they have made great strides in addressing some of the key issues in developing culturally relevant approaches to drug abuse treatment. With the present model, we hope to continue to develop an approach grounded in specific American Indian customs and knowledges. In our discussions, we often look on the AA program with great admiration and try to draw from its wisdom, yet we also ask questions about how its spiritual views may conflict with Cherokee spiritual views, how some Cherokees may confuse its emphasis on surrender with powerlessness, and how its rhetoric about low self-esteem, family dysfunction, and communication difficulties may not be discussed in larger cultural, political, and socioeconomic contexts. Our goal in developing the Gifts of the Seven Winds Treatment Approach for American Indians was to create a proactive preventative program with culturally specific intervention strategies to facilitate a sense of identity tied to tribal community.

Gifts of the Seven Winds Treatment Approach for American Indians

Gifts of the Seven Winds is a secondary prevention model aimed at decreasing the prevalence of alcohol abuse among Cherokee adolescents. This model is designed for Cherokee adolescents, their families, and communities. In phase one, the Seven Winds participants meet on a Saturday for eight hours for intensive psychoeducational and leadership sessions in the areas of drug and alcohol treatment and family communication in the larger context of a Cherokee value and belief system. In phase two, the Seven Winds group is responsible for building a sweat lodge on appropriate grounds and getting wood and stones, as well as other tribally appropriate materials, for the sweat ceremony. Participants are required to learn two Cherokee songs for the sweat. They are also required to complete psychoeducational assignments. In phase three, Seven Winds participants convene for another similar six-hour session, followed by a sweat ceremony and a traditional meal prepared by supportive community members. A "giveaway" occurs during this meal.

Selection, Phases, Activities, Techniques, and Assignments

Selection

Seven Winds' brochures, letters, and application forms are sent to tribal agencies and high schools with Cherokee populations. Counsellors, principals, and tribal leaders at these places are asked to nominate Cherokee students with leadership potential and to give them an application form. A parent or guardian is required to sign a letter of commitment to participate with their child in the sessions in order for the student to participate. Interested students and parents are asked to send completed nomination and application forms to Seven Winds facilitators for consideration for participation. While the program does not have rigid cut-off criteria for acceptance in the program, acceptees must demonstrate a firm intention to participate throughout the duration of the program, an intention to resist drug and alcohol misuse, and demonstrate leadership potential. Six to ten students coupled with their parents or guardians are selected for each site.

Phases

A Saturday is chosen to conduct the first eight-hour Seven Winds psychoeducation and leadership marathon session. It is recommended that facilitators conduct the first five activities described in the following sections on this day. In phase two, which takes about a month to two months, participants contact and solicit the aid of an appropriate tribal leader and plan and construct a sweat lodge in an appropriate area. In phase three, another Saturday is chosen to conduct the last eleven-hour Seven Winds psychoeducation and leadership marathon session. Facilitators conduct the last two activities, followed by the sweat ceremony and dinner with special recognition activities.

Facilitators

It is recommended that two facilitators oversee the operations for the program as well as conduct the sessions. We recommend that at least one of the facilitators should be a respected community member with a minimum of three years counselling experience working with at-risk/high-needs youth in a behavioural health program. If possible, there should be one male and one female facilitator for participant gender identification and for modeling healthy male and female interaction. At least one of the facilitators should be Cherokee and both should at least be able to speak words in Cherokee for hello, how are you, and thank you (o si yo, do I tsu, and wa do, respectively). Facilitators should be tribally sensitive and trained in open-ended questioning. Facilitators are responsible for writing a brochure that is disseminated in targeted communities. Facilitators are also responsible for writing a newsletter that is sent out to all Project Seven Winds' participants. Project Seven

Winds' newsletter consists of an overview of the first marathon session, an update on the work done in preparation for the purification ceremony, poems, stories, essays and drawings, pictures and short descriptions of recent accomplishments and plans of Project Seven Winds' participants, and reminders about the final day's activities. Facilitators also help coordinate and supply information to local and tribal newspapers and radio stations about Project Seven Winds' activities. They also oversee the final dinner and conduct the giveaway. Lastly, facilitators are responsible for getting gifts for participants for the giveaway. One of the gifts should be a certificate that documents and celebrates leadership qualities demonstrated during the Project Seven Gifts program and invites ongoing leadership performances. Also, facilitators provide each participant with a CD of Cherokee songs, including "Morning Healing Song" (*Ip se kea*), "Cherokee Morning Song," and "Wash My Spirit Clean."

Coordinator

It is also crucial that facilitators recruit a committed person or persons from the area of each site to coordinate several activities. They are responsible for distributing and collecting applications for potential participants, gaining commitments of full participation from the selected participants, securing a facility for Project Seven Winds to conduct its program, helping to coordinate all facets of the purification ceremony (e.g., finding a location and soliciting the appropriate persons to supervise the building of the lodge and securing appropriate water pourers and rock carriers), and supervising the catering of the dinner. They also help the facilitators with making the proper connections to local newspapers, writers of newsletters, and deejays for dissemination of the activities of Project Seven Winds.

Activities

While much "American Indian literature" makes reference to the sacred four directions, many tribal Elders from various tribes refer to seven directions. The directions often have colours, animals, natural resources, principalities, government, virtues, and vices associated with them. We have chosen to focus on specific meanings attached to the seven directions of the Cherokees (Mooney, 1982). While none of the meanings are foreign to any tribe, or for that matter any group of people, by using these "meanings" as guides, we are placing the treatment in a traditional Cherokee framework. Some of the specific techniques that follow the general framework emerged from and have been given by various American Indian traditions, ceremonies, and rituals; they are not specific to a single tribe. Following each description of the directions are sample questions that may be used during that phase of therapy. There are also some assignments given during the first Seven Winds' marathon session that participants should complete before the next session, such as learning Cherokee songs.

I. East—Red—Success and Triumph

The program begins by having the person who will be pouring at the sweat to lead Project Seven Winds' participants in a prayer and song. Then in a circle, facilitators and participants introduce themselves. Next, participants are presented with a box of cut-out animals. As the box is passed around, each participant chooses an animal with whose qualities they would like to emulate. Each participant describes those qualities to the group. There is a naked branch the facilitators bring to act as a Medicine Tree. After each description, the participants walk to the center of the circle and hang their animals on the tree. After each participant has hung his or her animal on the tree, one facilitator talks briefly about how our potentials are empowered and supported when we connect ourselves with others.

In part two of this activity, facilitators start with a dialogue revolving around the following information. Persons coming in for help with drug and alcohol misuse sometimes disclose the desperateness they feel regarding their problem as well as recount stories describing the destructiveness of their behaviour. It is easy for a counsellor to get caught up in the negative aspects of their stories. It is suggested that the counsellor offer empathy for the pain a person may express, but s/he should also work to create in the client a belief that there are reservoirs from which they can draw that will help the client succeed. One of the most predictive elements of treatment for positive outcome is the client's initial level of expectation (Price, Anderson, Henrich, & Rothbaum, 2008).

Cherokee people too have long expressed the importance of having hope in the possible triumphs of each new day. Cherokee ceremonial rituals typically acknowledge the east first. Lodges open to the east, letting the first rays of sunshine stream into the buildings. The east is associated with new beginnings. It is appropriate to honour traditional American Indian ways by beginning with wisdoms associated with the east.

After the aforementioned points are discussed, the participants are then asked for responses to the following questions.

Primary Group Discussion

1. (*sa quu i*) This direction symbolizes new beginnings. How do you view this point in your life as a possible new beginning? How does it feel? If you were to describe it as a landscape that stretches out in front of you, what does it look like?
2. (*ta li*) Tell a story about a time when you had to start over. What resources did you find in yourself or something beyond yourself to help pull through?
3. (*tso i*) Tell a story about when you were able to overcome the desire to misuse drugs or alcohol. How do you make sense of this? How does that success inform you in your current state of being?
4. (*nv gi*) What kind of person do you wish to become? Envision that person and describe him or her.

5. (*hi s gi*) In a role play, one person represents drugs and/or alcohol while another will play him or herself engaging in dialogue with the substance.
6. (*su da li*) Many religions, including American Indian religions, associate profound changes in life to yielding one's ego up to something larger than oneself. How do you feel about this?
7. (*g li quo gi*) To conclude, the participants sing the "Cherokee Morning Song."

II. North—Blue—Defeat and Trouble

After participants sing the "Cherokee Morning Song," the facilitators begin a dialogue on the following topic: For many people, the first few years of drinking and doing drugs may be associated with fun. But most people who continue to misuse quickly experience destructive consequences in almost every area of their lives. A melancholy or an agitated depression typically sets in. Alcohol is often used as a kind of medication for treating the sadness. Many times the alcohol does not really take the sadness away but actually exacerbates it. One may even speculate that some people drink because they are afraid to feel sad.

One of the beauties of the Cherokee directions is that it accepts melancholy as a part of life. Trouble and defeat and the accompanying melancholy are part and parcel of living. Melancholy is not unequivocally bad. Embracing it for brief periods of time may bring balance into our lives. One may feel sad and instead of quickly tricking oneself out of it or avoiding it, one can stay with it for a while. Now not too long, mind you. Melancholy can become a jealous lover if you stay with it too long. It may keep you in a shell and not let you interact with others. It can gain such a strong hold on you that you will want to stay in bed with it most of the morning and do next to nothing, including taking care of your kids. But it may be that melancholy only possesses those who try to avoid her or him entirely.

Melancholy may have something to teach us. It quiets us down and may even aid us in reflection. Indian people have sought it in vision quests and solitary journeys. It tells us about the deep ironies of life. Melancholy persons may at times have more insight than the rest of us. Go and be by yourself in the woods, near a river, on a hill and allow melancholy to visit you a while and help you think about your troubles and defeats in a profound way and garnish the insights and apply them to your life. Sometimes people bring a bottle of alcohol to share with melancholy. At first, it may be hard to get melancholy to talk without alcohol, but if you listen carefully to melancholy, you can usually hear melancholy's whisper increase in volume. For myself, I have learned to embrace him or her as a friend and then bid him or her good-bye after a little while. I have learned that I have the power to send melancholy away. He or she has a way of sticking around too long if you do not give him or her the slip too quickly. After talking to him or her, you get up and act silly, joke, and have fun. But remember the insights you gleaned from the quiet time with melancholy.

The participants are then given an opportunity for responses.

Primary Group Discussion

1. (*sa quu i*) When has blue melancholy come to visit you? Tell a story about melancholy's visit. How long did s/he stay? What relationship did you have with melancholy?
2. (*ta li*) How was drugs or alcohol invited into your life? Tell a story about an early visit it had with you.
3. (*tso i*) How did the civilness of its company change through your relationship with it?
4. (*nv gi*) How has it impacted your relationships with family, friends, work, and personal goals?
5. (*hi s gi*) What relationship does drugs and alcohol have with emotions such as melancholy and agitated depression?
6. (*su da li*) What emotions do drugs and alcohol take from you? Give you? For how long?
7. (*ga (li) quo gi*) Tell a story about when it may have invited trouble into your life.
8. (*tsa ne la*) What have you learned from your experiences with melancholy? Drugs and alcohol? Trouble?
9. (*so ne la*) The "Cherokee Morning Song" is sung again, with comments by the facilitator about how life goes on and changes even in the midst of our difficulties.

III. West—Black—Death

Participants form a circle sitting on folding chairs. The facilitator takes his/her chair out of the circle, stands in the center, pulls two people into the middle, and says, "My name is so and so" and shakes each of the persons' hands. Then the facilitator can ask questions of the two, but they do not have to answer truthfully. Next, the facilitator says, "It is nice to meet you, but I gotta blaze." At the word "blaze," everyone is to change chairs. Because there is one less chair than there are participants, one person is left standing in the middle. The game repeats itself and then comes to an end then the facilitator stops it unexpectedly, as death will come in the midst of our lives.

During part two of this activity, the facilitators engage in a dialogue based on the following information. The Cherokee stories call death the land of the darkening West. Many of the journey stories move toward this direction. In the story *Brass the Gambler*, maybe the most famous of Cherokee stories, the darkness of the west, or death, becomes a major influence upon Chooch's (boy in Cherokee) life from adolescence on. It quickens his steps in this life. Death challenges him to live while he can because opportunities to assert himself in this life are limited to a brief time. We never know when our end will come. We never know when we are in a last circumstance to make choices or do good things for someone or for ourselves. Death tells us that the end is coming and that we should make the most of the precious moments we have. Participants are given a chance to make responses.

Primary Group Discussion

1. (*sa quu i*) How do you feel about the fact that your current life on earth is coming to an end?
2. (*ta li*) What will people say about you at your funeral?
3. (*tso i*) What people need you to be alive the most? What do they need from you?
4. (*nv gi*) If you were to personify death, how would it look?
5. (*hi s gi*) As a deadening presence in your current life, what is it currently murdering?
6. (*su da li*) Now, some believe that the other side of death's face is friendly. It reminds us that we have only so long to do certain things before our time on this spinning ball is past. What does this face of death tell you to get busy doing before it is too late (relationships, goals, etc.)?

A conclusion to this activity is to have participants write letters to significant others as if writing from the other side, expressing regret of unfulfilled possibilities as well as hopes they have for them.

IV. South—White—Peace and Happiness

Participants situate themselves in two lines facing each other, with approximately five feet separating the two lines. They begin passing a nerf ball back and forth all the way down the lines and back. If the ball is dropped, it must go back to the person who tossed it first, and the process is recommenced. When this is done successfully a few times, a person in each line is blindfolded. Good communication is required to pass the ball down the lines and back. Peace and harmony is achieved when it is done successfully. Participants sit silently for a few moments before the next part of this phase.

During the second part of this exercise, facilitators have a dialogue based on the following information. Many Cherokee stories begin with the phrase, "Long ago when the world was young," and then they sometimes move into descriptions of an idyllic life before a character begins having challenging experiences. Integrating the experience of happiness and innocent periods into our lives is crucial. Everyone has been blessed with at least intervals in his or her life that have been somewhat happy. Many counsellors and clients seem to feel that they are working in session only if they are crying about the bad times. But one of the directions of the Cherokees beckons us to be happy and at peace. It would do our clients good if we spent more time helping our clients enter into those memories more often and help them take some of the materials from those times and bring them back into their present lives.

One medicine man the first author has worked with told him categorically that it is not enough to go back with a client to the time of traumatic events. He said it was vital to help clients to experience the pure healing energy that ran through the client's life before the trauma. The group will be given an opportunity for responses.

Primary Group Discussion

1. (*sa quu i*) Tell me a story about a time when you felt cared for and deeply loved.
2. (*ta li*) When was a time when you experienced the joy of giving something to someone?
3. (*tso i*) What are some of the things that you enjoyed most when you were happy?
4. (*nv gi*) Tell of a story when you were "in love" or at least infatuated with someone.
5. (*hi s gi*) What was the funniest thing that ever happened to you?
6. (*su da li*) What is innocence? What are you innocent about now? Are there any innocent joys left for you? How can you experience them?
7. (*ga (li) quo gi*) How could you bring peace into your life? How is peace and drugs and alcohol related or unrelated? What do you envision peace looking like in your life?
8. (*ta ne la*) How is acceptance of others and yourself related to peace in your life?

V. Above—Brown—Unascertained but Propitious

In this activity called Design X 3, participants are arranged in groups of three, sitting one behind another and facing the same direction. The facilitator explains the role each group member plays during the activity. 1) The back person in each line is given a design card. Only these persons are allowed to look at the designs. Without speaking, they draw (with their fingers) the design on the backs of the persons seated in front of them. 2) Middle persons may speak to the other members of their group but may not look at persons behind them nor over the shoulder of the persons in front of them. The goal for the middle persons is to describe the design drawn on their backs to the persons in front of them. 3) Without looking back or talking, front persons follow instructions received from middle persons and attempt to replicate the design given to their line's back person. Once all the groups have finished this stage of the activity, the facilitator allows the total group to compare group drawings with the original designs. The activity can be repeated by having group members change positions in the lines. Facilitators ask participants how they coped with the doubts they may have had about the effectiveness of their actions in the game because of their various handicaps.

The facilitators then engage in a dialogue based on the following information. For many people who misuse alcohol, this session, which deals with uncertainty, can stir up doubts and uncertainties that may precipitate drinking if appropriate closures are not utilized. Therefore, it is vital that the therapist offers the client a strong security base during this session and wraps things up appropriately in the end. Some clients we work with are persons who are addicted or who misuse drugs and alcohol. Some may say this is a contradiction. Their lives are out of control. But many are almost insanely jealous of their romantic partners and try to keep them under lock and key. Others are in constant power struggles trying to get things done the way they want things done. In some ways, those with drug and alcohol problems wrestle with control issues and find their outlet from the anxiety associated with control through alcohol and drugs. Cherokee spirituality is not based on learning indisputable facts or believing exactly the right way. Once a person has everything figured out, there really is not a lot of reason to be here anymore. And there are a lot of bored and uninteresting people who seem to think that they do have everything figured out. However, the notion of faith is not founded on certainty. Contrary to what a lot of narrow-minded people like to tell us about faith, it is inextricably bound up with doubt. Faith is faith only when it is overcoming doubt, not once it has frozen into an unquestionable certainty. Doubt opens us up to growth if it is mixed with faith. Without faith, doubt paralyzes us. We say, "I don't think I can do this." And we wallow in our anxiety and do not act. Or we can doubt but courageously step out into the dark with the faith that something good might happen. Faith must constantly overcome doubt in order for us to grow, but faith without doubt is arrogance and consequently stultifying. Participants then discuss the dialogue they have overheard.

Primary Group Discussion

1. (*sa quu i*) How do you cope with ambiguity or uncertainty? Why is uncertainty so difficult to cope with for you?
2. (*ta li*) What specifically are you uncertain about in this life? What uncertainty bothers you the most? As an assignment, write three questions about life that you are uncertain about and rate how much they bother you on a scale from ten to one.
3. (*tso i*) When has the control freak reared its head in your life to control a significant other?
4. (*nv gi*) How big was it? Was it male or female? Describe its looks.
5. (*h s gi*) How were your control issues connected to uncertainty and ambiguity? What are some ways you try to control and manipulate others?
6. (*su da li*) When has doubt about your view of the world or your lifestyle opened you up to growth? How have some of the doubts you have had about the way you have led your life affected you lately?

7. (*g (li) quo gi*) What are the doubts you have about your life right now? Do you trust us to understand them? How does it help to talk about them?
8. (*tsa ne la*) How can you be at peace without being certain about the future?

VI. Below—Yellow—Regression Into Defeat and Trouble

This activity is called Gadugi, which is a Cherokee word that was used to refer to "get togethers" to rebuild homes and barns. In this instance, it refers to getting together to support and rebuild each other after difficult times. One participant sits in the middle of the circle. Every person around the circle offers one positive adjective to the person in the center. The center person simply absorbs the kind word with *wa do* (thank you). Participants sing the "Morning Healing Song" (*Ip Se Kea*).

The facilitators ask participants how positive encouragers may have helped them during hard times and then enter into a dialogue based on the following information. No treatment program can ignore relapse prevention. The area of development most overlooked in all types of counselling is backsliding, falling off the wagon, or regression. One of the most dangerous times in phases of growth is when we make what seems to be a major change. It is dangerous because with every step we make up the ladder, a demon called pride meets us on that step and tempts us with self-righteousness. How many people have we known in drug and alcohol counselling who recover and simultaneously begin to lord their growth over others in preaching condescendingly or even condemning others for their faults, or they express feelings that they are now invulnerable. AA deals with this by having their members to always humble themselves by declaring themselves as alcoholics all their lives. For many, this is a brilliant technique, but some also view this as burdensome. The point is that "backsliding" is a crucial issue that should be dealt with directly and profoundly.

Marlatt and Gordon (1985) wrote that those who "fall off the wagon" often experience self-blame, guilt, anxiety, and depression, which leads to increased susceptibility to further drinking. They argue that future relapse is reduced when the person views the episode as a mistake resulting from specific, external, and controllable factors. Their *Relapse Prevention Therapy* entails helping clients identify circumstances that increase risks for relapse and helping them cope effectively if relapse occurs. This program agrees with the AA tenet that support from others is crucial to recovery. Participants then discuss the overheard dialogue.

Primary Group Discussion

1. (sa quu it) What is Relapse in the context of drug and alcohol use?
2. (ta li) How will you know if Relapse is coming around you again?
3. (tso i) How will you defend yourself?

4. (nv gi) What are four helpers or facilitators that might help you battle relapse?
5. (hi s gi) What relationship is there between Relapse and Failure? Are they the same thing? Explain.
6. (su da li) What do you need if Relapse gets the best of you?
7. (g (li) quo gi) Tell a story of a time when you were "knocked down" by an incident or crisis, but you got back up and persisted. How long did it take to get back on track? What helped you to get going again? How do you feel about yourself for having persevered?

VII. Center—No Color—Conscious Integration

Participants begin this activity by singing the Cherokee song, "Wash My Spirit Clean." This activity is called, Tso s da nv tli, or we are relatives. Participants stand in a circle. They are to first arrange themselves from shortest to tallest and from the darkest complexion to the lightest. Facilitators ask about how focusing on differences can sometimes lead to conflicts. Everybody is then to sit in a circle. The facilitators ask participants in what ways people may be equal or at least akin within the deepest recesses of their hearts.

The facilitators begin a dialogue based on the following information. The last direction is the center, or the human heart, and involves superseding individual goals, personal satisfactions, and feelings of superiority to reach awareness of interconnectedness. Every one of us has different temperaments that are relatively stable throughout our lives, but this does not mean that we cannot benefit from growing in all personality domains. For instance, some clients come in and tell us that they are not emotional. Maybe they primarily move through this life by using their heads. I would argue if they are too overweighed in the head, they live pretty sterile existences and might be happier if they allowed themselves to be more emotional. It would not hurt them to say kind encouraging things to their spouses and children, and they may experience a more profound connection in doing so. As far as the Cherokee directions are concerned, it may suggest that the integration of sadness, uncertainty, lack of control and allowing ourselves to feel vulnerable should be integrated with happiness, triumph, and success. Allowing ourselves to suffer and hurt may be prerequisite to happiness. Still many of us try to avoid sadness. Drinking and drug use is one of the most conspicuous symptoms of someone who fears vulnerability. The universal tribal wisdom of balance gives direction to feel and think as a whole human being. This entails a realization that each of us is all of us. We are one. We are never more individual than when we realize our oneness with everything, nor are we ever more egoless. Participants discuss the overheard dialogue.

Primary Group Discussion

1. (*sa quu i*) How are you like the rest of the people in this room?
2. (*ta li*) A group activity may involve having each person sit in the middle of the circle. Have each person offer the person in the middle a

compliment based on a strength seen during therapy. The person in the center accepts the honour.

3. (*tso i*) Have each person draw a line on a paper with one end being labeled emotion and the other reason. Have them mark an x on the place they feel they are in regard to the polar opposites. Then discuss.
4. (*nv gi*) Have clients consider the foundation they have worked on during therapy. Have them each tell what they have put into their life's foundation? How strong is it?
5. (*hi s gi*) How strong will the foundation be when the temptations to abuse drugs or alcohol come?
6. (*su da li*) How have you became more or less balanced during treatment? Participants hold hands and sing "Wash My Spirit Clean."

Sweat Ceremony

Sweat rituals have been demonstrated to accelerate group dynamics and contribute to multiple dimensions of well-being (Eason, Colmant, & Winterowd, 2009). Mooney (1982, p. 230), in reference to a field report collected in 1888, said that an eighty-year old Cherokee man recalled myth keepers and priests conducting purification meetings in the "asi, or low-built log sleeping house, to recite the traditions and discuss their secret knowledge . . . tell stories" and to give instruction to persons by appointment. Persons sat in a circle around the "hot" charcoal fire and one or two pine knots, which were placed on a large flat rock in the middle of the floor, were burned.

Today sweat ceremonies continue to be conducted by most tribes, though these ceremonies are more in line with Plains Indian ceremonies. Heated rocks are typically placed in the center of a low structure made of willow branches covered with tarps. Participants in the ceremony sit in a circle around the hot rocks that have water poured over them to release the steam. Humbling themselves amidst the nourishing and purifying steam, they offer prayer for the health of others. There are usually four rounds of singing, praying, and storytelling, according to how the person who pours decides. While this is a fairly common description, one should realize that there are as many different ways of doing sweats and experiencing them as there are people and lodges. Anyone who has visited many lodges knows this.

Purification is far from simple to define. There are those who will simply see the sweat ceremony as a means of getting rid of toxins in their bodies. However, some traditional American Indian people speak of energy flowing naturally through all things. Yet humans often block the energy, which causes illness and toxic relationships. For instance, our minds will get stuck in loops, repeatedly returning to the same images or ideas to the point of bringing worry, self-pity, and stagnation. We may ruminate on what others have done to us or how they have disappointed us. In order for the flow to resume its naturalness, a person must "let go." This may or may not involve forgiveness. The point is to let go and make ourselves aware of and available to the spirit—the energy that runs through us. The flow of energy can purify our bodies, minds, emotions, and spirits of toxins.

Purification is gaining freedom from the vanity of finding our esteem in our possessions, self-centredness, and judging others, or maybe it is cleansing ourselves from sins as Christians contend. The purified self is emptied of delusions as one is engaged in the eternal now. To live with a purified being is to accept one's life as it is and becoming one with others. The Lakota call it Metokweeosin. The purified person lives selflessly for others and enjoys it; he or she has a thankful and positive mind. Once in the sweat lodge, profound and sincere self-reflections, prayers, and meditations can begin to expunge the conscious as well as the subconscious pictures that are imprinted on our beings. It is recommended that prayer accompany the sweat ceremony because as long as the ceremony is regulated to mental activities, it can be as cold and unfeeling as many other rituals. Emotion usually accompanies prayer. When we look deeply, we see that we are much wider and deeper than all the problems and sins we carry around.

When persons are in the lodge, the pourer will explain the few rules that participants will abide by. They are typically that persons should be silent as the first Seven Grandfather rocks are brought in at the beginning of the ceremony and when the pipe is being passed around at the end of the third round. The pourer should also strongly encourage participants to leave the lodge if they feel that the heat or anxiety is too much for them to bear and that this is honourable. It is required that participants in the Gifts of the Seven Winds sweat learn three Cherokee songs, in the Cherokee language, which they sing during the phases described earlier and in the purification rite. Participants are also to verbalize the word, *tso s da nv tli*, or we are related, whenever they enter or leave the lodge. Prayers and stories along with additional songs may be sung during the ceremony.

Meal and Recognition Ceremonies

The facilitators are responsible for soliciting the services of several persons in the local Cherokee community to cook a traditional Cherokee meal for the participants and anyone else who comes to support the participants during the sweat ceremony. During the meal, facilitators present leadership certificates of recognition and small gifts to each participant. An Elder is asked to lead the group in prayer and song before the meal.

Conclusion

The Gifts of the Seven Winds Program seeks to integrate conventional group therapy with Cherokee values and healing rituals. The creation of the Seven Winds was achieved through collaborations with an Eastern Band Cherokee community. It is believed that such an effort has the potential of helping

Cherokee families to develop greater resilience against the onslaught of drug and alcohol misuses. In this approach, community involvement is strongly emphasized as well as relevant cultural issues pertaining to Cherokee families and Cherokee youth. Participants are asked to reflect upon and experience the historical and cultural context of the Cherokee community, its cultural revitalization, and healing movements that define the source and nature of alcohol/drug use among Cherokee people. The curriculum focuses on community rather than individual healing, holistic wellness rather than cognitive education, stories rather than problem solving, and strengths rather than problems and deficits.

References

Coggins, K. (1998). *The recovery medicine wheel: An alternative pathway to healingand wellness*, 2nd ed. Culpepper, VA: Ventajas.

Eason, E. A., Colmant, S. A., & Winterowd, C. L. (2009). Sweat therapy theory, practice and efficacy. *Journal of Experiential Education, 32*(2), 121–136.

Garrett, M. T., & Carroll, J. J. (2000). Mending the broken circle: Treatment of substance dependence among Native Americans. *Journal of Counseling and Development, 78*(4), 379–388.

Gutierres, S. E., & Todd, M. (1997). The impact of childhood abuse on treatment outcomes of substance users. *Professional Psychology: Research and Practice, 28*(4), 348–354.

Hawkins, E. H., Cummins, L. H., & Marlatt, G. A. (2004). Preventing substance abuse in American Indian and Alaska Native youth: Promising strategies for healthier communities. *Psychological Bulletin, 130*(2), 304–323.

LaFromboise, T. D., & Low, K. G. (1989). American Indian children and adolescents. In J. T. Gibbs, & L. N. Huang (Eds.), *Children of color: Psychological interventions with minority youth* (pp. 114–147). San Francisco, CA: Jossey-Bass.

LaFromboise, T. D., & Rowe, W. (1983). Skills training for bicultural competence: Rationale and application. *Journal of Counseling Psychology, 30*(4), 589–595.

Marlatt, G. A., & Gordon, J. R. (1985). *Relapse prevention: Maintenance strategies in the treatment of addictive behaviors*. New York, NY: Guilford Press.

Mitchell, C. M., & O'Nell, T. D. (1998). Problem and conventional behavior among American Indian adolescents: Structure and validity. *Journal of Research on Adolescence, 8*(1), 97–122.

Mooney, J. (1982). *Myths of the Cherokee and sacred formulas of the Cherokees*. Nashville, TN: Elder-Booksellers.

National Institute on Alcohol Abuse and Alcoholism. (2004/2005). Alcohol and development in youth—A multidisciplinary overview. *Alcohol Research and Health, 28*(3), 107–175.

National Institute on Alcohol Abuse and Alcoholism. (2006). National epidemiologic survey on alcohol and related conditions: Selected findings. *Alcohol Research and Health, 29*(2), 71–152.

Novins, D. K., Beals, J., Moore, L. A., Spicer, P., & Manson, S. M. (2004). Use of biomedical services and traditional healing options among American Indians: Sociodemographic correlates, spirituality, and ethnic identity. *Medical Care, 42*(7), 670–679.

Okwumabua, J. O., & Duryea, E. J. (1987). Age of onset, periods of risk, and patterns of progression in drug use among American Indian high school students. *International Journal of Addictions, 22*(12), 1269–1276.

Price, M., Anderson, P., Henrich, C. C., & Rothbaum, B. O. (2008). Greater expectations: Using hierarchical linear modeling to examine expectancy for treatment outcome as a predictor of treatment response. *Behavior Therapy, 39*(4), 398–405.

Radin, S. M., Neighbors, C., Walker, P. S., Walker, R. D., Marlatt, G. A., Larimer, M. (2006). The changing influences of self-worth and peer deviance on drinking problems in urban American Indian adolescents. *Psychology of Addictive Behaviors, 20*(2), 161–170.

Rodgers, K. B., Fleming, W. M. (2004). Individual, family, and community factors related to alcohol use among Native American adolescents. *Adolescent & Family Health, 3*(3), 140–147.

Spear, S., Longshore, D., McCaffrey, D., & Ellickson, P. (2005). Prevalence of substance use among white and American Indian young adolescents in a northern plains state. *Journal of Psychoactive Drugs, 37*(1), 1–6.

Wallace, J. M., Vaughn, M. G., Bachman, J. G., O'Malley, P. M., Johnston, L. D., & Schulenberg, J. E. (2009). Race/ethnicity, socioeconomic factors, and smoking among early adolescent girls in the United States. *Drug and Alcohol Dependence, 104*(1), 42–49.

White Bison. (2002). *The red road to wellbriety: In the Native American way*. Colorado Springs, CO: White Bison Inc.

4 Traditional Spiritual Healing

Wendy Hill

Throughout the years of engaging in spiritual healing work in many different Indigenous communities across Turtle Island/North America, I have gained some valuable insight into the spiritual power that all individuals have. Unfortunately, many people have been given limited understanding and resources to understand themselves, both spiritually and in other ways. Spiritual healing work is one of the many aspects of healing that I do for a person; spiritual healing is part of overall healing. If people do not believe they have control and power within themselves, then how can they feel responsible for their healing? Illness, pain, and emotional trauma are all linked in one way or another. The healing that is necessary for any individual to feel better is as individual as the person's fingerprint. There is no general approach to a person's healing. This is why the length of traditional healing sessions can vary; some people need only an hour, others need several hours. This may also be true for Western mental health services. The length of a healing session and depth of the healing depends on what the person has experienced and how willing he or she is to let go of the pain. If a person is shy or unwilling to admit to the events that have led to the emotional, mental, or physical problems, then the spirit cannot be healed. The knowledge and awareness of what an individual needs to bring healing can only come from a higher spiritual power. A healer is the person responsible for giving the help, whether it is through words or bringing the spirits into the space with the person to allow that experience to happen.

My work in the many Native communities as a traditional healer or traditional medicine practitioner has allowed me to witness many miracles, and these are the experiences that underpin what is shared in this chapter, along with the spiritual teachings and traditional knowledges I have learned. The name or word *healer* is a misnomer because it is not I who does the healing work. Any healing that happens comes from the *spirit world*; I am only a middle person and distraction to the spiritual healing work itself. It is the Creator and his spirit helpers who do the work of healing. As human beings, we are all very unique in everything about us; for example, our fingerprints and handprints are great indicators of our physical uniqueness. There are also our life paths and life experiences that are unique, even siblings will view life differently despite growing up in the same environment. In other words, people can witness the same experience in life, but we will all have a different view or feeling about that experience. This is true for the way in which people heal from different experiences that have caused pain. This pain first begins with the spirit and then the emotions, the mind, and, finally, the body. This process of experiencing pain from all types of harm depends also on where or how a person is first harmed; the pain might go the opposite direction if it is the body that gets physically harmed first. If the harm a person experiences creates an emotional or spiritual pain, then it will begin from the spirit.

As a healer, I have learned the spirit inside each person has needs. Some of those needs are to feel safe, have fun, be kind, etc., but the most important need of a person's spirit is to be at peace. When people have difficult experiences in childhood, they have very significant impacts because as children our spirit is very strong and ever present. Because of this spiritual strength in childhood, children have a great memory of how they were treated in the spirit world before birth and then put those expectations on family and people around them. The actions, events, and behaviours of others towards us in our lives on earth give us a message of safety or no safety. Generally, when people lose their sense of safety and begin to feel afraid, they start to lose faith in everything. This is when we know people will need some healing, because the lack of faith, the fear of others, and the past events have a great impact on our spirits. These experiences are very unique to each person, thus the method and timing in which each person heals are also unique.

My experience as a healer has led me to know that two people can have a very similar event happen to each of them that is harmful, yet each person will handle it differently. For instance, one person may take up drinking alcohol or abusing drugs and live a very self-destructive lifestyle, while the other one might not. The difference comes from within the individual, his spirit, and his relationship to a higher spiritual power, such as the Creator. Or the difference may come from a person's own strong mind of not wanting to feel defeated or controlled by past events. But one thing I know from my work as a healer is that the body has a memory for traumatic events. Thus even the individual who chooses not to be self-destructive in order to cope with traumatic memories will still carry triggers and a memory of a past event that was scary or harmful. My healing work with people varies with each individual; my ability to help a person depends on his or her trust and faith in me and in the Creator. Once we as human beings lose this sense of trusting others, that loss of trust becomes the obstacle that must be overcome. In order to be able to heal so that a person regains his or her trust in others, I as a healer must be that person who earns this trust. The presence of spirits from the spirit world in the healing session that I conduct allows me to help others with this process of earning trust by allowing others to feel the spirits' presence.

The memories that often cause the most emotional pain for people are the events that have the most significant lessons for life and healing. For example, when the Indian residential schools began in Canada in the 1800s, many Native children were intentionally stolen from their parents and communities by the federal government, and this event was traumatic for everyone involved. The parents and grandparents of those stolen children felt a great loss that created sadness and helplessness. This intentional assault on Native peoples in North America has had a great negative impact on the well-being of many Native communities and families. When children do not feel safe and loved, their spirits become very weak, and this is where many addictions, mental illnesses, and violence started within Native people. These events or memories, when they stay inside of us, can seem much larger and more difficult than when we bring them outside of us. When we speak about these memories of traumatic events and how we currently feel, it is like trying to do a puzzle in the dark. When we speak to others about memories of traumatic events and associated thoughts and feelings, we have a partner to help put the pieces together, and these people provide a different light by which we can see. This is some of the process that can bring healing: the knowledge that is shared from the spirit world of some of these events and what the purpose of these events were to teach us. For example, I worked with a person who had been sexually abused as a child in a residential school who was now eighty years old and wanting to heal from those experiences. She went to a Truth and Reconciliation Commission trial to tell her story of the residential school, and it was a traumatic event for her to go back to that time in her memory and tell that story. When she returned to her community after the trial, she came to see me for a healing session, and she was still emotionally traumatized; in our session, she returned to when she was an eight-year-old. My work with her was to bring her back to her current life as an eighty-year old. Through the help of her spirit guide and the help from the spirit world, we were able to bring her back to the present; she felt stronger and more capable of handling her past and functioning in her current life again. She was so wounded from her residential school abuse, that she could no longer function in her present life because she had opened that wound that she had been putting away for so long. This is something that many people have learned to do. When something horrible happens, they do not want to talk about it because they do not want to feel the emotions of the experience, so they avoid it. This avoidance is a coping skill, but it does not help us to deal with or to heal from these experiences. Instead, instead avoidance creates a monster of a memory.

Trauma is one of the biggest healing issues that Native peoples are dealing with in many communities. From my experiences, one of the most prevalent and most painful experiences that people are carrying is a history of sexual abuse, whether it is from a relative or anyone else; it often becomes a lifetime traumatic event. The justice system's process of dealing with sexual abuse is often too scary and painful for victims to go through to remediate the experience in any way. There is really no justice for many of the people who have survived rapes and sexual attacks as children or adults.

Another important aspect of sexual abuse for Native peoples is that, for many survivors, priests or nuns who were "representatives of God" were the perpetrators of such abuses. This experience that a trusted person in the community from a church could commit violent sexual acts against children was overwhelmingly emotionally and mentally numbing to many children who experienced this, and it ruined their faith in a higher spiritual power; healing from a loss in belief in spirituality is also the healing that many Native people need.

In my view, Indian residential schools were torture institutions where knowledge transmission and traditional Native life skills, values, beliefs, and practices were halted for Native children, which created a legacy of loss for all future Native generations. For example, transmission of traditional Indigenous values related to parenting skills were lost in residential schools; this is why we have so many Native children involved with child welfare systems today. Survivors of residential school were not taught how to be parents due to the institutional environment and isolation from their families and communities, where parenting skills were normally passed down from generation to generation. Thus when these survivors later had children of their own, they did not know how to parent them. A great deal of the emotional hurt that occurred in residential schools and subsequently in child welfare systems happened because the implicit messages that both residential schools and child welfare agencies gave Native children about their peoples and families was, "Your parents did not want you!" or "Your community does not want you or care about you!" These implicit messages are what many Native peoples carry today: the belief that they are not loved and cared for by their families and communities. Many Native peoples did not and still do not feel a sense of belonging in their own communities or in wider Canadian society. Belonging is a universal human need. In addition, my experiences as a healer have shown that many survivors of residential schools and child welfare systems experienced shameful and ridiculing messages regarding Native culture and identity. A result of this emotional harm perpetrated on children in residential schools and child welfare systems is that there are many Native people who are addicted to alcohol and substances, mentally unstable, violent, and incarcerated; these outcomes are the after-effects of the federal government and churches' attempts to "help" the Indigenous people through racist and colonial legislation that was intended to destroy. This history of destruction has happened not only here in North America but in many other countries all over the world. Today, because of mass communication, especially through the Internet, we as Native peoples are increasingly learning what harms have been done to Indigenous peoples worldwide and what harms continue in order to "fix or civilize" Indigenous peoples. This history and ongoing destruction of culture and identity also adds to the depression, frustration, anger, and helpless feelings that many individual Native people feel. As a healer, I work with these individuals to help them move from these overwhelming emotions to more stable emotions that are grounded in spirituality. My position and perspective as a healer is inherently spiritual.

When I work with people, the spirit world looks at the whole person, meaning the spiritual, emotional, physical, and mental aspects of who they are. For example, the time a person is born to the earth until the day he comes to see me, is what he or she talks to me about. What creates actual healing for the person in the session with me is the person knowing that the spirit world knows him or her and the life he or she has lived. The person may learn the different reasons of why he or she went through many of those events to give him or her meaning and purpose. Specifically, when a person goes through a very painful event, many times he or she can get stuck in the emotions and beliefs or thoughts that he or she had at the time of the traumatic event. But when the person starts to understand why he or she had to go through those events and what it taught him or her from his or her spirit guide's view, this brings healing from the pain. I will share a story regarding the residential school traumas and how one person shared with me what she learned. This lady was taken from her community when she was five years old. She was walking down a dirt road, carefree and innocent, as she had many times with her mother or a sibling. Her mother had sent her to an aunt's house to borrow some sugar. A man came from behind her in an older car and stopped in front of her. He started to yell at her and walked toward her. She did not know English, so she did not understand what he was saying to her. All she knew was this white-skinned, tall man in a suit and hat was coming at her. Her first instinct was to run. He caught her and hit her a few times in the face. This was the first time she ever experienced a hit to the face from an adult. He took her on a long ride, and when they stopped, she was at a huge building she had never seen before. She had fallen asleep from crying because he had hit her a few more times during the drive. She could not stop crying, and all she could think about was how her mother would be scared and wonder where she was. A few weeks later, the priest raped the little five-year-old girl. The sexual violence continued every week for the next eleven years, until she eventually left that place. She left a broken human being, so she started to drink alcohol not long after she left there. Soon she started to have sexual relationships with different men; she thought this was normal and what was expected of her. She eventually started to hate White people and any people of authority because of these horrific events. Soon she ended up in prison for fighting and assaults; she was angry and resentful about how her short sixteen years of life had unfolded. Time went on, and she got older and angrier. She had children and did not have a clue how to love them, teach them, or make a healthy family. All she knew was the abuse, mistreatment, shame, and mean and hurtful ways that she grew up with. Her alcohol abuse continued. That is how she raised her children, so they were also growing up with no love, kindness, knowledge, or pride, and they too started to drink alcohol at a young age. One day one of her children committed suicide. This event devastated her, and she stopped drinking during her son's funeral. A few days later, she started to ask her other children what they knew about her son's death. She quickly learned that her brother, her son's uncle, had sexually abused her son. This brother had been taken to a different residential school at the same time she herself had picked up back when they were children, and he brought the sexual predator behaviour home from the school. This crisis of her son's suicide was the event that forever changed her. She decided to try to stay sober and become more aware of what her children were experiencing and how they felt about life, death, and her as a mother. It was very difficult for her but she did it; she was on the sobriety wagon. She relapsed a few times in her initial year of sobriety, but ultimately she remained committed to not drinking. After a few years of sobriety, she decided to go to a treatment center to deal with her addictions and her history of trauma; this is when I met her and the spirit world gave her some direction of what she needed to do to get stronger to really start to deal with her traumatic past and to find purpose with her life. After years of learning some parts of Native culture and experiencing a sweat lodge (or spirit lodge) ceremony, she was a believer in spirituality. She began to remember some of the songs of her ancestors that she had forgotten when she was taken to residential school, and she began her journey to learn about the relationship between herself and the spirit world. Simply knowing that her spiritual ancestors had ways to help to heal the spirit through traditional ceremonies made her feel happier and better able to cope with her problems. She knew that spirituality is what she wanted to learn and share with other residential school survivors. She immersed herself in Native culture, and one day she went on a fasting ceremony, which is a ceremony in which Native ancestors connect humans on earth with the spirit world. During this time in her life, a message came for her from the spirit world, which was, "The Native peoples had to go through residential schools because other peoples, including the White people, have been going through sexual abuse from church figures and family for years. But no one talked about it because of the shame and fear that silenced the people. Because these people were supposed to represent "God" these victims would not, or felt they could not, tell anyone because no one would believe them. So it would be the Native peoples who would bring it to the surface for the world to hear and see and *deal* with this problem." This message is what healed her, because then she knew what she had to do. This is when the national and international media began to publicize stories about criminal charges of perpetrators of child sexual abuse. This story is one example of how healing can occur when the spirit world is utilized.

Peoples' relationship with the spirit world is what is necessary to help to heal the wounds of traumatized peoples, and it is my belief that the wound sits in the spirits of individuals. Spiritual healing is what enables individuals to understand themselves in the context of their spirit and their spiritual needs. Every race of people was given a way to unite with the spirit world and communicate with the spirits, however, with the loss of these cultural ways and spirituality comes a disconnection to this resource for healing. There are many mental health professionals such as counsellors, psychologists, and psychiatrists who enter Native communities to work; however, because they are not Native and do not understand Native cultures and identities, many of the Native peoples do not feel comfortable with them and thus do not utilize their services. The Native community members know that many of these mental health professionals have no idea how it feels to be Native and they never know unless they were born Native. Unfortunately, these usually are the only "professionals" whose services are offered to Native communities for any kind of healing. But this is not the type of healing service that Native communities really need because they are grounded in Western worldviews and practices. The reason these Western professional mental health services are ineffective is because culture and spirituality is connected to our Native identity, and cultural and spiritual aspects of healing are often neglected in Western services. The primary cause of Native peoples' "mental illnesses" is a loss of positive self-identity. When Native peoples can participate and practice their ancestral spiritual ceremonies, languages, songs, and way of life, in a positive light, this is when healing happens. Unfortunately, accessing these resources and practices can be very difficult for many Native peoples because of the past outlawing of this way of life by the Indian Act, and many Native communities have lost their ceremonies, songs, and languages; the result is an interruption of the transmission of culture through generations. The anger and hate that exists in many Native peoples is because of this great disconnection to cultural knowledge and the history of harmful and inhumane acts against Native peoples. In all human beings, our spirit is the part of us that needs to feel safe, loved, and happy, and it needs to be able to carry those emotions inside of us as well. Due to the experiences within the history of Indian residential schools, the spirit is the part of many Native peoples that has been neglected and not understood because spirituality has not been taught to anyone who went to residential school or their descendants; this is why many Native individuals struggle with emotions today.

Currently, the Western system of education for mental health professionals, including counsellors and psychologists, neglects spirituality. This lack of attention to spirituality is a problem for mental health professionals who want to help Native peoples, because for Native peoples, healing begins with the spiritual. Further, this lack of understanding of the integrity of spirituality to healing for Native peoples is a problem for Western-trained professionals because it needs to be understood that Native spiritual healers, traditional knowledge keepers, traditional healthy Elders are those who must be entrusted with the healing of Native individuals. Unfortunately, because healing in general is a major issue for Native communities, this lack of knowledge and understanding by Western professionals further adds to a sense of hopelessness for many individuals, families, and communities.

The infestation of sexual abuse, incest, physical, mental, emotional, and spiritual abuse is the most damaging outcome of the Europeans to the original inhabitants of North America. This legacy of abuse remains a major healing issue for Native peoples. The ceremonies and people that Natives need to heal are limited due to the history of colonization and the ending of the transmission of cultural knowledges, which include attacks on traditional medicine people/healers. From my position as one of those people blessed with an ability to help heal individuals' spirits, emotions, minds, and physical problems, I hope to restore faith and hope to Native peoples from their traumatic experiences.

The human body is the part of people that tells us what has happened in our lives and how we have thought about what has happened. Our body has a memory of what we experience from the time we are born until the end of our lives. Sometimes people will have a physical reaction to events, such as certain tones of voice, or characteristics of someone from the past that has hurt them. This physical reaction is called a body memory and over time for someone who keeps traumatic memories inside, it will take its toll on that person's physical health. Over time and as a result of intensely thinking about and reacting to traumatic events in one's life, the body eventually manifests this experience through physical pain in the body. Thus when a person comes to me with physical problems, the problems are usually linked to a traumatic event that has happened in his or her life and the attitudes or thoughts that he or she has carried in his or her mind regarding the trauma. When I begin to help such a person through hands-on healing in a healing session, it is the spirit of the Creator who brings the healing to the person; however, there is also a message from the spirit world about why this has happened and what the person needs to work on changing in terms of thoughts, attitudes, and behaviours in order to avoid recreating those problems in the same pattern that brought him or her to the current state of physical pain. I compare this message from the spirit world to a prescription that a medical doctor would write for the physical ailment, except this "spiritual prescription" does not include the taking of pills. My "prescription" is usually about the thoughts and actions of how the person is handling his or her current life circumstances. These thoughts and attitudes that people carry with them about what has happened to them and about their belief in themselves is what affects them the most. The belief about the self affects people's spirit the most because they need to have a positive but honest belief in themselves, others, and the Creator. How people have treated themselves as well as others is important, because people must begin with honesty in order to heal from trauma; people cannot pretend that they do not know how they have treated others or themselves. My responsibility is to help people understand their responsibility in receiving the help that they have come asking for. The spirit world, like the world on earth, has rules, and one such rule is that individual people are responsible for helping themselves. For example, I cannot help another person to heal unless he or she asks for help. In this way of helping others, an individual must first be aware of and willing to deal with his or her problems. The first step of healing is to acknowledge responsibility to health and life.

A lack of being responsible for one's own healing is a current problem in Native communities, because many people have learned to believe that it is the medical doctor, psychologist, counsellor, etc., who is responsible for fixing them. Many people just want to be fixed, and quickly, and this is an obstacle in terms of helping people to heal. For example, some individuals who come to see me for healing have expressed a belief that it is someone else (doctor/professional) who is responsible for their health. But when I tell people what the spirit world sees in them and wants them to change, this can seem too difficult for some. To make changes in their lives, people must show the spirit world that they do want to be healthy and have a better life. Health is not only about the physical body, it is also about the events in people's lives and how they affect their thoughts, emotions, and, especially, their spirits. To work on healing with the spirit world is to look at a person's whole life and to listen to the spirit world for advice regarding what he or she needs to change.

I will share a story of own my spiritual healing experience. I was recently diagnosed with breast cancer. The medical doctor tried to send me for surgery to have my breasts removed the day following my mammogram. I was very scared, but at the same time, I could hear a spirit voice telling me that everything was going to be okay. I refused to have the surgery and told the doctor that I would instead go home to speak to my family and see what we should do as a family. I immediately began to pray, asking the Creator to guide me and help me to deal with this disease. I believed that the Creator was in control of everything and that nothing "just happens," so I asked the spirit world for help and guidance on how to handle this disease. After praying and consulting with my family, I asked my doctor to let me have one month to try a different way to find a cure or healing from this disease, and he reluctantly agreed. During that month, I prayed very hard and cried very much, begging the spirit world for help and health. I asked my friends and family to pray for help for me. After three weeks, I received a dream about the help I would receive from the Creator. I did what was shown to me by the Creator; I took the traditional medicine and did a ceremony for the healing that I was asking for. The next visit to my doctor confirmed that I had received healing from this medicine and ceremony; the doctor sent me for an ultrasound and more blood work to check the growth of the cancer and everything was gone. The healing I received came from a spirit animal that had shown me that the Creator was choosing this spirit to bring the healing for me. The faith that I have in the spirit world and the Creator is what helped me to stay calm and receive the help and message that I needed. This is the change I had to make and the message the spirit world gave to me: "The breasts are for nurturing, and you have not nurtured yourself. You must find the time to do things for yourself so that you feel nurtured. You must make time for you and your needs also; life is about balance, make time for yourself and for others in an equal way." This is one example of how spiritual healing works; I took a medicine to help with the physical part, but

I also had to change how I thought and felt about myself and carry through with the actions of taking care of myself and nurturing myself.

This chapter has shared experiences from the position as traditional healer in order to educate Western mental health professionals who want to support Native peoples in healing from trauma. There remain many stories to share of the miracles I have seen that have made my faith in the healing power of spirituality very strong. I know that spirituality has helped me and many others. The Creator is the one behind any healing, and the person chosen as a healer to work with the spirit world must have a strong belief and relationship with the spirits. Spirituality is the key ingredient to any healing that happens for Native peoples; inherent to this process is the belief that the Creator can heal all things.

Part 2

South

Innovative Integration in Psychological Practice

5 Indigenous North American Psychological Healing Ways and the Placement of Integration and Decolonization

Glen McCabe

Indigenous North Americans, referring to the Métis, First Nations, and Inuit in Canada and American Indians and Alaska Natives in the United States, have been seeking help from traditional healers and Elders for as long as anyone in their communities can remember (Angel, 2002; Peat, 2005. They reside in different countries and in different political jurisdictions within these countries, but tend to experience the same social, emotional, and mental health issues and also seek similar resources for help in efforts to deal with their problems.

Currently, Indigenous North Americans are seeking help from traditional helpers and from mainstream counsellors at unprecedented rates. At the same time, Indigenous North Americans still experience high rates of mental health complaints (Cockerham, 2000). Also, they experience higher than normal rates of violent and accidental deaths, family breakdown, and criminal incarceration (French, 1997; Saul, 2014). Added to this is a substantial interest among non-Indigenous people in the healing practices of Indigenous healers and Elders. Many of the people who use traditional healer services claim that they feel helped by the interventions they experience. In addition to this, Indigenous people are pursuing the services of mainstream mental health practitioners at a significant rate, while honouring their traditional beliefs and methods (Mehl-Madrona, 1997; Peat, 2005). Many also claim to feel helped.

These phenomena have given rise to increased attention from researchers and clinical practitioners both inside and outside the Indigenous community. Much of the attention has been focused on the kinds of techniques used by traditional Indigenous helpers and on the similarities and differences that they bear when compared to mainstream interventions. In this brief chapter, I will try to outline the nature of a model of psychotherapy that is used by Indigenous North Americans that was the central focus of a qualitative research project I undertook about a decade ago. This model, as you will see, on first look bears a considerable resemblance to methods used by European and North American practitioners, which might lead one to suggest that the model that was described by the people I spoke with in my research is an integrated one made up of methods used in both the mainstream and

Indigenous communities and grounded in the same theoretical understanding associated with these techniques.

Since the model described here is made up of conditions that are also highly prized in many mainstream therapies, you could with some justification assume that there is a culturally hybridized therapy, or integrated model, if you like, that might be emerging and evolving from the interaction between these two communities. As one will, hopefully, see by the end of this chapter, there is some truth in this assumption, but perhaps it is a somewhat limited truth.

The Helpful Conditions

Twelve therapeutic conditions are presented here under separate headings. They are personal readiness, spirituality, sacred ceremony, sacred teachings, authenticity, role modeling, life lessons, safety, respect, empathy, challenges, and self-knowledge. I have seen these conditions present in my own clinical practice over the years as well as in my research efforts.

Readiness for the Healing Path

The people I spoke with indicated that they believe that a person who wants to be helped has to be ready to engage in the work needed and to receive and act on the transformational pressures and challenges this can bring. Some Indigenous traditional healers will not accept clients if they are not completely compliant with the prescribed treatment plan. Kaufert and O'Neil (1989) found that, "Native healers expect absolute compliance from their Native patients and often will not accept patients who do not bring this submissive attitude to the traditional healing encounter" (p. 57). Indigenous people accept that if one has problems and wants help, a willingness to share feelings and accept change as it comes are necessary for healing to take place. The point is that until a person is ready, no effective work can be done.

Spirituality

A belief that there is a greater being or a spirit that actually has a presence in the lives of people when they ask for it is one of the major fundamental conditions of the traditional healing experience. In the words of one traditional Elder who participated in my research, "We have a connection to the universe, and that connection then connects us to the Creator, the one who creates all things." Rod McCormick (2000), an Indigenous Canadian counselling theorist, asserts that spirituality is essential for people who seek help from a traditional healer. He furthermore suggests that the basic Indigenous belief is that it is, "only through getting beyond the self that humans are able to connect with the rest of creation" (p. 26). According to this idea, doing healing work in the Indigenous community without some belief in the concepts of creation and spirituality would be a futile effort. Psychological wellness in Indigenous communities is often perceived as spiritual wellness (Restoule, 1999).

Ceremonies Are Essential

Healers that I spend time with and the participants in my research agree that ceremonies, which are closely connected to spirituality, are essential in the healing process. Sweat lodge ceremonies, sharing circles, healing circles, and pipe ceremonies are seen to be requirements of the Great Spirit for healing work to begin. Ceremonial practices and activities ground the intangible spiritual into reality and also contextualize the spiritual teachings and other important aspects of healing work within the practical experience of a person seeking help. Ceremonies are seen by healers and users of healer services to be indispensable in the overall healing environment.

The Sacred Teachings

Indigenous spirituality is expressed through sacred teachings, which are lessons about morality, maturity, and treatment of the world (including people) around us. The teachings come from the Gichi Manitou (Great Spirit) and are often connected to symbols in the physical world of human experience, such as animals and plants (Angel, 2002; Bopp, Bopp, Brown, & Lane, 1984). The teachings can be used as assessment tools or as gauges, if you like, to measure progress and the place a person is at in his or her current experiencing of self. The healer provides the sacred teachings during the course of counselling work for their clients to consider and to try to apply in their lives.

The Therapeutic Alliance

Traditional healers and their clients depend on the development and maintenance of a working therapeutic relationship. There seems to be a deeply rooted need for a positive and fully functional relationship between the client and the Indigenous counsellor. Just as the therapeutic alliance does in the non-Indigenous community, it provides an opportunity to work in an immediate context referencing transference and countertransference issues and places the connection between the client and the counsellor in a prominent position in the counselling process. In general, the therapeutic alliance is considered to be the most significant and measurable helpful condition (Martin, 2010). It may well be so in the Indigenous world as well as in the non-Indigenous world.

Safety

Safety, understandably, bears a very close connection with the therapeutic alliance. In fact, it is one of the builders of the therapeutic relationship. The people who see traditional Elders emphasized the need to feel safe and secure in the healing environment (McCabe, 2007). Many have said the issue is especially important since they have been abused in the past (McCabe, 2003). The feeling of safety for people who have been abused can be difficult to develop and needs to be worked at with awareness and diligence. One person I spoke with, in a very heartfelt way, said, "Well, first of all, I think (the healers) have given me a secure place to do my healing, . . . being allowed that time and that ability to just cry or to talk about my feelings in a completely safe environment." He felt the healer must create the safe environment and the safe relationship. Abuse of this is considered a very deep transgression in the Indigenous counselling environment (McCabe, 2007).

Authenticity

Authenticity in the healer is absolutely crucial to the positive outcomes that people look for in their healing work. The healer also expects that clients will be genuine in their attempt to heal their emotional wounds, but the healer does not judge clients when they falter on the healing path. There are basic expectations in this area. Healers should be real and not play roles or present facades. Healers are expected to be open and sincere, as well as able to demonstrate legitimacy. Healers are expected to have faith in their personal experiences and their ability to help others. Client participants in my study placed a huge emphasis on this point. Clients asserted that healers must be genuine (McCabe, 2003).

Role Modeling

Role modeling is a very powerful therapeutic tool in the healing process. It, like many of the helpful conditions, is crucial as a factor in the therapeutic alliance. Rod McCormick (2000) has found that role modeling was a positive feature in providing counselling services to Indigenous people. LaDue (1994) points out that, "The potentially most harmful problem facing Native communities today is the loss of our Elders" (p. 105). One of the major contributions of Elders and healers in Indigenous communities in North America is to demonstrate for others how to live a good life. They do this through their lifestyles, attitudes, and ability to deal with life's problems (Kulchyski, McCaskill, & Newhouse, 1999). One person told me, "Everybody just loves to be around the healer because she exudes beauty and calmness and love. So I feel like that's what I want. That's what I want to be like too. She is a great role model."

Unconditional Acceptance

Unconditional acceptance expresses the need for recipients of healer services to be accepted by the healer regardless of the mistakes of the past and their current lifestyles. Indigenous clients often perceive difficulties in their lives as being compounded by ongoing social rejection and marginalization. Indigenous people who are already on the healing path have told me that if they felt the least bit judged by a counsellor, they would disconnect from that person quickly. What is of some concern is that they also said that when this has happened to them, it took quite a bit of time to regain enough trust before seeing another person for help.

Empathic Understanding

Empathy is considered by many to be one of the most powerful psychotherapeutic conditions, especially by those who adhere to the humanist school of therapy. Indigenous people have told me that they perceive the feeling of being understood as one of their central needs in traditional healing. One person told me, "it's a feeling that somehow you know (the healer) understands you. And this person is there for you." Another said, "Somehow something resonates, kind of vibrates the heart." This kind of experience with a healer tends to cause the client to go further with their exploration and self-understanding.

Challenges

A healer's willingness and inclination to ask meaningful questions and gently point out inconsistencies in a person's behaviours and attitudes and their expressed wish for healing seems very important to Indigenous clients. The client is encouraged by the healer to look honestly, and perhaps even critically, at him or herself. Many of the Indigenous people I have spoken with about this indicate that the presentation of a simple, straightforward question can help to stimulate them to start dealing with their issues more honestly. Healers feel this helps a person to address and resolve his or her emotional pain and move from there into more productive and satisfying behaviours and thinking patterns (McCabe, 2007).

Lessons of Daily Living

This is related to the sacred teachings, but it is a different view. This category relates to everyday experiences and how to deal with them. It shows that when a person experiences success in daily life, there is a tendency to want to repeat the behaviour. Clients and healers alike demonstrated that they placed a high value on this aspect of the teachings (McCabe, 2003). The importance of learning lessons from daily lived experience is the increased presence of pro-social behaviour, sensitivity, and assertiveness; letting go of the "bad stuff" and learning about what self-care means; accepting the reality of life; the value of discipline; letting go of the need to control; and, finally, the letting go of the need to compete and compare oneself to the successes or failures of others.

Insight Into the Inner and Unknown Self

Healers and clients of healers have pointed out to me that they believe there is an inner and unknown self and that to understand and accept oneself, insight is required. Duran and Duran (1995) agree that this is germane to psychological wellness and point out that they see the modern experience of Aboriginal people as being largely understandable in terms of inner conflict and unresolved emotional urges. They have identified that there is much value in tapping into the inner experience of a person in order to find out what may be otherwise unknown to the client. McCormick (2000) outlines an existential view of how Aboriginal people have tended to drift toward alcoholism and drug abuse. Duran and Duran (1995) also connect this to colonization and acculturation. They say, "The last five hundred years have been devastating to [Indigenous] communities; the effects of this systematic genocide are currently being felt by our people" (p. 6).

An Integrated Model

This model of counselling on first appearance might lead one to believe that this is the same as any mainstream model. However, this is not necessarily true for several reasons. This model, no doubt, contains features of mainstream psychotherapy models, even what are referred to as faith-based models, but one must take into account two serious differences. First, one must consider that the experiencing and understanding of conditions such as empathy and unconditional positive regard are interpreted very differently by Indigenous people in comparison to non-Indigenous people. Second, how these two concepts are realized in counselling can be very different. Third, the faith-based experience is founded on a different interpretation of spirituality. For example, it has been my experience that Indigenous North Americans tend to experience empathy as a very powerful element akin to mind reading. I have had people react in very negative ways, saying that no one can understand the life of another and that a person must be very careful when speaking to another about his or her emotional state. It seems that the use of empathy is important, but is to be used very gently and subtly. To do it any other way would likely be very threatening for an Indigenous person.

Another example of this difference would be authenticity. Many Indigenous people believe that a helper from the mainstream population might find it difficult to achieve legitimacy due to being perceived as coming from a different culture and also because of the potential of being an oppressor, even if it is not his or her intention. From this view, authenticity, although crucial to the healing process, may elude the non-Indigenous helper regardless of his or her intentions and honesty.

In the context of spirituality, this area is of greatest distinction between traditional healing and mainstream counselling work, as the underpinnings are very different. The scientific mind of mainstream people believe in things being linear and separate (Peat, 2005; Suzuki, 1997), while the Indigenous healer believes that all things are intertwined and dependent on each other. This moves the whole understanding of healing and wellness as a different condition altogether from the conceptualization of the non-Indigenous person. In the mainstream, the scientific perspective asserts that in order to understand a phenomenon one must isolate it and study it. In Indigenous traditional thinking, all phenomena must be seen as totally connected and immersed in each other in order to be understood. This is extended to the world of psychological healing in the same way as one would view biology or astrophysics.

From this standpoint, it is plain that these psychotherapy models are similar but different at some very basic levels. When therapists ask me about what would be helpful in preparing them to work in an Indigenous community, I often tell them that living in an Indigenous community for a couple of years would be useful. They usually react by saying that they cannot do this due to time and commitment restraints but, short of this, I do not know what would assist them in their wish to be helpful and effective in their work with the Indigenous community.

In short, the model described briefly in this chapter is an integrated one, but it is not simply a model that uses aspects of both cultures. It is fundamentally different in some respects, while at the same time, recognizable as having similar elements to mainstream approaches. This makes it virtually impossible to simply apply the conditions and techniques that a mainstream counsellor would use without any further consideration or the expectation of having the desired impact.

One of the answers to this dilemma is connected to practitioner identity and self-understanding (Martin, 2010) in conjunction with understanding and knowledge of the Indigenous community (McCabe, 2007). A counsellor who knows him or herself well and has good understanding and acceptance of Indigenous ways will be able to make important distinctions between what to apply, how to apply it, and when it is best used. These are not simple things to achieve because they mean looking in detail at one's own identity and cultural context, as well as at that of the people one is trying to help.

A Decolonizing Model

One of the central discussions in and around the Indigenous community that has emerged recently centres on the idea that work with Indigenous people should be driven by a decolonization ethos (Saul, 2014), particularly in the context of emotional and psychological healing (French, 1997; Gone, 2010; McCabe, 2007; McCormick, 2000). The same argument has been made in regard to activities such as research with Indigenous people (Smith, 1999). Smith (1999) suggests that old methods and ways of doing research with Indigenous people anywhere in the world need to be deconstructed and replaced with ways that address the issues of oppression and colonization without doing further damage.

It was in this frame of reference that I undertook the research noted earlier. My sense of the work was that it could and should be an emotionally healing influence as much as it was an academic exercise. I believed that if it were helpful in that regard, then it would, by definition, be a decolonizing influence. I used qualitative phenomenology as the method of choice because I believed it to be a potentially strong decolonizing approach. It is typically reliant on narratives offered by participants, and at its heart, there is a focus on determining the embedded "truth" that the participant offers through a broad and open narrative. This, I believe, can also be applied as a directive in doing healing work with Indigenous people anywhere in the world.

Healers from different communities can help each other by working cooperatively and supportively with each other, but only once there is confidence that more damage will not be done. Clinical psychology, psychiatry, and mental health services in general may have failed the Indigenous peoples of North America until now, but it does not have to stay that way. Respected and proven traditional healers and Elders are clinical practitioners in their own right and use sound and worthy methods of prevention, intervention, and after care as perceived by the members of their own communities. This should be enough to legitimize their work. Practitioners from outside the Indigenous community can work together with traditional healers and Elders to learn and assist and to have a positive influence rather than running the risk of doing further damage, even though unintended.

In Closing

There has been a growing body of research and commentary related to Indigenous North American healing ways. Some of this has been broadly based and looks at the general issues of diversity and some of it has been directed more specifically toward the need for decolonization. The reasons for this increased attention are likely many and varied, but one central factor is that the use of Indigenous healing ways has become of interest to both Indigenous and non-Indigenous people. People in both these spheres who use traditional healing ways often claim that it has helped them (McCabe, 2007). Another reason for the increased interest in traditional healing is that issues of social and psychological disruption among Indigenous North Americans have not abated, but rather seem to have increased (Lawrence, 2003). In contrast to this, Indigenous people are seeking out the help of mainstream counsellors in increasing numbers (France, McCormick, & Rodriguez, 2013).

As is indicated earlier, I have conducted research into the healing and wellness practices of Indigenous North Americans. It has focused on determining what factors seem to contribute to the improved emotional and psychological states that people claim they experience as a result of using the services of traditional healers. It has shown that even after living lives of emotional pain with only their hope to keep them going, Indigenous people in Canada and the United States continue to seek help with their efforts to mend their emotional wounds and social problems.

This research has resulted in the gathering of rich commentaries about the healing journeys of people who have found something within themselves that they thought did not exist there. The healers themselves spoke of their own healing journeys in a manner similar to those of their clients. In this sense, the healer is just like the clients he or she serves. Very often, both have been through darkness to find light and to know how to better deal with the vagaries of life as they experience it.

In this brief chapter, I have talked about twelve of the conditions that seem to be inherent in the work of some Indigenous people. However, this is only part of the story. What is yet to emerge will further tell the tale and free people from the bonds of emotional suffering and pain. This work is an ongoing process, and I expect that other outcomes will emerge that give more detail and scope to the results and will greatly expand the discussion of healing among Indigenous people around the world and likely the non-Indigenous community as well.

For a hundred years there have been slow and gradual changes in the prospects of Indigenous North Americans (Saul, 2014; Wilson & Morrison, 1995). My father's generation began the Indian-Métis Friendship Centre movement in the 1960s. In cities such as Winnipeg, Toronto, and Edmonton, there were groups emerging to bring Indigenous people together to share ideas and enjoy the company of the community. This was an important step in recharging the positive social fabric of the urban Indigenous community in Canada. From there many things have been underway that are connected to healing and wellness in the Native experience.

My sense of this whole process is that the suffering and healing of one is linked to the suffering and healing of the many. Wherever this path takes us and whatever is revealed as we travel it, there can be little doubt that the human desire for centering will cause us to continue the journey and to maintain our hope, enhance our safety, and reduce the power differentials that exist within the fabric of communities all around the world. This may result in a fully integrated model of therapy that works for all people, or it may not, but the work we do on bringing healing and wellness to each other is essential and is absolutely connected to the time and energy we devote to our collective wellness.

References

Angel, M. (2002). *Historical perspectives on the Ojibwa Midewiwin: Preserving the sacred*. Winnipeg, Canada: The University of Manitoba Press.

Bopp, J., Bopp, M., Brown, L., & Lane, P. (1984). *Scared tree: Reflections on Native American spirituality*. Silver Lake, WI: Lotus Press.

Cockerham, W. C. (2000). *Sociology of mental disorder*, 5th ed. Upper Saddle River, New Jersey: Prentice Hall.

Duran, E., & Duran, B. (1995). *Native American postcolonial psychology*. New York, NY: State University of New York Press.

France, H., McCormick, R., & Rodriguez, M. (2013). The red road: Spirituality, the medicine wheel, and the sacred hoop. In H. France, M. Rodriguez, & G. Hett (Eds.),

Diversity, culture and counselling: A Canadian perspective, 2nd ed. (pp. 292–309). Calgary, Canada: Brush Education.

French, L. A. (1997). *Counseling American Indians*. Landham, MD: University Press of America, Inc.

Gone, J. (2010). Psychotherapy and traditional healing for American Indians: Exploring the prospects for therapeutic integration. *The Counselling Psychologist, 38*(2), 166–235.

Kaufert, J. M., & O'Neil, J. D. (1989). Biomedical rituals and informed consent: Native Canadians and the negotiation if clinical trust. In G. Weisz (Ed.), *Social science perspectives on medical ethics* (pp. 41–63). Philadelphia, PA: Kluwer Academic Publishers.

Kulchyski, P., McCaskill, D., & Newhouse, D. (1999). *In the words of elders: Aboriginal cultures in transition*. Toronto, ON: University of Toronto Press.

LaDue, R. (1994). Coyote returns: Twenty sweats does not an Indian make. In K. Nanette (Ed.), *Ethics alive: Feminist ethics in psychotherapy practice* (pp. 93–111). New York, NY: The Hawthorn Press.

Lawrence, B. (2003). Gender, race and regulation of Native identity in Canada and the United States: An overview. *Hypatia, 18*(2), 3–31.

Martin, D. G. (2010). *Counseling and therapy skills*, 3rd ed. Prospect Heights, IL: Waveland Press.

McCabe, G. H. (2003). *Finding the healing Path: The therapeutic conditions of Aboriginal traditional healing*. (Unpublished doctoral thesis). Winnipeg, MB: University of Manitoba.

McCabe, G. H. (2007). The healing path: A culture and community-derived indigenous therapy model. *Psychotherapy: Theory, Research, Practice, Training, 44*(2), 148–160.

McCormick, R. M. (2000). Aboriginal traditions in the treatment of substance abuse. *Canadian Journal of Counselling, 34*(1), 25–32.

Mehl-Madrona, L. (1997). *Coyote medicine: Lessons from Native American healing*. New York, NY: Fireside Press.

Peat, F. David. (2005). *Blackfoot physics*. Boston, MA: Red Wheels/Weiser.

Restoule, B. (1999). *Healing in Ojibway First Nations communities: Investigating the relationship among acculturation, health and identity*. (Unpublished doctoral thesis). Kingston, ON: Queen's University.

Saul, J. R. (2014). *The comeback*. Toronto, ON, Canada: The Penguin Group.

Smith, L. (1999). *Decolonizing methodologies: Research and indigenous peoples*. Dunedin, NZ: University of Otago Press.

Suzuki, D. (1997). *The sacred balance: Rediscovering our place in nature*. Toronto, Canada: Greystone Books.

Wilson, C., & Morrison, R. (1995). Taking stock: Legacies and prospects. In R. Morrison, & C. Wilson (Eds.), *Native peoples: The Canadian experience*, 2nd ed. (pp. 607–629). Toronto, Canada: McClelland and Stewart, Inc.

6 Counselling Indigenous Peoples in Canada

Suzanne L. Stewart and Anne Marshall

The Assembly of First Nations (2002) defines Indigenous peoples as comprising three distinct cultural groups: First Nations (status and non-status Indians), Métis, and Inuit. The term Indigenous is often used interchangeably with Aboriginal, Native, and Indian. Among the many cultural minority groups within Canada, Indigenous peoples are among the fastest growing populations. According to 2011 statistics, Indigenous peoples represent approximately 4 percent of Canada's total population or about a total of 1,409,100 people (Statistics Canada, 2015a). About 50 percent of the Indigenous population is under the age of twenty-four and 40 percent are under the age of sixteen (Statistics Canada, 2015a). Thus the population is growing with a high concentration of youth. Since the 1970s, there has been a large migration of Indigenous peoples from rural areas and First Nation reserves to cities. Currently, over 600,000 self-identified Indigenous people live in cities—54 percent of the total Aboriginal population—and the numbers are expected to grow according to demographic trends (Statistics Canada, 2015a). The Indigenous population is becoming increasingly urban; in 2006, 54 percent lived in an urban centre, an increase from 50 percent in 1996 (Indigenous and Northern Affairs, 2010). From 2001 to 2006, the Indigenous population in Canada increased by 196,475; over this period, the Indigenous population grew by 20.1 percent, a rate five times that of the non-Indigenous population

Mental health is a vital aspect of overall health for Canadian Indigenous peoples. However, Indigenous cultural understandings of mental health and healing are distinctly different from understandings that have prevailed in most North American mental health provider settings, including in counselling contexts. Counsellor training in Canada and the United States is based almost exclusively on a Western paradigm of health that differs from an Indigenous worldview (Gone, 2004). These differences in paradigmatic worldviews can form a barrier to effective helping for Native peoples who seek counselling services from formally trained counsellors, including those who may be trained in cross-cultural or multicultural approaches. Further, Duran (2006) suggests that counselling Indigenous individuals from a non-Indigenous perspective (i.e., Western perspective) is a form of continued oppression and colonization, as it does not legitimize Indigenous cultural views of mental health and healing. "A postcolonial paradigm would accept knowledge from differing cosmologies as valid in their own right, without their having to adhere to a separate cultural body for legitimacy" (Duran & Duran, 1995, p. 6).

Some counselling educators, researchers, and practitioners are increasingly recognizing the inseparability of cultural foundations and mental health needs and are attempting to undertake more effort to explore traditional cultural conceptions of mental health and healing. For example, Indigenous mental health and healing training, education, and practice have been incorporated into many postsecondary-training programs across the country (Stewart, 2009). In order to address more culturally relevant knowledge regarding mental health and healing, this paper will present a brief history of Indigenous peoples and what its implications are for mental health and healing, an overview of key issues for Indigenous clients, and two models of Indigenous counselling.

Indigenous Peoples in Canada

A Brief History of Indigenous Health in Canada

According to oral tradition, prior to first contact with Europeans in the 16th century, the incidence of health problems among Indigenous peoples in what is now called Canada was low (Waldram, 2004). However, contact brought a dramatic increase in physical and mental illness to Aboriginals (Kirmayer, Brass, & Tait, 2000). Over seven million Indigenous peoples are estimated to have inhabited North America prior to contact in 1492, with almost 90 percent of these people dying as a result of indirect and direct effects of European settlement by 1600, and infectious disease brought from Europe was the major killer, followed by a change in traditional diet to one of European foodstuffs (Young, 1988). Today there continue to be health problems, such as diabetes and obesity, in Native communities related to diet and epidemiology (Kirmayer et al., 2000).

Implementation of federal policy has destroyed Indigenous cultures through the creation of land reserves, residential schools, and bureaucratic control. Indigenous settlements were chosen by non-Native governments, who forced First Nations off of their traditional lands and onto other territories, often grouping bands together that had previously no history of living together (Dickason, 1997). These groupings were forced to make new social structures and sustainable ways of life. Indigenous groups were moved to lands with little or no natural resources, i.e., lands not deemed liveable for settlers (Royal Commission on Aboriginal Peoples, 1994). Referring to a damaging example of this relocation for the Inuit peoples, Kirmayer et al. (2000) write, "The disastrous 'experiment' of relocating Inuit to the Far North to protect Canadian sovereignty—a late chapter in this process of forced culture change—revealed the government's continuing lack of awareness of cultural and ecological realities" (p. 609).

Prior to contact with European explorers, North American Indigenous communities had effective methods for preventing and treating illness and injury (Young, 1988). For example, Bopp and Lane (2000) have recorded how the Nuxalk peoples of British Columbia effectively survived the small pox epidemic by creating and following a plan to "avoid complete annihilation" (p. 7): community members were ordered by leaders to scatter from villages in pairs and to remain "in shouting distance" apart, and if one partner died, the other was to bury them (p. 7). If the remaining person then became ill, he or she was to bury him or herself in a shallow grave until dead. After one year of this separation, surviving members were to return to their villages. All the Nuxalk then gathered near the river, and it was estimated that of the thirty thousand peoples who were alive before the epidemic, two hundred and forty seven remained. Thus the Nuxalk peoples survived and treated a major illness.

Through the colonization, bureaucratization, missionization, and education processes of the Canadian colonial governments, the control of healing and other health practices was largely transferred from Indigenous peoples to programs and institutions sponsored by the Canadian government (Waldram, 2004). According to Waldram, while this new system helped to mitigate some of the devastating health problems brought from Europe (such as influenza, tuberculosis, and small pox, which developed through the early contact period), it failed to protect the health and well-being of Indigenous peoples in the following ways. First, the health care services provided by the Canadian federal government had no foundation in the traditional knowledge and cultural values and practices of Indigenous peoples. The government's health care practices were unfamiliar and frightening for many Indigenous peoples and further undermined their trust in and identification with their own practices and resources, which was also supported by the assimilationist education provided through residential schools (Truth and Reconciliation Commission of Canada, 2015). These healthcare services also took some Indigenous individuals away from their communities, sometimes for extended periods, when they required certain types of medical treatment, such as for tuberculosis or pneumonia. Second, Robbins and Dewar (2011) write that traditional healers were ridiculed and persecuted by the dominant culture and by governmental legislation; in reaction, traditional healers were forced to practice their traditions such as Potlatch, Sundance, and shamanic healing in secret. As a result, many Indigenous peoples no longer accessed the benefits of their traditional healers' skills and knowledge, either because they did not know how to access these services or because they had been taught to mistrust, fear, or condemn their own healing traditions (Robbins & Dewar, 2011). Through this process of eliminating the practice of traditional healers, a great deal of very valuable cultural knowledge has been lost. Third, the Western perspectives that dominate mental health interventions have roots in modernism, a worldview that values objective truth, rational thinking, and the constancy of measurement (Sue & Sue, 1990). This focus on Western perspectives to mental health means that Aboriginal communities only had access to certain Western types of treatment and prevention programs, mostly those-which focus on individuals and diagnostic labels rather than on the type of healing and human and community development and interdependence needed to restore Indigenous individuals, families, and communities to a level of health and wellness (Smith, 1999). Lastly, Indigenous peoples lost control over the institutions and processes which were supposed to protect the health of their people (Alfred, 1999; Waldram, 2004). Indigenous peoples were taught, through missionization and residential schools, that the dominant society knew best which services and programs they needed. Even now, as many Indigenous communities are negotiating with the Canadian government for the transfer of health programs to their control, they are often being given administrative responsibility for existing programs but very little real power to actually recreate culturally based health and social service programming in order to move towards maximum health and well-being (Waldram, 2004).

Current Health Concerns

Kirmayer et al. (2000) explain that cultural discontinuity and oppression are linked to high rates of alcoholism, suicide, depression, and violence for many Indigenous groups today, particularly youth, yet many communities continue to grow and even thrive despite such challenges. The history of health and colonization, beginning in the 1500s and continuing into current times show a clear connection between mental health and colonization; Kirmayer et al. (2000) link specific health problems, such as obesity, diabetes, low self-esteem, depression, and suicide to this colonial history and oppression. There are social origins for the mental health distress currently being experienced in Native Canadian communities. These social origins include government policy that created residential schools and poverty and economic marginalization. Kirmayer et al. (2000) write that residential schools are a major source of cultural extermination for Aboriginal peoples; from 1879 to 1973, the Canadian government mandated church-run boarding schools to provide education for all Native children. Aboriginal children were forcibly removed from homes and relocated to residential schools, often geographically far from their families, with siblings usually sent to separate schools, in order to fulfill the policy goal of systematically breaking down Aboriginal culture and family (Truth and Reconciliation Commission of Canada, 2015). In residential schools, Aboriginal children were denied all ties to their cultures, including language and customs. In short, their identity as Aboriginal was completely taken away. Physical and sexual abuse by teachers and clergy was rampant in residential school life, and the government and churches only recently acknowledged these atrocities (Truth and Reconciliation Commission of Canada, 2015).

Poverty and economic marginalization, as part of Aboriginal colonial history, contributes to the current legacy of mental health problems. Effects of poverty are third-world living conditions, especially on many reserves, and high rates of chronic health problems that exist in today's communities. Kirmayer et al. (2000) state that

> the effects of poverty are seen in the poor living conditions on many reserves and remote settlements that lead to chronic respiratory diseases, recurrent otitis media with hearing loss, and tuberculosis; in the past, these necessitated prolonged hospitalizations that further subverted the integrity of families and communities.
>
> (p. 610)

This economic marginalization is seen as a creation of the social order in which Native peoples are embedded within Canadian society. Further, it is suggested by Kirmayer and colleagues that the presence of mass media in such communities today makes the values of consumer capitalism central and creates feelings of deprivation for those community members where none previously existed. Kirmayer and colleagues note that health research in Indigenous communities does not always allow for differences in incidence and prevalence of specific mental health problems among and between communities, but rather tends to generalize information to all Native communities. Kirmayer and colleagues suggest that in Indigenous contexts today, there are constant transformations of forms of community and that this sort of evolution is at the root of recovery, or "revitalization and renewal" (p. 611). Further, it is the "mediating mechanics," or what are described as individual and self-perceptions, contributing to social and mental health problems that are closely related to issues of individual identity and self-esteem (p. 611). The collectives of communities influence these factors. For example, the wide variation of suicide rates across Native communities indicates that it is important to consider the nature and health of overall communities and how these communities respond to the ongoing stresses of colonization and governmental control, including sociopolitical marginalization.

The mental health implications of this colonial history are significant for Indigenous communities and individuals (Duran, 2006; Kirmayer et al., 2000; Waldram, 2004). These implications include high rates (compared to non-Indigenous populations) of grief and loss, depression, family violence, sexual abuse, substance abuse, addictions, trauma, and suicide. Of these issues, trauma and suicide will be discussed in detail because of their saliency within communities and because of their prevalence as presenting problems within counselling with Indigenous clients (Duran, 2006).

Trauma has been documented in the literature as a major healing issue in many Indigenous communities across Canada (Bopp & Lane, 2000; Caron,

2012, 2004; Menzies, 2009; Wilson, 2004). Bopp and Lane (2000) write that trauma for Native individuals and communities is a complex and intergenerational phenomenon that has its roots in the colonial history that has taken away and destroyed many traditional Native cultural practices. Bopp and Lane define trauma as, "the psychological, physical, and mental effects associated with a painful experience or shock" (p. 25). Experiencing trauma events puts an individual or community in a position of being overwhelmed emotionally with the traumatic experience. This overwhelm is dealt with in many different ways by different people and communities. People often turn to substance abuse, violence toward others or the self, suicide, and many other forms of self-destructive behaviour; these effects are often described as indicators or consequences of psychological trauma (Tedeschi & Calhoun, 1996).

In a report based on a health study with the Nuxalk Nation of British Columbia, Bopp and Lane (2000) write that psychological trauma can occur from a single event or a series of prolonged events and that trauma can occur to individuals as well as communities. Regardless of the specifics of the traumatic events, the trauma itself creates certain characteristic effects on individuals and the way that they understand their environments and relationships. "Trauma affects whole communities by undermining social, cultural, economic, and political structures and relationships as well as the capacity of that community to interact in a healthy balanced way with the society around it" (Bopp & Lane, 2000, p. 26). When trauma is ongoing, or occurs more than once, a sense of helplessness and hopelessness often sets in for the individual or the community. Bopp and Lane conclude that healing support for Indigenous communities and individuals dealing with psychological trauma must address these core aspects of trauma.

Karmali et al. (2005) conducted a population-based observational study that describes the epidemiological characteristics of severe psychological trauma among status Indians in the Calgary health region. They discovered that in their sample, severe trauma—such as suicide or accidental death—occurred about four times more among status Indians than non-Indigenous groups. Further, the large difference in rates between status Indians and non-Indigenous groups was present for specific causes, such as suicide, assault, and car accidents.

In addition to understating epidemiological characteristics of trauma and rates of trauma in Indigenous communities, issues of morbidity and accurate depictions of the real effects of trauma must be documented and understood in qualitative and quantitative terms, and they must include all Aboriginal peoples and not only status Indians (Caron, 2004). There is a need for qualitative information because there exists ample evidence to suggest that suicide is a problem, but not enough data to describe what this means to individuals and communities involved. Also, health care services, including mental health services, must be more accessible and more culturally appropriate for Native communities dealing with psychological trauma, and such qualitative data could be used to improve such services. Caron (2004) suggests that traumatic injury and death are easily preventable health problems, but that it would take the support of the healthcare community and greater society to work collaboratively with Indigenous groups to deal with the psychological effects of trauma. For example, the overall First Nations men's death rate for mortality from avoidable causes is two times higher compared to non-Aboriginal men, and for First Nations women, it is 2.5 times more likely: "The age-standardized avoidable mortality rate per 100,000 person-years at risk for First Nations men was 679.2, while it was 337.6 for non-Aboriginal men. The rate was 453.2 for First Nations women, compared with 183.5 for non-Aboriginal women" (Statistics Canada, 2015b).

Substantial research on Indigenous suicide shows high levels of suicide in some, but not all, communities. As discussed earlier, Indigenous peoples in general do not have the same health status as non-Natives in Canada; however, when it comes to suicide, the difference is especially dramatic. Indigenous youth, as a national population, commit suicide approximately five times more often than non-Indigenous youth (Health Canada, 2015); "For First Nations females, the suicide rate is 35 per 100,000 compared to only 5 per 100,000 for non-Aboriginal females. The suicide rate for First Nations males is 126 per 100,000 compared to 24 per 100,000 for non-Aboriginal males" (p. 1).

Studies by Bagley, Wood, and Khumar (1990) and Bohn (2003) identified regional variations in Indigenous community suicides, indicating that Health Canada's generalized statistics may not fit for specific communities. Chandler and Lalonde's (1998) research further elaborates on this within-group difference as linked to Aboriginal self-government and cultural identification and practices. In the 1980s, the federal government initiated a process meant to transfer healthcare responsibility to First Nations and Inuit governments. The rationale for this decision by the government was that Indigenous peoples best understood their community's healthcare and service delivery needs and thus should be in control of these services (Health Canada, 2003). In 1994, Health Canada conducted a study on the success of this transfer of healthcare services programme and found that transferring management control led to a decrease in health problems and issues within communities and more culturally sensitive healthcare delivery (Health Canada, 2006). In addition, health care, including dealing with suicide, became a priority that could be acted upon. Seminal research by Chandler and Lalonde (1998) examined suicide in the context of self-government and local control of health care, education, and other infrastructure. In studying suicide among British Columbia's nearly two hundred Aboriginal communities, they found that while some communities had suicide rates eight hundred times greater than the national average, in other communities, suicide was practically non-existent. Chandler and Lalonde further identified six protective factors that help make sense of the differing suicide rates across some Native communities. These factors are discussed as cultural continuity and could be considered an index of community-level success in renewing or reclaiming cultural tradition: 1) land claims, 2) self-government, 3) education services, 4) police and fire services, 5) health services, and 6) cultural facilities. More specifically, Chandler and Lalonde found that communities with some form of self-government had the lowest rate of youth suicide. Land claims were the second and education the third most important factors in predicting a low suicide rate in the communities studied. Communities possessing three or more cultural continuity factors experienced substantially fewer suicides than communities without such factors present. Thus these factors are important to consider regarding the mental health of communities in terms of suicide rates. Further study is currently needed to examine other correlates of mental health such as depression, self-esteem, addictions, and family violence with such factors of cultural continuity.

Challenges of Current Counselling Services

Specific challenges arise when a Western mental healthcare system is imposed on Indigenous individuals and communities. First, Western and Indigenous notions of mental health are different; second, counsellors trained in Western notions of mental health do not effectively service Indigenous mental health populations; and third, using a Western paradigm of mental health in an Indigenous context is a form of continued oppression of Indigenous peoples.

Related to the first point, counsellor training that is based on Western notions of health and healing does not match Indigenous conceptions of well-being. Western-based counselling approaches are culturally inappropriate in Indigenous contexts because the many values and ways of being and doing are different (Duran, 2006). A Western approach would not be effective with Indigenous clients if it did not take into account the context of the client's life. Often, health policies and programs designed by non-Indigenous individuals or institutions have been inappropriate for dealing with Indigenous problems because the philosophies and ways of living that underpin each approach are very different from Western healing (Vicary & Bishop, 2005). Indigenous healing is different because it employs a holistic model, which is defined as a whole person that includes a mind, body, and spirit approach to well-being (Waldram, 2004, 2008). Western approaches to counselling such as constructivism and family systems are often considered more culturally appropriate in Indigenous contexts because they take into account contexts of the individual; however, they are not based on Indigenous worldviews or paradigms that reflect notions of interconnectedness, spirituality, and Native rules of behaviour (Blue & Darou, 2005). Western culture in Canada emphasizes a hierarchical and individualist worldview, which is in opposition to Indigenous beliefs. Western approaches to counselling are largely based on individualism, such as the person-centred approach (Duran, 2006). McCormick (2000) maintains that the European-Western paradigm is built on a model of creation containing a hierarchy of God, humans, and nature, including concepts of domination of humans by God, of animals by humans, and of humans exploiting the land. An Indigenous counselling model, in contrast, according to McCormick (2000), would be based on connectedness, equality, and harmony between people and nature.

Sue and Sue (1990) suggest that mental health approaches in general could benefit from the worldviews of Indigenous healing methods. These are usually informal and naturally existing help-giving methods present in all traditional Indigenous cultures that focus on interdependence or connectedness in healing. For example, in traditional Dene communities in Canada's north, grandparents not only took care of grandchildren so that parents could do valuable work for the community, such as hunting and craft making, but those grandparents also passed on cultural knowledge that was vital for individual and group survival as a distinct people (personal communication, Stewart, 2006).

Related to the second point that counsellors who receive training only in Western approaches to mental health and healing are not meeting the needs of Native clients seeking counselling services, there is currently an under-use of mental health services, such as counselling, by ethnic minority groups, including Indigenous peoples (Sue & Sue, 1990). Some researchers have suggested that this under-use stems from the fact that counselling approaches are not culturally sensitive to the Indigenous clients' values, beliefs, or worldviews: "Counselors may lack basic knowledge about the client's ethnic and historical backgrounds; the client may be driven away by the professional's counseling style; the client may sense that his or her worldview is not valued" (Trimble & Thurman, 2002, p. 61).

King (1999) conducted a survey with an urban Indigenous adult population in Denver, Colorado, to identify their mental health needs. King concluded that mental health provider agencies are not meeting the current needs of urban Native adults, who stated a preference for Native health service providers or at least providers who are sensitive to cultural community needs. Over 90 percent of the adult respondents said they would use mental health services if Native persons trained in mental health services or non-Natives who had training in Native sensitivity as well as mental health services made those services available. Community health was also a theme in King's data. The study's author's recommendations were that all levels of Indigenous community mental health are in dire need of mental health services that are grounded in an Indigenous paradigm. Mental health is underpinned by community health, according to King, and community-level interventions that fit the Indigenous culture of the community, such as prevention and education, are needed to address the mental health of individuals sampled in this community. Blue (1977), Blue and Darou (2005), and McCormick (1997) have also studied and written about how and why Indigenous peoples utilize services only when these services are grounded in a First Nations helping model. These researchers have worked in Canadian contexts and conducted interviews with Native clients in counselling.

To address the third point, Western perspectives on mental health continue the oppression of Indigenous peoples because they delegitimize Indigenous views of health and healing. According to the Aboriginal Healing Foundation (2002), conceptions of traditional health and healing are integral to current efforts by Canadian Indigenous peoples to face the legacy of suffering and dislocation brought on by the history of colonialism. For example, in 2000, the Champlain District Mental Health Implementation Task Force in Ontario began the implementation of mental health reform in two specific First Nations communities (Akwesasne and Golden Lake). This reform is marked by recognizing the need to support First Nations' capacity to design, deliver, and control their own mental health services and to respect traditional contemporary Indigenous approaches to healing and wellness (Poushinsky & Tallion-Wasmund, 2002). Further, the reform recommends that within First Nations communities, there must be at least one or a combination of three streams of available mental health services: traditional mental health services provided by traditional healers and healers through ceremonies, Indigenized mental health services (Western mental health paradigms that have been converted and delivered by Natives), and Western mental health services delivery to Natives by non-Natives.

The intent and results that have underpinned much health research has been a tool of power and control over First Nations. Many mental health treatment applications have been designed to dominate and control people with mental illness. Foucault (1971) initially explored the process of social control. He wrote that when the (Catholic) church lost control of much of the general Western population in the 1800s, the medical profession seized an opportunity to control the masses. The movement of the medical profession at the time evolved into the present-day mental health care system in the Western world, including Canada. In this perspective, mental health care practitioners can be seen as possessing and exerting social control through the process of labeling in diagnosis and the sometimes subsequent taking away of a person's rights when he or she is deemed not of sound mind.

Indigenous Mental Health

In 1991, the government of Canada published the "Agenda for First Nations and Inuit Mental Health." It includes a description of mental health within a framework of holism and positive psychology as they are embedded in community and cultural identity:

> Among the First Nations and Inuit communities, the term mental health is used in a broad sense, describing behaviours that make for a harmonious and cohesive community and the relative absence of multiple problem behaviours in the community, such as family violence, substance abuse, juvenile delinquency and self-destructive behaviour. It is more

> than the absence of illness, disease or dysfunction—it is the presence of a holistic, psychological wellness which is part of the full circle of mind, body, emotions and spirit, with respect for tradition, culture and language. This gives rise to creativity, imagination and growth, and enhances the capacity of the community, family group or individual identities to interact harmoniously and respond to illness and adversity in healing ways.
>
> (p. 6)

This holistic description of mental health makes an important point about the interrelatedness of spiritual, mental, social, and community aspects of health. Health as possessing an interrelated quality along with notions such as community and identity allows for an examination of mental health through a systemic lens that is grounded in an Indigenous paradigm.

Mussell (2005) writes that mental health in the context of Indigenous counsellors and policy makers is about focusing on the mental health issues that exist as the most serious detriments to the survival and well-being of Native peoples. Part of an Indigenous worldview is the notion of holistic health, which marks how people view themselves, their families, and their communities in a forward-thinking manner.

> Holistic health is the vision most First Nations peoples articulate as they reflect upon their future. At the personal level this means each member enjoys health and wellness in body, mind, heart, and spirit. Within the family context, this means mutual support of each other . . . From a community perspective it means leadership committed to whole health, empowerment, sensitivity to interrelatedness of past, present, and future possibilities, and connected between cultures.
>
> (p. 26)

An integral concept to the notion of holistic health is the concept of interdependence, as pointed out by Mussell. For Indigenous peoples, mental health problems result from lack of balance and interdependence among the four aspects of human nature identified earlier. When balance, or harmony through interconnectedness, is restored through paying attention to the needs of the four aspects of the self, the family, or the community, health is achieved in Indigenous worldviews.

> The medicine wheel model is a conceptual and practical framework for the holistic philosophy of mental health. Absolon (1994) defines the medicine wheel as a paradigm that is relevant to the needs for assessment purposes in healing work, an expression of a First Nations Worldview, that views healing as a process that achieves a balanced relationship with the self, Mother earth, and the natural world."
>
> (p. 25)

Originating with the Plains Natives, the Medicine Wheel is an ancient and widely used concept in Indigenous North American cultures, that models health and wellness for multiple aspects of a person or community (Mussell, 2005). When considering the Medicine Wheel, it is important to note that the term medicine as it is used by various First Nations people does not refer to drugs or herbal remedies (Thunderbird, 2005). Storm (1972) explains that medicine in Plains culture refers to the personal characteristics and strengths of individuals that come to them through a particular animal reflection that occurs though the wheel. The characteristics of this reflection on an individual are determined by the nature of the animal itself (e.g., bear eagle, wolf, pheasant) and also by the location of the individual him/herself.

Storm, a Plains Native and teacher of the lessons of the Medicine Wheel, explains the philosophies of the circle. The Medicine Wheel is seen as demonstrating that we need multiple perspectives through its construction of the circle as a non-linear structure (Storm, 1972). She writes that the Medicine Wheel, as a circle, can be best understood in terms of a mirror that reflects all aspects of life and world. "Any idea, person, or object can be a Medicine Wheel, a Mirror, for man" (p. 5).

Teachings in contemporary Indigenous communities based on the Medicine Wheel create an epistemological paradigm that employs a holistic foundation for human behaviour and interaction; it informs a framework for mental health through a discussion of its four quadrants, each one a separate representation of north, south, east, and west (Thunderbird, 2005). For example, in the Sault Nation, the construction of the wheel is meant to help people seek strong, healthy bodies (represented by the north-facing quadrant), strong inner spirits (represented by the south-facing quadrant), healthy minds (east quadrant), and inner peace (west quadrant) (Four Directions, 2005).

The Medicine Wheel embodies how Indigenous mental health can be conceptualized in a theoretical and pragmatic model for healthcare delivery (Poushinsky & Tallion-Wasmund, 2002). The Dze L K'ant Native Friendship Centre Society (2006) in Smithers, British Columbia, employs a holistic healing model based on the Medicine Wheel in their counselling programmes. The Medicine Wheel model is described as one of the centre's tools for reaching the goal of mental health counselling, which is to "help Aboriginal and non-Aboriginal clients with serious forms of mental illness by supporting their ability to function in social relations and manage their daily lives" (p. 1). The centre's model embeds practices of "mental health support" and "being in sound mind" through the acknowledgement of the four aspects of each person's personal "will" as depicted by the Medicine Wheel (Dze L K'ant Native Friendship Centre Society, 2006, p. 2). Mussell, Nichols, and Adler (1993) have also created a Medicine Wheel as a working tool for mental health practitioners that depicts the same four components of mental health. Each component is linked to specific needs that individuals must meet in order to achieve balance, or health, in all parts of self, with a person's will in the centre, which represents the power to make decisions and act upon them. The needs of the intellectual aspect of self consist of concepts, ideas, thoughts, habits, and discipline. The needs of the spiritual aspect of self involve a sense of connectedness with others and creations of the Great Spirit. The needs of the emotional aspect include love, discipline, recognition, acceptance, understanding, privacy, and limits, while the physical aspect's needs consist of air, exercise, water, sex, food, clothing, and shelter. The ability of a person to meet these needs is through his or her own personal power, through his or her sense of will.

France and McCormick (1997) also developed a healing circle based on Medicine Wheel teachings; while this model may appear dated in terms of current literature, it is worth exploring and utilizing, as it is seminal and groundbreaking in terms of bringing an Indigenous paradigm into the practice of Western counselling psychology. France and McCormick (1997) call this healing circle a helping circle, and it models a training programme of a peer counselling service for First Nations university students. France and McCormick's First Nations Peer Support Network was created because they saw a need to make counselling services more accessible and culturally appropriate for First Nations students. The programme is based on local Indigenous philosophies and practices and employs several traditional cultural tools, including the Medicine Wheel, along with contemporary counselling approaches.

The purpose of the First Nations Peer Support Network is to provide an informal helping and support service using volunteers from the First Nations community to work with other First Nations people (France & McCormick, 1997): "What we hope will make the support network effective, is to combine both established helping practices with the traditional 'spirit' that makes First Nations people unique" (p. 27). The programme is implemented through a training model that is based on the circle of the Medicine Wheel, which is called the Helping Circle. The students training to become peer supports sit in a circle, which is opened with a prayer or excerpt of Native philosophy. A stone is passed to each person in the circle as a symbol of his or her opportunity to speak and share a personal story. In the Helping Circle, the facilitator should model the target skill and provide the participants an opportunity to practice the skill. "The facilitator may choose to let all of the participants use the skill as a group or allow individuals to volunteer to use the skill" (p. 28). The authors explain that the First Nations helping approach must be based on the four principles as depicted in the Medicine Wheel. In the phases of the training for their programme, the four dimensions of the self are explored. Further, the circle, as a model, embodies a non-linear perspective and represents a cultural view of helping as counselling and teaches this to the students by using the metaphor of the wheel with its emphasis on holism. France and McCormick (1997) write, "Helping generally does not move in a direct 'line.' In this sense, helping is cyclical as compared to a linear line or moving direct from a statement of the issue to a solution" (p. 31).

In contrast to the Indigenous models that are based in the medicine or the circle, most mental health treatments in Canada have been predominately viewed in non-Indigenous ways that disregard ideas such as holistic health and healing. Mental health interventions typically utilize a range of Western-based perspectives from the *Diagnostic and Statistical Manual of Mental Disorders'* (Fifth Edition) pathological model to person-centred therapy, where the focus is on the individual and not on interdependence with others as it would be in an Indigenous model. Duran (2006) writes that much of the Western paradigm of mental health is marked by beliefs in logical positivism, linear thinking, and individualism that promote illness instead of Indigenous wellness: "Western trained therapists are trained to think within a prescribed paradigm that targets pathology" (p. 19).

Future Directions

Future approaches include community-based counselling interventions that are based on cultural models of health and healing. Health and healing from an Indigenous paradigm can better serve Indigenous clients and non-Indigenous clients whose needs are not being met by the current Western system of counselling and psychotherapy. Working in collaborative ways with both Indigenous communities and non-Native communities is one way to begin integrating multiple worldviews and practices. Paying closer attention to the ethics of cross-cultural interactions in counselling and how Western approaches can be used to empower, rather than oppress, Indigenous clients and communities is key.

Conclusion

It is important to have awareness of health problems currently facing Indigenous communities; it is from the point of understanding that the profession of counselling can take a turn to focus not on further explaining these dysfunctions but to instead identifying healing solutions with the counselling context. Culturally based mental health and healing is a major issue for Indigenous peoples in Canada, as there is currently a health crisis in some communities. The reality of high rates of psychological maladjustment, such as alcoholism, suicide, depression, and more, suggests there is a need to look closely at the health and healing resources within communities. Taking a community-based lens and applying it to counselling services is one way to begin this process that honours both Western and Indigenous notions and practices of healing. Working collaboratively with individuals, families, organizations, communities, and nations allows both counsellors and clients to share their healing resources to address the erstwhile unmet needs of both the people and the profession.

References

Aboriginal Healing Foundation. (2002). *The healing has begun: An operational update from the Aboriginal healing foundation*. Ottawa, ON: Aboriginal Healing Foundation.

Absolon, K. (1994). Building health from the medicine wheel: Aboriginal program development. A resource paper for *Native Physicians Association Conference* at Winnipeg.

Alfred, T. (1999). *Peace, power and righteousness: An indigenous manifesto*. Don Mills, ON: Oxford University Press.

Assembly of First Nations. (2002). *Top misconceptions about Aboriginal peoples*. Retrieved from http://www.afn.ca

Bagley, C., Wood, M., & Khumar, H. (1990). Suicide and careless death in young males: Ecological study of an Aboriginal population in Canada. *Canadian Journal of Community Mental Health, 29*, 127–142.

Blue, A. W. (1977). A study of Native elders and student needs. *United States Bureau of Indian Affairs Education and Research Bulletin, 5*, 15–24.

Blue, A. W., & Darou, W. (2005). Counseling First Nations peoples. In N. Arthur, & S. Collins (Eds.), *Culture-infused counselling: Celebrating the Canadian mosaic* (pp. 303–330). Calgary, AB: Counseling Concepts.

Bohn, D. K. (2003). Lifetime physical and sexual abuse, substance abuse, depression, and suicide attempts among Native American Women. *Issues in Mental Health Nursing, 24*, 333–352.Bopp, M., & Lane, P. (2000). *The nuxalk plan*. Lethbridge, AB: Four Worlds International.

Caron, N. R. (2004). Getting to the root of trauma in Canada's Aboriginal population. *Canadian Medical Association Journal, 172*(8), 1023–1024.

Caron, N. R. (2012). Getting to the root of trauma in Canada's Aboriginal population. *Canadian Medical Association Journal, 172*(8), 1023–1024. doi: 10.1503/cmaj.050304.

Chandler, M. J., & Lalonde, C. (1998). Cultural continuity as a hedge against suicide in Canada's First Nations. *Transcultural Psychiatry, 35*, 191–219.

Dickason, O. P. (1997). *Canada's First Nations: A history of founding peoples from earliest times*. Toronto: Oxford University Press.

Duran, E. (2006). *Healing the soul wound*. New York: Teachers College, Columbia University.

Duran, E., & Duran, B. (1995). *Native American postcolonial psychology*. Albany, NY: State University of New York Press.

Dze L K'ant Friendship Centre and Society. (2006). Medicine wheel model for mental health. Retrieved from http://www.bcaafc.com/centres/smithers/Mental.html

Foucault, M. (1971). *The order of things: Archaeology of the human sciences*. New York: Pantheon Books.

Four Directions. (2005). *Native American Indian General Service Office Newsletter, 4*, 2. Retrieved from http://www.naigso-aa.org/index.htm

France, H., & McCormick, R. (1997). Helping circles: Theoretical and practical considerations of a using a first Nations peer support network. *Guidance & Counselling, 12*(2), 27–31.

Gone, J. (2004). Keeping culture in mind. In D. A. Mihesuah, & A. C. Wilson (Eds.), *Indigenizing the academy* (pp. 124–142). Lincoln, NE: University of Nebraska Press.

Government of Canada. (1991). *Agenda for First Nations and Inuit Mental Health*. Retrieved from http://www.hc-sc.gc.ca/fnih spni/pubs/ads/literary_examen_ review/rev_rech_6_e.html

Health Canada. (2003). *Acting on what we know: Preventing youth suicide in First Nations*. Ottawa, ON: Health Canada.

Health Canada. (2006). *Health Promotion: Mental Health Promotion For People With Mental Illness*. Retrieved from http://www.phac-aspc.gc.ca/publicat/mh-sm/mhp02-psm02/1_e.html

Health Canada. (2015). *Mental Health and Wellness—First Nations and Inuit Health*. Retrieved from http://www.hc-sc.gc.ca/fniah-spnia/promotion/mental/index- eng.phpIndigenous and Northern Affairs. (2010). Fact Sheet—Urban Aboriginal Population in Canada. Retrieved from https://www.aadnc aandc.gc.ca/eng/1100100014298/1100100014302

Karmali, S., Laupland, K., Harrop, A. R., Findlay, C., Kirkpatrick, A. W., Winston, B., Kortbeek, J., Crowshoe, L., & Hameed, M. (2005). Epidemiology of severe trauma among status Aboriginal Canadians: A populations-based study. *Canadian Medical Association Journal, 172*(8), 1007–1011.

King, J. (1999). Denver American Indian mental health needs survey. *American Indian and Alaska Native Mental Health Research, 8*(3), 1–12.

Kirmayer, L. J., Brass, G. M., & Tait, C. L. (2000). The mental health of Aboriginal peoples: Transformations of identity and community. *Canadian Journal of Psychiatry, 45*(7), 607–617.

McCormick, R. (1997). Healing through interdependence: The role of connecting in First Nations healing practices. *Canadian Journal of Counselling, 31*(3), 172–184.

McCormick, R. (2000). The relationship of Aboriginal peoples with nature. Paper Presented January 15 at the *National Consultation on Vocational Counseling*, Ottawa, ON.

Menzies, P. (2009). Homeless Aboriginal men: Effects of intergenerational trauma. In Hulchanski, J. David; Campsie, Philippa; Chau, Shirley; Hwang, Stephen; Paradis, Emily (Eds.), *Finding home: Policy options for addressing homelessness in Canada* (e-book), Chapter 6.2. Toronto: Cities Centre, University of Toronto. www.homelesshub.ca/FindingHome.

Mussell, B. (2005). Perceptions of First Nations Males (Part III). In W. J. Mussell (Ed.) *Warrior-caregivers: Understanding the challenges and healing of First Nations men*. Ottawa, ON: Aboriginal Healing Foundation.

Mussell, W. J., Nichols, W. M., & Adler, M. T. (1993). *Meaning making of mental health challenges in First Nations: A freirean perspective*, 2nd ed. Chilliwack, BC: Sal'i'shan Institute Society.

Poushinsky, N., & Tallion-Wasmund, P. (2002). First Nations and mental health. *Foundations for Reform, Section 17*. Champlain District Mental Health Implementation Task Force.

Robbins, J. A., & Dewar, J. (2011). Traditional indigenous approaches to healing in the mordern welfare of traditional knowledge, sprituality and lands: A critical reflection on practices and policies taken from the Canadian indigenous example. *The International Indigenous Policy Journal, 2*(4), 1–17.

Royal Commission on Aboriginal Peoples. (1994). *The high arctic relocation: A report on the 1953–55 relocation*. Ottawa, ON: Minister of Supply and Services.

Smith, L. T. (1999). *Decolonizing methodologies: Research and indigenous peoples*. New York: Zed Books.

Statistics Canada. (2015a). *Aboriginal Peoples: Fact Sheet for Canada*. Retrieved from http://www.statcan.gc.ca/access_acces/alternative_alternatif.action?l=eng&loc=/p ub/89–656-x/89–656-x2015001-eng.pdf

Statistics Canada. (2015b). *Health Report, August 2015. Avoidable Mortality Among First Nations Adults in Canada: A Cohort Analysis*. Retrieved from http://www.statcan.gc.ca/daily-quotidien/150819/dq150819b-eng.pdf

Stewart, S. (2006). Personal Communication with Elise Doctor of Yellowknife Dene First Nation. December, 20, 2006.

Stewart, S. (2009). Sharing narratives on an indigenous academic's evolution: A personal experience of cultural mental health stories as research. *First Peoples Child & Family Review, 4*(1), 57–65.

Storm, H. (1972). *Seven arrows*. New York: Harper and Row.

Sue, D. W., & Sue, D. (1990). *Counseling the culturally different*. New York: John Wiley & Sons.

Tedeschi, R. G., & Calhoun, L. G. (1996). The posttraumatic growth inventory: Measuring the positive legacy of trauma. *Journal of Traumatic Stress, 9*(3), 455–471.

Thunderbird, S. (2005). *Medicine Wheel Teachings*. Retrieved June 15, 2005 from http://www.shannonthunderbird.com/medicine_wheel_teachings.htm

Trimble, J. E., & Thurman, P. (2002). Ethnocultrual considerations and strategies for providing counseling services for Native American Indians. In P. Pedersen, J. Draguns, W. Lonner, & J. Trimble (Eds.), *Counseling across cultures* (5th ed., pp. 53–91). Thousand Oaks, CA: Sage.

Truth and Reconciliation Commission of Canada. (2015). *Honouring the Truth, Reconciling for the Future: Summary of the Final Report of the Truth and Reconciliation Commission of Canada*. Retrieved from www.trc.ca

Vicary, D., & Bishop, B. (2005). Western therapeutic practice: Engaging Aboriginal people in culturally appropriate and respectful ways. *Australian Psychologist, 40*(1), 8–19.

Waldram, J. (2004). *Revenge of the Windigo: The construction of the mind and mental health of North American Aboriginal Peoples*. Toronto, ON: University of Toronto Press.

Waldram, J. B. (2008) *Aboriginal Healing in Canada: Studies in Therapeutic Meaning and Practice*. Ottawa, ON: National Network for Aboriginal Mental Health Research.

Wilson, A. (2004). *Living well: Aboriginal women, cultural identity and wellness*. Winnipeg, MB: Manitoba Aboriginal Women's Health Community Committee.

Young, T. K. (1988). *Health care and cultural change: The Indian experience in the Central Subarctic*. Toronto: University of Toronto Press.

7 Lessons From Clinical Practice

Some of the Ways in Which Canadian Mental Health Professionals Practice Integration

Olga Oulanova and Roy Moodley

There is an emerging trend among individuals of diverse cultural backgrounds residing in North America to seek alternative, complementary, and traditional healing approaches to address their ailments (cf. Moodley, Sutherland, & Oulanova, 2008; Moodley & West, 2005). In the mental health domain, the situation is no different. Members of ethnic minority groups turn to alternative forms of healing as a response to the frequently inappropriate and inadequate mental health services offered to them by mainstream providers. This help-seeking behaviour appears to be motivated in part by a reaction against the pervasiveness of Western biomedicine with its focus on psychopathology and the failure of the Western mental healthcare model to address maladies in a holistic manner (Moodley et al., 2008). Research publications from varied settings confirm this trend, revealing that traditional healing continues to play a vital role in the lives of very diverse populations (cf. Berg, 2003; Dein & Sembhi, 2001; Kurihara, Kato, Reverger, & Rai Tirta, 2006).

Given this tendency to seek out alternative forms of help, it is not surprising that in many North American Aboriginal communities' traditional healing approaches, such as talking circles, drumming, smudging, and Medicine Wheel teachings, continue to subsist (cf. Beals et al., 2006; Gurley et al., 2001; Kim & Kwok, 1998). After all, these healing tools have been in use for hundreds of years and represent potent ways of fostering and restoring wellness for Indigenous peoples (cf. LaFromboise, Trimble, & Mohatt, 1990; McCormick, 1996; Poonwassie & Charter, 2005). However, it is surprising that these traditional forms of healing are often used concurrently with mainstream healthcare services (cf. Oulanova & Moodley, 2010; Waldram, 1993). Indeed, an examination of the literature reveals that both in the Aboriginal communities and in many other ethnic minority communities in North America, more and more people are seeking out the services of traditional healers alongside conventional treatments, thereby engaging in dual interventions (Moodley & West, 2005). In fact, examining the extensive fund of research on Indigenous helping modalities conducted in the domains of mental health, nursing, medicine, and anthropology, it is apparent that this phenomenon is not limited to North America. In many parts of the world, these healing practices currently coexist with Western conventional healthcare services (Hurdle, 2002; Vicary & Bishop, 2005; Waldram, Herring, & Young, 2006). Given the pervasiveness of traditional healing practices and the ability of these approaches to attend to an individual's health needs on numerous levels, multidisciplinary researchers argue that competent mental health services for individuals from diverse ethnic and cultural backgrounds may in fact require some form of integration of these healing modalities or, at a minimum, collaboration with Indigenous healers (cf. Al-Krenawi & Graham, 1999; Constantine, James Myers, Kindaichi, & Moore, 2004; Duran, 1990; Kirmayer, Simpson, & Cargo, 2003; McCormick, 1997; Sima & West, 2005).

An overview of the literature reveals that some clinicians have responded to this call for integration of traditional forms of healing with mainstream services. Indeed, many patients seek out traditional healing interventions at the same time as Western interventions to complement inadequate mainstream healthcare services (Moodley et al., 2008; Moodley & West, 2005). A number of mental health professionals simultaneously resort to both of these helping modalities in their clinical interventions (cf. Heilbron & Guttman, 2000; Oulanova, 2008; Robbins, 2001). This is an intriguing phenomenon given the significant discrepancies between the traditional Indigenous and Western conceptualizations of what constitutes wellness and how healing is believed to occur. Indeed, how does a clinician simultaneously draw on such seemingly different approaches? Which specific elements of traditional healing can be used alongside mainstream interventions? And what is the background and training of mental health professionals who practice such integration? These are some of the questions that we will consider in the present chapter. Although theoretical discussions about integration of traditional healing practices with conventional mental health services are abundant, there is little academic writing that actually documents such efforts. As a result, the present understanding of integration remains theoretical in nature and fails to inform clinical practice in a meaningful way. This chapter aims to address this pressing need to divulge what such integration looks like in clinical practice by exploring the coexistence of traditional Indigenous forms of healing with mainstream healthcare services. However, to establish a foundation for the subsequent discussion of our findings, we will first briefly outline some key differences between these two approaches, particularly focusing on the domain of mental health care.

Aboriginal Traditional Healing and Western Counselling: An Overview of Key Differences

Scholars and clinicians have called attention to some key differences in the core beliefs underlying Aboriginal traditional healing and Western counselling approaches. These discrepancies are most evident in the following domains: the conceptualization of wellness and healing, the place of spirituality, the nature of the therapeutic relationship, and the role of the client's environment. We will next provide a brief overview of each of these.

While in the traditional Aboriginal worldview, health is conceptualized in a holistic manner, wherein the spiritual, physical, emotional, and mental components are regarded as inseparable, in the Western mental health tradition, the focus is often exclusively on the mental and emotional elements (Duran, 1990; France, 1997; Garrett & Carroll, 2000; Ross, 1992). Therefore, an Aboriginal person may seek the help of a healer to address problems in any, or all, of the following domains: spiritual, physical, emotional, and mental. On the contrary, in the West, one commonly obtains services of different helpers for each of these concerns (Morse, Young, & Swartz, 1991). For spiritual issues, one may speak to a priest; for ailments of the body, a physician; for emotional difficulties, a counsellor; and for mental needs, a psychiatrist. This is in stark contrast to the Aboriginal view on health and the outlook on help seeking.

Reflecting this holistic understanding of health, spirituality forms a critical part of overall well-being for Aboriginal peoples (France, 1997; Lewis, Duran, & Woodis, 1999; McCabe, 2007). For example, Aboriginal healing usually involves interactions with the spirit world through healing ceremonies (Morse et al., 1991). These ceremonies are frequently conducted outdoors, thus reinforcing the connection with the natural elements and with the spirit world. In contrast, spirituality appears peripheral to conventional Western mental health care. Consequently, mental healthcare providers are unlikely to explicitly address clients' spiritual concerns in the course of psychotherapy. In mainstream mental health clinics, the treatment is carried out within the boundaries of the institution and without any explicit involvement of the spirit forces.

An additional difference lies in the dynamics of the therapeutic relationship. Traditional Aboriginal healing sessions tend to be didactic in nature, offering the client wisdom that has been accumulated in the community, usually in the form of storytelling (Morse et al., 1991). For example, a traditional healer may share with the client the Medicine Wheel teachings, and in the course of helping, the healer would relate these traditional teachings to the client's presenting concern. In contrast, the role of the Western counsellor or psychotherapist is typically less directive.

Lastly, while Western health care focuses on the individual client, healing in the Aboriginal context emphasizes relatedness by aiming to restore harmony and balance within the spiritual, physical, emotional, and mental aspects of the individual, as well as between the individual and the community (Duran, 1990; Garrett & Carroll, 2000; McCormick, 1996; Poonwassie & Charter, 2005). There is an accent on interdependence and connectedness in the Aboriginal conceptualization of wellness. Therefore, the traditional helping approach is systemic in nature, extending beyond the narrow focus on the individual.

Aboriginal Traditional Healing and Western Counselling: A Call for Integration

Western scholars and clinicians have suggested that given the central place of traditional healing practices in the lives of Indigenous peoples, it may be necessary to incorporate elements of traditional healing when counselling Aboriginal clients (cf. Duran, 1990; Heinrich, Corbine, & Thomas, 1990). As discussed previously, many clients already do this on an individual level by concurrently using Western mental health services and Indigenous healing practices (cf. Beals et al., 2006; Gurley et al., 2001; Kim & Kwok, 1998; Wieman, 2006). However, the earlier discussion of the significant differences between the worldview informing Aboriginal traditional teachings and that underlying Western counselling practice highlights the challenges inherent in mental health professionals engaging in such integrative efforts and drawing on these seemingly distinct approaches to helping. Despite these challenges, a number of Canadian mental health professionals routinely integrate Aboriginal healing practices with counselling interventions (Oulanova & Moodley, 2010). The present chapter will draw on our research inquiry into this phenomenon to explore how integration of Aboriginal and Western approaches to healing is being accomplished in the Canadian context.

Methods

Intrigued by what integration of Aboriginal traditional healing practices and Western counselling interventions may actually look like in clinical practice, we interviewed nine Canadian mental health professionals (psychologists, counsellors, and social workers) who reported routinely integrating these two seemingly distinct helping approaches in their work with clients. Participants resided in Ontario, Saskatchewan, Alberta, and British Columbia and were of diverse backgrounds: three were Ojibwa, one was Ojibwa and Odawa, two were Métis, one was Dene, and two participants were of European descent. Their work settings included private practice, urban Aboriginal health centers, government organizations, a college counselling center, and a regional hospital. Using a semi-structured interview approach, the interviewer (first author) invited participants to speak about their path to practicing integration and to describe their integrative efforts. All interviews were audio-recorded, transcribed, and analyzed for themes in accordance with the Grounded Theory guidelines (Strauss & Corbin, 1990).

Results

A Grounded Theory analysis of the interviews revealed a number of themes that, taken together, depict the integrative process practiced by the participants. Since a detailed description of the emergent themes has been published elsewhere (Oulanova, 2008; Oulanova & Moodley, 2010), we will next offer a brief summary of these themes. This summary will serve as a foundation for the subsequent discussion of the case studies, which are the focus of this chapter.

Our analysis of participants' accounts revealed that the following factors influenced their paths to practicing integration: *ancestors*, *Aboriginal community*, and *mainstream education* (Oulanova & Moodley, 2010). For example, having traditional healers among their ancestors and receiving teachings from community Elders affected participants' own path to practicing in an integrative manner. While the aforementioned factors taught participants skills and particular approaches, all these teachings were filtered through participants' Aboriginal identity, their personal journey, personality characteristics, their perception of calling/destiny to become a healer, and their perception of being an advocate for Aboriginal peoples (Oulanova & Moodley, 2010). In terms of assessing when to incorporate traditional healing into their clinical interventions, participants reported that they use indirect cultural assessment, ask clients directly about their experience with traditional healing, practice from a client-centred orientation, and resort to intuition (Oulanova & Moodley, 2010). Lastly, participants' integrative efforts consist of the following components: incorporating *traditional elements* (e.g., using smudging and drumming with clients), working from a particular *approach* (e.g., employing holistic and culturally based interventions), and *referral and collaboration* (e.g., consulting with and referring to Elders and traditional healers) (Oulanova & Moodley, 2010). Figure 7.1 provides a visual illustration of the influential components on the participants' (referred to as "mental health professional") journeys to practicing integration, as well as portrays the components of participants' actual integrative efforts. The arrows pointing from the three circles toward the "mental health professional" box represent the key aspects of participants' experiences which taught them skills and particular approaches relevant for their clinical work. The arrows leaving the mental health professional box and pointing to the other three circles represent participants' self-described integrative efforts. In reality, these integrative efforts are closely related since one individual often practices all three forms of integration. For example, a mental health professional may approach a client's concern in a holistic manner, refer the client to an Elder during the course of therapy, and conduct part of the therapy outside the constraints of the office.

In this chapter, we will offer three case studies which illustrate how the aforementioned themes manifested in the clinical work of the participants. Although not intended as a comprehensive representation of integrative efforts, our subsequent discussion will thereby serve to demonstrate some of the ways in which integration of Aboriginal and Western approaches to healing take place in the Canadian mental healthcare context. By means of these case studies, we will discuss the following aspects of integration: traditional healing medicines inside the therapy room, naturalistic healing outside the therapy room, and holistic counselling.

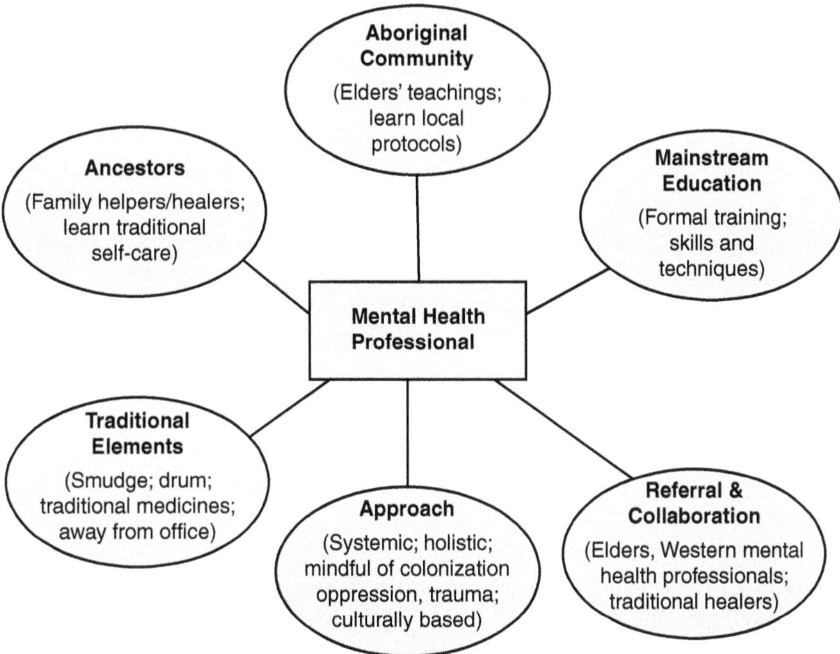

Figure 7.1 This figure illustrates the factors which influenced participants' paths to practicing integration and the components of their integrative efforts.

Traditional Healing Medicines Inside the Therapy Room

Traditional healing medicines are physically present inside the therapy rooms of Canadian mental health professionals who practice integration in a number of ways. For example, some clinicians provide visual access to traditional healing elements in their offices. These healing elements include medicines used to smudge, a shell to burn the medicines in, an eagle feather, and drums. Such visual access enables the client to initiate integration when the client feels the need for an integrative intervention, rather than the therapist instigating such efforts. This visual access to traditional medicines also creates an archetype of a home, thereby representing a form of hospitality. However, once in the therapy room, how are these traditional medicines incorporated into conventional counselling interventions? In other words, how do mental health professionals actually combine these helping modalities in working with clients? These questions are critical in understanding *how* integration of Aboriginal traditional healing practices and counselling interventions take place in clinical practice, and we will explore these issues through the following case study illustration.

Case Study 1: Frank

Frank is a Métis man in his fifties who has been working in the mental health field for over fifteen years. He has practiced in rural and urban communities in the Prairie Provinces in Canada, in settings such as school and university counselling centres as well as in private practice. In terms of formative experiences on his path to becoming a helping professional, he received teachings from an aunt who was a traditional healer. Growing up, his aunt instructed him in healing practices and shared traditional stories. In addition, he obtained direct experience with many Aboriginal healing practices. For example, as an adolescent, he took part in sweat lodge ceremonies held in a remote rural community. Finally, Frank has always been an approachable person, and his personality seemed particularly suited for counselling work: "I sort of fell this way; the wind sort of pushed me this way. But I think, I think the source of the wind was my personality."

In terms of his clinical work, Frank's approach in every session is to ask a lot of questions and thereby inquire about the clients' involvement with Elders and traditional healers, and their views on health and illness and on traditional ways of healing. Such open discussion generates possibilities for including traditional practices in the counselling session: "The answers that will best work for the client can be found within the client. The integration that best suits that client will flow from that dialogue." A crucial element that enables Frank to practice in an integrative manner is that he does not perceive a dichotomy between traditional practices and Western counselling:

> I do not see a real conflict between Western and traditional Aboriginal practices. My understanding is that Aboriginal practices were not practiced as a religion, but that it was a matter of finding what works in any given situation. Both traditions may be described as scientific in a sense.

One of the traditional healing tools that Frank frequently uses in therapy is drumming. Specifically, he has used drumming alongside Eye Movement Desensitization and Reprocessing (EMDR), which is an integrative standardized psychotherapy approach primarily used for the treatment of trauma (Foa, 2000; Levin, Lazrove, & van der Kolk, 1999). He has integrated these two approaches when providing counselling to adolescent clients. He has also used the drum in working with a teenage client who was in a suicidal crisis. In that situation, Frank used the drum to facilitate therapeutic dialogue and enable the client to articulate her experiences:

> She would not talk to me until she started beating the drum, and once she started beating the drum, it loosened her, she was able to talk to me and tell me her deepest feelings while she was beating the drum.

As the case illustration suggests, an important component of Frank's integrative work involves including traditional healing elements such as drumming in his counselling interventions. However, it appears that integration begins even before particular healing tools are explicitly introduced into the session. By openly displaying traditional healing tools, such as a drum, in the office, Frank communicates respect for and belief in the validity of Indigenous approaches to healing. McCormick (2005) offers additional insight into this when he suggests, "one of the roles of therapy for traditional Aboriginal society has been to reaffirm cultural values" (p. 298). Indeed, exhibiting healing tools such as a drum or an eagle feather in the office is one way to validate Aboriginal traditional ways of helping. Kirmayer et al. (2003) further affirm the important role of traditional practices in Aboriginal mental health by explaining that, "Recuperating these traditions [traditional methods of healing] therefore reconnects contemporary Aboriginal peoples to their historical traditions and mobilizes rituals and practices that may promote community solidarity. More broadly, the recovery of tradition itself may be viewed as healing" (p. 16). Displaying Indigenous healing elements in the office setting and incorporating them into clinical interventions communicates to clients that traditional ways of healing are valid and important approaches to helping. This in itself seems to represent a significant component of the healing process.

Naturalistic Healing Outside the Therapy Room

Some healing work carried out by Canadian mental health professionals who practice integration takes place outside of the therapy room constraints. In contrast to the conventional Western approach to counselling, wherein the therapy session is usually limited to the office, these clinicians take clients out on the land or to the water. This approach is congruent with our previous discussion of the differences between the core beliefs underlying mainstream Western and Aboriginal traditional approaches pertaining to conceptualization of wellness and how healing takes place. Indeed, in the traditional Indigenous view, connection to the land and one's physical environment constitutes an important part of the healing process. The following case study illustrates how some Canadian mental health professionals navigate such holistic and naturalistic healing outside of the therapy room.

Case Study 2: Amelia

Amelia is an Ojibwa woman in her early thirties who has been working in the mental health field for five years. She has provided mental health services in a range of settings, including a large urban centre and a remote rural community in British Columbia. Her clinical experiences included working in the addictions field, counselling residential school survivors, and working in private practice where she sees both Aboriginal and non-Aboriginal clients for a variety of concerns.

Amelia grew up with Aboriginal healing traditions actively practiced in her family. For example, her father was very knowledgeable about traditional herbal remedies, and her mother shared with Amelia traditional women's teachings of her community. In addition to her parents passing on traditional teachings to her since a young age, she attended a community band school where Aboriginal teachings were integrated with the Western mainstream curriculum. As a result of her upbringing and early education, Amelia acquired knowledge about elements of traditional healing such as how to use medicines, traditional protocols for sacred ceremonies, and an understanding of traditional women's teachings. In her clinical work, Amelia draws on her knowledge of and experience with traditional healing practices to offer her clients the possibility of integrative interventions. Such interventions commonly involve conducting part of the session outside of the constraints of the therapy office. For example, Amelia may talk to a client about ways to take care of him or herself that involve using nature for grounding. At times, she may actually accompany a client in this process:

> So sometimes the clients ask to be taken down to the river, or if I see that it would be really appropriate because I know enough about this person. If they are river people, let's say, we can go down there towards the end of the session. If they had a huge release, and I want to do some grounding with them.

In this way, Amelia conducts part of some therapy sessions outdoors, assisting clients to use the natural environment, such as the river, as a healing tool.

Our conversations with other mental health professionals practicing integration revealed that Amelia's approach is certainly not unique. Several participants stated that they conduct sessions outdoors, recognizing the therapeutic potential of connecting with the land or the water. A number of scholars have written on the subject, highlighting the important role that the physical environment plays in the well-being of Aboriginal peoples (McCormick, 2005; Zapf, 2005). For example, Zapf (2005) explains that inherent in Aboriginal traditional healing practices is a close connection with the land, which in turn represents "a source of energy and knowledge" (p. 638). In his research, McCormick (2005) found that nature characterized "a large part of what facilitates healing for Aboriginal people" in terms of "being in or with nature and using the natural world for self-healing" (p. 295). Participants' accounts resonate scholarly writing in this domain in conveying that being present with the client outside of the office constraints can facilitate healing in important ways.

Holistic Counselling

Canadian mental health professionals who practice in an integrative manner emphasize that an important component of their work consists of attending to clients' concerns in a holistic and systemic manner. This entails specifically addressing spiritual, physical, mental, and emotional elements of the individual, while taking into account the influences of the client's family and community. We will explore what this multidimensional approach to healing looks like through the next case illustration.

Case Study 3: Alex

Alex is a man of Ojibwa and Odawa heritage who had worked as an artist for a number of years prior to deciding to pursue a career in the mental health field. He is in his fifties and has been employed as a counsellor in an Aboriginal social service agency in a large urban centre for seven years.

Alex was raised in a small Aboriginal community in Ontario. He grew up in a "traditional way," with ceremonies such as smudging routinely practiced in his family. In terms of his path to becoming a professional helper, Alex obtained a degree in mental health and thereby received specific training in counselling interventions. In addition, Alex largely draws on his family teachings, as well as the traditional knowledge that he had acquired while apprenticing with an Aboriginal Elder. He apprenticed with this Elder for one year, during which time his tasks included tending to the fire for sweat lodge ceremonies, as well as learning about and picking traditional herbal medicines.

Alex routinely draws on the teachings of the Medicine Wheel, works from a circular approach, and ensures that he attends to the physical, spiritual, emotional, and mental needs of his clients. For example, if a client comes in and states that he has nowhere to live, Alex begins by addressing the physical needs (e.g., asking questions such as "Are you eating well? Are you taking care of your body?"). Once they have explored the physical component of the client's concerns, Alex moves into the next segment of the Medicine Wheel and invites the client to explore his or her spiritual needs. He proceeds in this manner until the circle is completed and they had discussed all the dimensions. As part of his interventions, Alex often shares with clients his understanding of the Medicine Wheel teachings and relates these traditional teachings to the client's presenting concerns. As a helper, he believes that he is required to attend to all of these components in order to assist the client to attain "balance." Alex's approach entails using the Medicine Wheel teachings in an explicit way with clients (i.e., providing specific teachings related to the Medicine Wheel), as well as allowing the Medicine Wheel and the holistic outlook inherent in its teachings to inform the way that he approaches the client's concern in each session.

As the case illustration suggests, some individuals integrate traditional practices into their work in less explicit ways than using traditional medicines in the session, or conducting therapy outside the constraints of the office. For some, integration signifies counselling Aboriginal clients from a particular culturally based approach, such as drawing on a systemic and holistic outlook. Scholars and clinicians offering recommendations for service providers who work with Indigenous clients (cf. Canales, 2004; Mitchell & Maracle, 2005; Poonwassie & Charter, 2005) have indeed endorsed such an approach with this client group. A holistic understanding of the person is an essential feature of the Aboriginal traditional worldview, and an attendance to all four dimensions of one's well-being therefore permeates Indigenous traditional ways of healing (Canales, 2004; Ross, 1992).

Conclusion

Drawing on illustrative case examples of three Canadian mental health professionals who integrate Aboriginal and Western approaches to healing in their clinical work, we explored how integration of these helping modalities is being accomplished in clinical practice. Although the present chapter began with an overview of significant discrepancies between the core beliefs underlying Aboriginal traditional healing and Western counselling approaches, our research with mental health professionals who draw on both of these helping modalities suggests that such integration is indeed feasible. Similarly to some clients who engage in dual interventions by accessing the services of traditional healers concurrently with mainstream mental health interventions, the interviewed clinicians draw on both of these helping modalities in their clinical practice. As the case illustrations imply, mental health professionals who are grounded in the Western mainstream mental healthcare model, as well as in the Aboriginal traditional conceptualization of health and wellness appear to skilfully navigate these two helping modalities. Importantly, the three case studies illustrate that mental health professionals arrived at working in an integrative manner as a result of a number of influences, such as receiving traditional teachings from their communities and growing up in an environment where traditional healing was routinely practiced. Therefore, it is not advisable for a mental health worker practicing exclusively from a mainstream orientation to incorporate elements of Indigenous practices. In cases where a client's involvement in traditional practices appears beneficial and the client expresses interest, it is best to refer the client to a professional who routinely practices integration.

References

Al-Krenawi, A., & Graham, J. R. (1999). Gender and biomedical/traditional mental health utilization among the Bedouin-Arabs of the Negev. *Culture, Medicine, and Psychiatry, 23*, 219–243.

Beals, J., Novins, D. K., Spicer, P., Whitesell, N. R., Mitchell, C. M., Manson, S. M., & the American Indian Service Utilization, Psychiatric Epidemiology, Risk, and Protective Factors Project Team. (2006). Help seeking for substance use problems in two American Indian reservation populations. *Psychiatric Services, 57*(4), 512–520.

Berg, A. (2003). Ancestor reverence and mental health in South Africa. *Transcultural Psychiatry, 40*(2), 194–207.

Canales, M. K. (2004). Taking care of self: Healthcare decision making of American Indian women. *Healthcare for Women International, 25*, 411–435.

Constantine, M. G., James Myers, L., Kindaichi, M., & Moore, J. L. (2004). Exploring indigenous mental health practices: The roles of healers and helpers in promoting well-being in people of color. *Counseling and Values, 48*, 110–125.

Dein, S., & Sembhi, S. (2001). The use of traditional healing in South Asian psychiatric patients in the U.K.: Interactions between professional and folk psychiatries. *Transcultural Psychiatry, 38*(2), 243–257.

Duran, E. (1990). *Transforming the soul wound*. Delhi, India: Arya Offset Press.

Foa, E. B. (2000). Psychosocial treatment of posttraumatic stress disorder. *Journal of Clinical Psychiatry, 61*(supplement 5), 43–48.

France, M. H. (1997). First Nations: Helping and learning in the Aboriginal community. *Guidance and Counseling, 12*, 3–8.Garrett, M. T., & Carroll, J. J. (2000).

Mending the broken circle: Treatment of substance dependence among Native Americans. *Journal of Counselling & Development, 78*(4), 379–388.

Gurley, D., Novins, D. K., Jones, M. C., Beals, J., Shore, J. H., & Manson, S. M. (2001). Comparative use of biomedical services and traditional healing options by American Indian veterans. *Psychiatric Services, 52*(1), 68–74.

Heilbron, C. L., & Guttman, M. A. J. (2000). Traditional healing methods with First Nations women in group counselling. *Canadian Journal of Counselling. Special Issue: Counselling First Nations People in Canada, 34*(1), 3–13.

Heinrich, R. K., Corbine, J. L., & Thomas, K. R. (1990). Counseling Native Americans. *Journal of Counseling and Development, 69*(2), 128–133.

Hurdle, D. E. (2002). Native hawaiian traditional healing: Culturally based interventions for social work practice. *Social Work, 47*(2), 183–192.

Kim, C., & Kwok, Y. S. (1998). Navajo use of Native healers. *Archives of Internal Medicine, 158*(9), 2245–2249.

Kirmayer, L., Simpson, C., & Cargo, M. (2003). Healing traditions: Culture, community and mental health promotion with Canadian Aboriginal peoples. *Australasian Psychiatry, 11*(Supplement), 15–23.

Kurihara, T., Kato, M., Reverger, R., & Rai Tirta, I. G. (2006). Pathway to psychiatric care in Bali. *Psychiatry and Clinical Neurosciences, 60*, 204–210.

LaFromboise, T. D., Trimble, J. E., & Mohatt, G. V. (1990). Counseling intervention and American Indian tradition: An integrative approach. *Counseling Psychologist, 18*(4), 628–654.

Levin, P., Lazrove, S., & van der Kolk, B. (1999). What psychological testing and neuroimaging tell us about the treatment of posttraumatic stress disorder by eye movement desensitization and reprocessing. *Journal of Anxiety Disorders, 13*(1–2), 159–172.

Lewis, E. W., Duran, E., & Woodis, W. (1999). Psychotherapy in the American Indian population. *Psychiatric Annals, 29*(8), 477–479.

McCabe, G. H. (2007). The healing path: A culture and community-derived indigenous therapy model. *Psychotherapy: Theory, Research, Practice, Training, 44*(2), 148–160.

McCormick, R. (1996). Culturally appropriate means and ends of counselling as described by the First Nations people of British Columbia. *International Journal for the Advancement of Counselling, 18*, 163–172.

McCormick, R. (1997). An integration of healing wisdom: The vision quest ceremony from an attachment theory perspective. *Guidance and Counseling, 12*, 18–21.

McCormick, R. (2005). The healing path: What can counsellors learn from Aboriginal people about how to heal? In R. Moodley, & W. West (Eds.), *Integrating traditional healing practices into counseling and psychotherapy* (pp. 293–304). Thousand Oaks, CA: Sage.

Mitchell, T. L., & Maracle, D. T. (2005). Healing the generations: Post-traumatic stress and the health status of Aboriginal populations in Canada. *Journal of Aboriginal Health, 2*(1), 14–23.

Moodley, R., Sutherland, P., & Oulanova, O. (2008). Traditional healing, the body and mind in psychotherapy. *Counselling Psychology Quarterly, 21*(2), 1–13.

Moodley, R., & West, W. (Eds.) (2005). *Integrating traditional healing practices into counselling and psychotherapy*. Thousand Oaks, CA: Sage.

Morse, J. M., Young, D. E., & Swartz, L. (1991). Cree Indian healing practices and Western healthcare: A comparative analysis. *Social Science and Medicine, 32*(12), 1361–1366.

Oulanova, O. (2008). *Navigating two worlds: Experiences of Canadian mental health professionals who integrate Aboriginal traditional healing practices*. Master's Thesis: University of Toronto, Toronto.

Oulanova, O., & Moodley, R. (2010). Navigating two worlds: Experiences of counsellors who integrate Aboriginal traditional healing practices. *Canadian Journal of Counselling and Psychotherapy, 44*(4), 346–362.

Poonwassie, A., & Charter, A. (2005). Aboriginal worldview of healing: Inclusion, blending, and bridging. In R. Moodley, & W. West (Eds.), *Integrating traditional healing practices into counseling and psychotherapy* (pp. 15–25). Thousand Oaks, CA: Sage.

Robbins, R. (2001). The dream catcher meditation: A therapeutic technique used with American Indian adolescents. *American Indian and Alaska Native Mental Health Research, 10*(1), 51–65.

Ross, R. (1992). *Dancing with a ghost: Exploring Indian reality*. Markham, ON: Octopus Publishing Group.

Sima, R. G., & West, W. (2005). Sharing healing secrets: Counsellors and traditional healers in conversation. In R. Moodley, & W. West (Eds.), *Integrating traditional healing practices into counselling and psychotherapy* (pp. 316–325). Thousand Oaks, CA: Sage.

Strauss, A. L., & Corbin, J. (1990). *Basics of qualitative research: Grounded theory procedures and techniques*. Newbury Park, CA: Sage.

Vicary, D. A., & Bishop, B. J. (2005). Western psychotherapeutic practice: Engaging Aboriginal people in culturally appropriate and respectful ways. *Australian Psychologist, 40*(1), 8–19.

Waldram, J. B. (1993). Aboriginal spirituality: Symbolic healing in Canadian prisons. *Culture, Medicine, and Psychiatry, 17*, 345–362.

Waldram, J. B., Herring, D. A., & Young, T. K. (2006). *Aboriginal health in Canada: Historical, cultural, and epidemiological perspectives*, 2nd ed. Toronto, ON: University of Toronto Press.

Wieman, C. (2006). Western medicine meets traditional healing: The experience of Six Nations Mental Health Services. *Crosscurrents: The Journal of Addiction and Mental Health, 10*(1), 10–11.

Zapf, M. K. (2005). The spiritual dimension of person and environment. *International Social Work, 48*(5), 633–642.

Part 3

West

Trauma and Contemporary Indigenous Healing

8 Injury Where Blood Does Not Flow

Eduardo Duran and Judith Firehammer

Trauma and how it is perceived in some of the traditional Native worldview has some fundamental differences. As the title of this chapter illustrates, there is a different root metaphor to how injury where blood does not flow is understood and it is to some of those differences that the authors hope to expand upon. The intent of this discussion is to deal with the treatment of psychological trauma, soul wounding, spirit injury, and heart sickness from a non-Euro-American–centric understanding as much as language limitations allow. In this manner, the authors hope to allow the reader to experience a different understanding of root metaphors and to some extent a different life-world. Short comparisons between Western and Indigenous approaches to understanding injuries where blood does not flow will serve as an avenue of comparison between the life-worlds.

It is important to understand that trauma can impact the personal as well as the collective relationship to the life-world, especially when the purpose of systemic trauma is designed to destroy that life-world. Effects of trauma as manifested in internalized violence/oppression symptoms will be analyzed from the historical perspective of the "Indian agent," who continues to be a psychological factor in the daily violence and internalized oppression of many Native communities. Warrior psychology will also receive a new yet ancient discussion because the authors believe that in order to truly understand the underlying psycho-spiritual factors that interact in historical trauma and effects, we must go to the source of the trauma. The source of the trauma is the ceremony of war, and because war is a ceremony, we must adhere to ceremonial metaphor in the treatment of trauma. Dealing with "warrior injury where blood does not flow" through a different cultural lens will hopefully facilitate further understanding on the part of the reader. Final thoughts on research and clinical methodology will be offered at the end of the discussion in order to bring awareness to principles of cultural competency.

Much of what we do in the field of psychotherapy is done from a very individualistic way of understanding the life-world. Not only is our work individualistic, it is also separated from the natural world, thus allowing our psychology to objectify people and problems they present within the realm of psychotherapy. In a pre-Cartesian life-world, this objectification of the life-world would not have been possible. In reality, there are cultures in the world today that have yet to buy into the notion that there are dualities between themselves and the life-world. It is this lack of epistemological duality that presents many Western researchers and clinicians with difficulty. The problems that face clinicians and researchers usually have an adverse effect on the person and/or community needing help in healing the effects of historical trauma.

Therefore, in order to deal with trauma from a culturally responsive perspective that is clearly different from a Western one, it becomes necessary to discuss that approach by utilizing metaphoric language that can transcend our notions of how everyone may fit into a Western mindset. Unfortunately, our field has failed extensively in the area of understanding how cultures other than the Euro-American one perceive disease models and the treatment of different illnesses, although progress has been made in the recent past. One major problem standing in the way of progress in the area of cultural competency/responsiveness is that most cultural competency has to be validated by a Western empiricist method that may be totally foreign to the people and community that we are attempting to address either through research or clinical practice. A fundamental question that can be asked is: are we trying to help people from different cultures or are we trying to acculturate and assimilate them into the Euro-American way of being in the life-world? Evidence from the research world offers more than a clue, and it is unfortunate that acculturation and assimilation still play a role in clinical practice and research (Duran, 2006).

Comparison of Native and Western Approaches

It may be of some utility to make some comparison of cultural models. It is important to differentiate between therapies that are ceremonial and those which are not if we are to gain root understanding of competency required to work with cultural groups who do not subscribe to Western forms of thought. It must also be understood that all forms of healing can have commonality if the healer is open to searching for the root metaphor and, in this manner, become more effective regardless of his or her theoretical orientation.

Some of the work that has been done in the area of trauma treatment has Freudian theory as its fundamental lineage and emotional problems caused by trauma are the focus of treatment (Horowitz et al., 1997). The idea that trauma causes fixation and that it may produce some sort of neurosis is well known, and this theory has validity in present-day treatment settings. Classic trauma theory can be useful in cross-cultural settings if the metaphor is shifted to one that makes sense to the community in which it is being used.

In Native American healing circles, trauma theory is thought of in a way that has spiritual meaning. For example, the practitioner does not tell the patient that s/he is fixated on an oedipal issue, and s/he needs to have several years of analysis to overcome the neurotic symptoms. Instead, the practitioner may say that there has been a spiritual intrusion at a certain point of the patient's life, and the appropriate balancing ceremony needs to occur. There are many different ceremonies across the vast number of tribes in the United States. Ceremonies have tribal-specific interventions that make sense to the worldview of the patient. Currently in Indian country, there are also pan-Indian ceremonies that incorporate different ceremonial metaphors from different tribes that have great utility in urban areas where most of the Native people in this country live. It is within this understanding of the cosmological universe that the patient is transported across time in order to "resolve," heal, exorcise, and harmonize the injury that occurred where blood does not flow. A key difference between the tribal and psychoanalytic model is that of time and intensity. In classic psychoanalysis, the journey may take years. On the other hand, the journey within tribal ceremony takes less time and is more dependent on spiritual intensity within a ritualistic paradigm.

One of the most popular therapies utilized presently for trauma and almost every possible diagnostic category is cognitive behavioural therapy. This form of therapy has risen to the top of therapist's armamentarium in large part because of the acceptance of the empirical science supporting the treatment model, which in turn makes this model one which is paid for by American insurance companies. One of the key components of the theory is that difficulties are caused by thoughts that have become distorted and makes the person feel symptoms of anxiety, depression, or anger (Beck, 1995). Cognitive behavioural therapy attempts to change cognitions that may be interfering with the person's life, and by changing the thoughts, the symptoms are alleviated (Meichenbaum, 1977, 1997).

Interestingly enough, traditional Native healers also utilize changing of thoughts as an intervention. There is a traditional Native teaching that integrates thinking good thoughts, and this is used as a general intervention in individuals and communities and can be categorized as an inoculation against the mind becoming stressed. If the person is thinking good thoughts, then these will counter negative thoughts and emotions and replace them with positive ones. It is apparent that cognitive behavioural techniques are part of Native healing. One of the key differences between the Western-based treatment and the Native method is that in the Native-based approach, the whole community participates and the technique is only a part of a larger life-changing intervention that will be discussed later.

Another widely used Western method is Eye Movement Desensitization Reprocessing (EMDR). This method, developed by Shapiro (1989), attempts to desensitize traumatic memories through eye movements. EMDR has been effective in the short term but therapeutic gains are not maintained over a six-month period (Devilly, Spence, & Rapee, 1998). In Native traditional healing, there are similar techniques that are used by healers. Patients are fanned with feathers from eagles or other birds considered sacred in patterns that may appear to be similar to EMDR. The rationale for the technique is different from the rationale for EMDR since it is theorized in the Native setting that spiritual energy is being harmonized in a manner that will neutralize the negative effects of trauma on the patient. The fanning along with the smoke that is used forms a therapeutic environment for the patient in which they are encompassed by a sacred container. Within this container, the patient can experience the trauma and then be able to establish a different relationship with the different spirit energies that continue to give the patient symptoms as well as with the spirit of the trauma itself.

In the aforementioned comparative examples, it is apparent that there are similarities in the techniques. The underlying theory or rationale for the techniques is different when comparing the Western and Native traditional approaches, and the differences emerge from long-established cultural root metaphors. These cultural root metaphors guide and dictate how the life-world of the culture impacts all the cognitions, behaviours, and general life of the person in that particular culture. Therefore, just providing technique-based interventions without the subjective understanding of the life-world of the patient and community will decrease the effectiveness of the intervention and at times cause more problems to the community because of the loss of faith in Western-based empirically validated interventions (also known as best practices).

Implications of Historical Trauma

If we are to make significant gains in the area of cultural competency, it is critical that we begin to embrace a philosophy of epistemological hybridity (Duran, Firehammer, & Gonzalez, 2008). The type of hybridity that is needed is one in which we as a discipline become empowered in a manner in which we are able to let go of paternalistic mindsets that keep us mired in outdated paradigms and therapeutic fundamentalisms. An example of the paternalistic mindset is when we refuse to integrate any form of treatment that has not been approved by Western empirical methods rooted in logical positivism. Many of the present "culturally approved" therapies fall within the positivistic paradigm and continue to alienate people in Native communities.

Two cultural metaphors that need to be explored in order to bring added cultural understanding and bridging are healing and curing. Within Native therapeutic theory, there is the notion that suffering may be an important ingredient in the process of life development (Duran et al., 2008). On the other hand, especially in the American cultural context, people are expected to attack their illnesses and be rid of them quickly without questioning what the illness or discomfort may be trying to teach them as far as their life's developmental journey. Western medical models are philosophically rooted in adverse reactions to presenting problems, i.e., get rid of the illness or problem facing the individual or community (cure the problem). In traditional Indigenous worldviews, the person with the issues is taught to bring harmony through relationship to the problem or sickness.

This understanding of suffering includes traumatic events. Within Native traditional healing, it is not enough to be rid of the symptoms that are present because of trauma. A key component to healing is a deep understanding of why the trauma may have occurred and what type of life lesson is embedded in the suffering and the event itself. In Western therapeutic circles, the task is to be rid of symptoms either by using some of the mentioned therapy methods, or by medicating the symptoms away through pharmacological or illicit drug use. In such cases, there may be a therapy that has empirical validity, as far as effectiveness, but these interventions may fall short of bringing the balance and harmony to the life of a Native American person who is seeking existential understanding more than relief of symptoms.

Another root epistemological belief system is the Native philosophy that we do not exist separately. This belief system has direct implications to the understanding of trauma and the treatment aspect of trauma. Many of the tribes in the United States and in other parts of the world have a deep understanding of what is known as the collective soul wound and has recently become better known as intergenerational or historical trauma (Duran, 2006). In essence, historical trauma is a collective trauma that has been suffered by a group of people because of historical events that were destructive to the physical, spiritual, and psychological life-world (Danieli, 1998). Some of the collective health problems in Indian country can be attributed directly to the collective traumatic historical events that led to the trauma (Duran, 2006).

Interestingly enough, researchers have collected empirical data that sheds new light on historical trauma. The research serves as a form of validation to a reality that the Native community has known for decades. This type of research can be very useful to Native communities because the research can start paving the way to bring in the type of help needed instead of systemic interventions based on medically diagnosed symptoms alone. The research indicates that a high prevalence of historical trauma is routinely manifested in ways that undermine the collective health of communities in Indian country (Whitbeck, Adams, Hoyt, & Chen, 2004).

Recently, Native communities have begun to deal with the effects of collective trauma by developing collective community healing ceremonies. Whole tribal communities are invited to these collective healings, and the collective history is revisited. One of the profound results of these community therapeutic interventions is that individuals as well as the communities realize that the problems are not inherent to the culture. Instead, the problems facing the community have a socio-historical component that must become part of the therapeutic process if the community is to move forward in a healthy way. The community therapy involves the creation of a community genogram that follows the history of the tribe back to creation and all of the traumatic events are listed in the genogram. Therefore, the community becomes aware of the trauma that may have occurred three hundred years ago and how this may be impacting the community and individuals at the present time.

After the community collective genogram becomes part of the community awareness, members of the community will stand in front of the community and bear witness to the trauma that they have specific knowledge about. This becomes especially intense if there are people in the "community healing" event who may be descendants of the perpetrators of the trauma. As part of the process, there is a ceremony of forgiveness and reconciliation, which is healing to both the injured and those who caused the historical injury. Ceremonies are being developed to deal with these situations across communities and tribes in order to have the healing needed from collective trauma.

Once the community healing ceremony is completed, there must be opportunity for individual healing, addressing problems and symptoms associated with individual trauma. These therapies must be done with the mindset that socio-historical factors are crucial to the trauma as well as the healing. The individual needs to understand that some or all of the individual trauma may also be directly linked to the collective traumatic events. For example, there are instances where people seek help for violent behaviour. It is critical to take the patient through their history and explore where and how the violence was first experienced as a collective historical event. By taking the patient through this socio-historical journey, the patient is able to objectify the violence and not identify with it. Much of the time in therapeutic circles, Native patients are diagnosed as violent and left with the impression that this is who they are as defective Native people. Even though the therapy may have passed the test of evidence-based treatment, it is obvious that the therapy can ironically serve to pathologize Native patients and ensure that Native patients continue to blame themselves and perpetuate a cycle of dysfunctional living and suffering (Duran, 2006).

There is a critical spiritual root metaphor that must be addressed in the actual defining of trauma from a non-Western cosmology. Most Western approaches view trauma as an event that harms the person physically, and this carries over into the psychological realm. There are also instances where the trauma is purely psychological and proceeds to bring symptoms to the person who suffered the trauma. In Native psychology and cosmological life-world, there is an additional component to the physical and psychological, namely, the spiritual aspect of life. In addition to believing that there is a spiritual component, it is believed that no trauma or injury can occur without it having an impact on the spiritual aspect of the personality. The fact that there is a spiritual injury in the trauma episode moves the discussion into the realm of spirits and sorcery. Spirits and sorcery are more than metaphors for most Native people who still live in a traditional life-world. Spirits and sorcery are real entities or psychological energies/complexes that influence the lives and environment of all beings.

Sorcery is a word that does not get much attention in our discipline, and this fact is one of the challenges in working with Native people and other groups who subscribe to a more spiritual understanding of the world. Simply applying the language of psychology to a worldview that understands trauma from a different standpoint can only add to the trauma via the therapeutic intervention. If the therapist is not willing to shift his/her metaphoric view of the world towards that of the patient, then the therapy will not be as effective as it would be if the worldview of the patient is the center of the treatment process. Simple logic dictates that the trauma is compounded when the patient is not understood in his or her psychological life-world, and the ability to heal is greatly impaired (Duran, 2006). Professionals who choose not to change their view of the world when working with Native people are part of ongoing neocolonialism, and their work has been characterized as clinical racism (Duran, 2006). This type of activity by professionals continues to add to the existing historical trauma that impacts the lives of Native people.

Even though the logic of perpetrating the trauma circle via therapeutic intervention is obvious, it occurs on an ongoing basis in health settings in Indian country. Most therapists working in Native communities (which have belief systems that are not congruent with the Euro-American psychological community) get all of their training from institutions that are not cognizant of how the Native psyche experiences psychological injuries where blood does not flow. If a person or community is experiencing several generations of historical trauma, then the lack of understanding from the treatment professional will only add to the historical trauma and solidify the feelings of alienation and lack of identity on the part of the patient. Alienation is part of the dynamics of not having a voice for your experience of the world and being told that what you believe is not valid—this is traumatic and causes injury where blood does not flow.

When the identity of the patient is attacked via the treatment process, there is further depersonalization and therefore makes it that much more difficult to make a therapeutic alliance, which is the *sine que non* of the healing endeavour. If the personality of the patient is split by the violence and trauma imparted by the lack of understanding of the therapist, the already split ego becomes even more fragile, and the patient will more than likely drop out of treatment and seek self-medication in search of some form of relief. In reality, this may bring about a demise of the person and traumatize the community with new hopelessness by reinforcing the belief that things can only continue with no relief in sight.

Oppression resulting from violence is a factor that impacts how a person and/or community reacts to trauma. Historical trauma is an ongoing process that manifests as internalized violence and oppression in Native and other communities as the effects of the trauma are internalized. The fact that people and communities live in an ongoing traumatic/oppressive life-world has brought on a process of desensitizing that allows the person to at times become unaware of smaller trauma and only react to the more dramatic and devastating traumatic events. Because of the process of desensitizing the community/individual, it becomes very difficult to develop strategies that would address the ongoing daily healing from historical and other cumulative traumas. Essentially, the community/individual is in a situation in which most interventions are of a crises management nature.

The long-term effect of living in "crisis mode" is that it keeps us from being able to create a more meaningful life-world and quality of life. Many of the chronic symptoms experienced at such high levels in Indian country can be attributed to the ongoing trauma of oppression as well as the historical aspect of trauma (Duran, 2006). It is important to understand that oppression can have two sources—one is from the historical oppressor and the other source is the internalized oppression. Much of the oppression in Indian country is of the second type, where Native people have taken on the values of the oppressor, and the oppression is passed on to individuals and communities in a cyclical fashion that perpetuates a destructive psychology in the life-world (Duran, 2006).

Archetypal and Spiritual Understanding of Trauma

After working with many patients who had been traumatized and soul wounded, it became apparent that there are other factors or forces that need to be addressed in understanding trauma. Patients we have seen had been involved in medical and/or psychotherapy, and in many cases, the patients continue to suffer from symptoms related to soul wounding. Most trauma treatment strategies focus on the physical and psychological processes, and many of the patients that we have worked with do not get better.

When seeing that many patients were not getting better from the symptoms that cause so much suffering, a simple question needed to be asked: could there be something else causing the ongoing symptoms? After some reflection and going over some of the teachings that were passed on to us from Elders, we realized that there is a spiritual component in trauma that must be addressed if the patient is to find relief from his or her suffering. The following archetypal theory has emerged out of the teachings:

1. When a perpetrator of trauma has intent to do harm, the intent has both a psychological and spiritual aspect to it. The actual violence is carried out on the body and/or mind as the perpetrator targets the victim.
2. The physical damage to the body is dealt with immediately by body mechanisms as they begin the healing process through blood clotting, bruising, and other biological processes. The psychological damage can be dealt with through psychotherapy.
3. As the violence is enacted, the spirit of the perpetrator is literally projected into the victim in a manner that is best understood as a spiritual

act or as sorcery. What led us to this understanding is the fact that many people who are victims suffer from guilt. The guilt experienced by the victim is not rational, and cultural understanding and analysis suggests that the guilt felt by the victim is the projected energy from the perpetrator. Victims and most humans have an aspect of their psychology that can be categorized as introverted or extroverted. Violent energy that has been introjected by the victim will eventually give symptoms that will manifest in a manner consistent with the psychology of the person.

4. Introverted people will internalize the violent energy that has been projected into them by the perpetrator. The violent energy/spirit of the perpetrator will begin to develop a life of its own in the unconscious of the person and will also begin to manifest through symptoms of depression, anxiety, and other discomforts. These symptoms are to bring attention to the underlying psychological problem. These discomforts are messages to the person that healing needs to occur at a deep spiritual level. Unfortunately, most victims do not realize that the symptoms are an attempt to move them towards healing, and instead they begin to make efforts to get rid of the internalized violent energy. The ego that does not understand the situation attempts to get rid of symptoms by getting rid of the perpetrator that mostly remains unconscious. Therefore, the introvert attempts to literally get rid of the projected perpetrator by unconsciously killing the perpetrator. Unfortunately, attempts at killing the perpetrator are misdirected, and instead the death of the victim is attempted through self-destructive behaviours such as addiction, physical illness, and suicide. All self-destructive behaviours are a form of suicide which in reality is an unconscious effort at killing the spirit energy of the perpetrator that has been projected into them. In treatment, the person must be alerted to the reality that is occurring in their unconscious in order for them to be able to address the situation in accordance to Native traditional teachings and healing processes.
5. Extroverted people also attempt to deal with the internalized perpetrator by projecting their symptoms. In this case, the person may also resort to addictions and other maladaptive behaviours. The difference with extroverts is that in an attempt to kill the perpetrator, their violence turns outward, and they become perpetrators of violence towards their loved ones and other community members. When the extrovert commits violence, that violence is an attempt to destroy the internalized perpetrator as seen through the projection of the person's unconscious processes. In other words, killing a relative is the equivalent of killing the internalized perpetrator. The problem with both the introverted and extroverted attempts at killing the internalized perpetrator is that the original spirit energy projected into them continues to live and develop within their psyches/spirits.

Internalized Indian Agent

Many of our communities presently suffer from violence and oppression that is perpetrated by people who are in authority or in power in various governing, health, and tribal agencies. It has become apparent to these authors that many of the behaviours that continue to traumatize some of the people working in agencies designed to help and assist our communities have a pattern that can be recognized in history. It is well known that many of the tribes became wards of the government and were subjected to oppressive treatment at the hands of the man placed in charge of the tribe—the Indian agent.

The Indian agent (civilian appointed to take over the military's role in controlling Native people) literally controlled the day-to-day life-world of Native people and had at their right hand the army as an enforcer of policy. Control of the life-world was quickly gained by having complete control over food and shelter. Violence was perpetrated on Native people when they were given rations of poor and rotten food with portions in keeping with a close-to-starvation diet. Shelter and the most basic needs for warmth, such as blankets and fire, were also acquired only at the mercy of the Indian agent. If some of the Native people's behaviour was not to the approval of the agent, there were consequences that threatened the existence of individuals as well as the community. Through controlling behaviour, the Indian agent was able to gain control of consciousness and began the process of changing Indigenous consciousness by brute force. The objective of the Indian agent was to destroy Native cultural forms, which represented what he perceived to be the "Indian problem." Therefore, the Indian agent exercised a malevolent influence, which became a model for those placed in authority at that time.

Some of the members of the community who were forced to capitulate in order to preserve their lives became like the Indian agent and at times, their actions were more brutal than the Indian agent. The psychology of internalizing violence and oppression is well understood within the theory of the Stockholm syndrome. The pattern became ingrained as communities struggled to survive, and those patterns continue to express themselves into the present day. The internal Indian agent manifests in the form of bureaucratic violence that threatens their economic way of life.

Through the control of community economy and ways to make a living, the modern Indian agent continues the violence and oppression that began over one hundred years ago. Much of the violence that is experienced in workplaces and community settings is not direct physical violence. Instead, violence in tribal settings is experienced within harsh bureaucratic policies and oppressive work environments. Supervisors and other bureaucrats at times take it upon themselves to make life difficult for those who do not subscribe to their Western bureaucratic or supervisory style. For example, the violence often manifests itself in threats against the economic survival of the community member who may be trying to improve life conditions. When the economic survival of the individual is threatened or taken away, then the violence becomes physical. This type of violence can be characterized as bureaucratic domestic violence and can be directly traced to the effects of historical trauma and internalized oppression as expressed by the original Indian agent.

An interesting aspect of the internalized Indian agent is manifested in tribal or work situations in which traditional structures are being upheld or revived by some of the bureaucracy. Just like in the original setting where the Indian agent was brought in to eradicate the Native life-world, the present internalized agent is also committed to eradicating the Native life-world. The "hang around the fort Indian" psychology (a term used for tribal people who were quick to side with the Indian agent as a way of survival; it is used by Native people today to describe Natives who have been co-opted by the oppressor) is rewarded in these situations and the Native person who wants to adhere to traditional values is systematically abused. If they do not conform, then they are subject to termination by the local bureaucratic entity and an ensuing bureaucratic domestic violence. When others in the community or agency workforce observe the consequences suffered by those who resist the modern Indian agent, they usually react with fear and conform to the requirements of the modern Indian agent whose function is to eradicate any awareness or attachment to the Native soul.

It is well known that many tribal programs realize that in order to be effective, they need to be culturally relevant. Cultural relevance is usually kept at the lip-service level with an obvious superficiality. Such efforts frequently serve as a foothold for maintaining the watchful eye of the Indian agent who has been put in a position of authority by those who have already lost their identity and connection to traditional culture through the intergenerational bureaucratic violence that is part of the legacy of historical trauma.

As long as the Indian agent is maintained in power, there is little hope for our communities, because in order to succeed, the members of the community have to emulate the Indian agent. Consciously or unconsciously, a choice is made since there is no way that one can emulate the Indian agent and maintain one's identity and soul. In essence, the Indian agent has become a sorcerer vampire, a parasite whose livelihood depends on robbing Native people of their souls and identity, perpetrating bureaucratic violence that can easily hide in the pages of policies and procedures of *Robert's Rules of Order*. In this manner, the Indian agent can publicly absolve himself of any wrongdoing and violate individuals again by making them feel as if they are not performing adequately and that it is really their fault that the community cannot accomplish their goals.

Over time, the Indian agent has become expert in the ongoing oppression. Native communities must become aware of this ongoing psychology and begin to address it whenever they find it. Courage will be required in the healing endeavour and, by addressing historical trauma and its effects, communities can begin to deal with the issue of the Indian agent. Healing historical trauma will continue to provide the critical analysis needed to exorcise ourselves from these malevolent forces, and in that way, we will began a new narrative that is more in keeping with teachings about living a good life in the current life-world.

Warrior's Soul: Treatment Issues With Native Veterans

The authors feel that to bring awareness to some of the healing factors that need to be addressed in the healing of historical trauma we must examine what happens in the ceremony of war. After all, war initiated historical trauma, and we need to reflect on some of the spiritual issues therein. In most ancient and modern tribal cultures, there are methods in which warriors/veterans are readmitted into the society after having to go and commit acts that go against natural law. Many tribal cultures regard the act of war as being contra life and out of harmony with natural order. Therefore, there has to be a method whereby order and harmony is re-established after it has been insulted and disturbed (even though this section is derived from working with Native veterans, the authors have found utility with veterans from other cultures).

It is important to analyze events and their effects and see what actually happens at the soul level when a warrior has to commit acts that go against the soul or psyche, as is the case in war. Life is sacred. All cultures, religions, and ideologies subscribe to some sort of idea regarding the sacredness of life. The warrior takes his/her life and places it against another life or lives in the path of doing his/her duty. From a Native perspective, in the point of contact between opposing warriors there is a spiritual understanding that is usually not in the realm of ego awareness. An energy or spirit of violence comes into play between the two people involved in the situation, and the outcome usually requires one of the warriors to die or be injured. Regardless of how the situation is resolved, both warriors are wounded where blood does not flow. Recent news from the Iraq War attests to the fact that post-traumatic stress disorder (PTSD) is rampant and warriors are returning with soul injuries as well as the physical traumas.

Presently, in the American culture, there are no ceremonies performed before or after going to war except in some instances where the veteran is part of a tribal tradition that understands natural law and the balancing that needs to occur through ceremony. Therefore, most veterans are left to fend for themselves in a system that has no understanding of the spiritual aspect of what occurs in war. Tribal wisdom understands that war has a spirit and is a living entity. It is this spiritual entity that needs to be balanced and restored in ceremony. War is in itself a ceremony and natural order requires that a healing ceremony be performed to restore balance.

These spiritual aspects are considered very serious, and some tribes believe that the actual identity of the person is at stake as her/she goes to war. For example, if you are part of such a tribe and you are part of taking human life, you stop existing as a member of that tribe, as you are swallowed by the *esprit de corp* of a military group and consumed by the spirit of war. When we realize that most tribal names actually translate into "human being," then the warrior taking a life ceases to be a human being. This is a far cry from saying that you have PTSD, which is a reductive, sterile, clinical term that means very little to the soul of the warrior/veteran. Once the warrior ceases to be a human being, there has to be a way to restore him/her back to being human, otherwise s/he will remain without identity and take on other identities, such as the several diagnoses that most veterans are given.

There exists a relationship between the energy of lethal violence and human beings participating in this dance called war. When we look at some ancient traditions that understand what happens at the time of death, it makes sense to think that the spirit that leaves the dying person's body may be a bit confused if the person is killed suddenly, as is frequently the case in modern warfare. The disembodied spirit may not know it has died and serious confusion may result from sudden displacement. In this confusion, the departing spirit may attach itself to the closest person or to the one that has been the cause of its departure. This phenomenon can be clearly understood if one is to ask most veterans what they are dreaming. Many report that they dream of the people that they have killed. In addition, the veteran also carries images of his/her friends who were killed since the spirits of the dead attach themselves to the closest person to them in order to try to make sense of the death process. The images of the dead are a deep part of veteran dream life, and they cause a tremendous amount of suffering through symptoms. Most of the symptoms are clinically known as anxiety, depression, suicidal ideation, severe thought disorders, and PTSD.

Veteran dreams clearly indicate that there is a huge elephant in the middle of the therapist's couch, and no one pays attention to it. The images are not subtle, as most veterans know, yet for some reason these are not usually part of the "best practice" model. For the Native veteran, unless the spiritual aspects of trauma are dealt with, the meaning and efficacy of treatment will suffer. Veterans then find a way of self-medicating, and other self-destructive behaviours are enacted to stop the dream-world visitors that haunt them continuously.

The first task of the treatment is for therapist and veteran to gain awareness of the process described in this discussion. Veterans need to have a cathartic process that allows them to talk about their deeds and acknowledge that these were not wholesome actions. The awareness that there may be a spiritual implication is also part of the initial stage of restoring harmony and balance. Awareness of the suffering that has occurred to others as part of the veteran's participation in war is critical so as to humanize the enemy that is haunting the veteran.

The next step in the process is to make peace with the internalized enemy who keeps appearing in dreams, fantasies, and PTSD reactions. Again, tribal traditions teach that in order to restore harmony, one must make amends to the offended individuals. Amends should be made through asking the images, and dreams of the dead, for forgiveness. In addition, an offering must be made to restore relationships in the sacred realm. This offering could be tobacco or food offered in a ceremonial fashion to the souls of the dead. Many cultures have special days during the year where this is done. In the United States, some cultures celebrate "all souls day" as part of reconnecting with the dead and keeping relationships in balance. This aspect of restoring the warrior's soul is critical if the warrior is to bring harmony back into his/her life-world.

Another activity that helps restore balance is by offering help on behalf of the communities that have been offended as part of the war that the veteran was involved in. There have been veterans who have gone back to the part of the world in which they committed the violation and have offered peace offerings to the Elders of the village, town, or area. At times, this is not possible and here is where intent can be useful; veterans can be assisted in therapy to offer help to someone with the intention and motivation that this help is on behalf of the suffering they have caused through proxy. There are tribal-specific ceremonies that can be used as well as therapeutic ceremonies that can be invented spontaneously by the warrior and healer within a strong therapeutic alliance. The main issue is that the ceremony is one of reconciliation with the enemy and must be performed; otherwise, the veteran will continue to be haunted. There are too many instances where, in order to stop the haunting, a warrior will commit suicide as a final offering to the spirit of war.

Veterans should be reminded that participation in war as warriors is an activity that is part of the present human condition, and being a warrior has traditional positive qualities which have mostly nothing to do with taking the lives of others. The main purpose of a traditional Native warrior was the nurturing of the tribe and family, chiefly through self-sacrifice. Traditional warriors' main objective was "that the people may live," which is metaphorically different than what is required of the modern warrior. Because of the nature of war, forces beyond our control are enacted, and these create severe problems in the lives of our warriors. The problems usually make themselves conscious once there is distance from what occurred and the individual is out of the craziness of the war zone. Once the veteran is out of the war, or even before s/he enters that realm, there should be instruction as to the effects of natural law on events such as the ceremony of war.

Once the veteran is out of the intensity of war, the problems begin to manifest themselves, although at times this can start in the battle zone. Just because forces may be out of ego-centred control does not mean that the veteran is helpless and at the mercy of the symptoms that plague the veteran once s/he is home. Therapists can guide veterans through a deep process, as described in this section, which will allow the veteran to become aware of the spiritual nature of war and to deal with the internalized entities who have lodged themselves where blood does not flow.

Hopefully, the discussion in this section has made the reader cognizant that there needs to be a different approach when working with Native and other populations who may not subscribe to the Western understanding of cosmology. It is a significant fact that Western approaches can further traumatize patients who are traumatized by invalidating the very identity of their patients. Resulting adverse reactions, such as violence and suicide, should be enough of a red flag to providers who are encapsulated by theoretical and clinical narcissism.

The situation is exacerbated when such providers hide behind the pseudo-science that provides us with "evidence-based therapies" that are supposed to be the answer to the patients'/community' complaints. Practicing science in this manner invalidates the centuries of traditional Native science and practice, which is at the core of healing in many Native communities. An example of invalidation of Native culture is when insurance companies hide behind "medical necessity" without any consideration for the cultural needs of the patient. What is sad is that physicians are hired to do this harmful task in order to protect the insurance company from complaints. The doctors working in this capacity are paid to save the company money, and in so doing, they traumatize the patient and community, creating a new phase of historical trauma in our society.

The trauma towards the community or individual has a dual-prong approach when our profession insists on utilizing methods that are foreign to the culture. It invalidates the life-world of both the individual and community. This type of invalidation ensures that the people involved will not be able to make their way out of the generations of trauma because additional bureaucratic injury is absorbed by the community through the actions of individuals who are in charge of helping the community. After several of these failed interventions, there is a loss of hope that occurs in the community towards any intervention because it is seen as "more of the same." Once the funding dries up, the well-intentioned researchers leave, causing further trauma by abandoning the community.

Culture, Evidence-Based Treatment, and Research

Treatment that is based on empirically derived data is prone to be one-sided and represents the interest of the researcher who is asking a question with a predisposed answer. Basing treatment in this manner can best be characterized as a social conditioning process.

> From a multicultural/social justice perspective, it is suggested that such an approach to counselling is largely designed to ensure that clients become productive and conforming members of society in ways that enhance the corporate structures that operate behind the scene. These structures represent supraordinate societal forces that significantly dictate what people in the general citizenry are conditioned to believe are

> appropriate ways of thinking and acting in the world . . . It is further asserted that this general psychological ideology influences both the empirically tested interventions counsellors are required to use, for reimbursement by third-party payers, and the assumptions and beliefs that underlie the diagnoses counsellors make of clients' mental health status.
>
> (Duran et al., 2008, p. 293)

Presently, the method that predominates in the "therapeutic industry" and our profession is cognitive behavioural theory–driven clinical practice. When examined from a multicultural research perspective, there is merit in this clinical approach (MacDonald & Gonzalez, 2006; Renfrey, 1992; Trimble, 1992). Regardless of the background of the researcher, or if the research is termed multicultural, it is critical that we examine if the actual methods are in themselves culturally competent and responsive. The reason for the additional critical approach to this type of research is that, from a social justice perspective, it should be emphasized that clinical work should not be implemented as "off the shelf" until cultural metaphor modification occurs (Duran et al., 2008).

Unless theory, practice, and research are deeply rooted in the life-world metaphor of the culture, effectiveness will be limited at best and more trauma will occur at worst. This being the case, it is not worth the risk to continue doing our work in the same manner that we have for over a century. If we continue merely offering what is acceptable to third-party payers with the approval of business executives and the whims of the American mainstream economy, we are falling into the practice of promoting another generation of historical trauma dressed in a neocolonial empirical mask. At the individual and community level, it matters little as to how ethical and statistically significant our practice is because the impact will be harmful and extend the ongoing pain that has become part of intergenerational experiences in the life-world of the individual and community.

Are we doomed to ongoing failure? Is there a way out? These should be the questions that we ask if we are to take a critical review of our practice as clinicians and researchers. Fortunately, there is hope. If research methods take into account ways of knowing the life-world of the community under study, the results should be more amenable to having results that will actually reflect the needs of the community (Allen et al., 2006; Duran et al., 2008; Fisher & Ball, 2002; Mohatt et al., 2004).

In essence, we already have methods that can continue to evolve in a manner that will provide answers to the suffering that continues because of trauma suffered by individuals and communities. What is needed presently is a commitment by our profession that will not allow our practice to be dictated by business and administrative decisions made by people who never have and never will treat a victim of trauma or have no sense of the cosmology of Native people. Our discipline must make commitments towards changing the way we treat our patients from diverse groups who do not necessarily subscribe to Western linearity. We must release our narcissism and be able to meet patients and communities at least part of the way.

One of the key guiding principles to ethical and moral practice is "first do no harm." Imposing a foreign worldview via diagnosis, treatment, and research to individuals and communities violates this principle, and we must stop this type of practice. It is difficult to recreate and reinvent ourselves once we have been doing things in a prescribed manner for many years. Many of our colleagues will continue on the same path, and they will continue to reap rewards from a system that is geared towards business as usual. That said, it does not detract from some of us sitting idly on the sidelines watching and keeping silent. It is critical that we bear witness and call on our brothers and sisters to take a critical look at their practice and research results as well as methods.

In order to ensure that the future evolves in a manner that is conducive to healing trauma in communities that are disenfranchised from the academy, we need to change the academy itself. The academy needs to become aware and responsive to the diverse world that we are a part of. Fixing the discipline of psychology will be a virtual "cake walk" compared to changing the deeply rooted narcissism and clique in our academic settings. It is critical that we commit to these changes if we are to impact not only the current suffering from trauma but also avoid imposing additional trauma through our antiquated clinical and research practices.

It is hoped that this discussion will lead to a self-critique within our discipline. In order for us to acquire the skills and abilities to help those who have been traumatized, it becomes increasingly important that we heal from the traumas that have plagued us as a collective group of healers via the root metaphors that have been imposed on our practice through a variety of means. We must take back the responsibility for understanding and learning new and different ways of understanding our life-world. Merely continuing to perpetuate the status quo will ensure that we continue the process of wounding our patients, our communities, and ourselves where blood does not flow.

References

Allen, J., Mohatt, G. V., Rasmus, S. M., Hazel, K. L., Thomas, L., & Lindley, S. (2006). The tools to understand: Community as co-researcher on culture-specific protective factors for Alaska Native. *Journal of Prevention and Intervention in the Community, 32*, 41–59.

Beck, J. S. (1995). *Cognitive therapy: Basics and beyond*. New York: Guilford.

Danieli, Y. (1998). *International handbook of multigenerational legacies of trauma*. New York: Plenum Press.

Devilly, G. J., Spence, S. H., & Rapee, R. M. (1998). Statistical and reliable change with eye movement desensitization and reprocessing: Treating trauma with a veteran population. *Behavior Therapy, 29*, 435–455.

Duran, E. (2006). *Healing the soul wound: Counseling with American Indians and other Native peoples*. New York: Teachers College Press.

Duran, E., Firehammer, J., & Gonzalez, J. (2008). Liberation psychology as the path toward healing cultural soul wounds. *Journal of Counseling and Development, 86*(3), 288–295.

Fisher, P. A., & Ball, T. J. (2002). The Indian family wellness project: An application of the tribal participatory research model. *Prevention Science, 3*, 235–240.

Horowitz, M. J., Marmar, C., Krupnick, J., Wilner, N., Kaltreider, N., & Wallerstein, R. (1997). *Personality styles and brief psychotherapy*, 2nd ed. New York: Basic Books.

MacDonald, J. D., & Gonzalez, J. (2006). Cognitive-behavior therapy with American Indians. In P. A. Hays, & G. Y. Iwamasa (Eds.), *Culturally responsive cognitive-behavioral therapy: Assessment, practice, and supervision* (pp. 23–46). Washington, DC: American Psychological Association.

Meichenbaum, D. (1977a). Dr. Ellis, please stand up. *Counseling Psychologist, 7*(1), 43–44.

Meichenbaum, D. (1997b). *Treating post-traumatic stress disorder*. Chichester, England: Wiley.

Mohatt, G. V., Hazel, K. L., Allen, J. R., Stachelrodt, M., Hensel, C., & Fath, R. (2004). Unheard Alaska: Culturally anchored participatory action research on sobriety with Alaska Natives. *American Journal of Community Psychology, 33*, 263–273.

Renfrey, G. S. (1992). Cognitive-behavior therapy and the Native American client. *Behavior Therapy, 23*, 321–340.

Shapiro, F. (1989). Eye movement desensitization: A new treatment for post-traumatic stress disorder. *Journal of Behavioral Experimental Psychiatry, 20*, 211–217.

Trimble, J. E. (1992). A cognitive-behavioral approach to drug abuse prevention and intervention with American Indian youth. In L. A. Vargas, & J. D. Koss (Eds.), *Working with culture: Psychotherapeutic interventions with ethnic minority children and adolescents* (pp. 246–275). San Francisco: Josse-Bass.

Whitbeck, L. B., Adams, G. W., Hoyt, D. R., & Chen, X. (2004). Conceptualizing and measuring historical trauma among American Indian people. *American Journal of Community Psychology, 33*, 119–130.

9 Historical Perspectives on Indigenous Healing

Allison Reeves and Suzanne L. Stewart

Historical Context of Indigenous Health

Since colonization, systemic racism, dispossession, and threats to cultural identity within Indigenous communities in Canada have led to many social and health problems that were, prior to contact with Europeans, largely unknown (Gunn Allen, 1986; Moffitt, 2004; Paul, 2000). The colonial legacy within Canada's Indigenous history dates back to the first European settlers following Cabot's landing on Canada's eastern shores in 1497. Throughout our more recent history, federally imposed policies, such as the Indian Act (relegating Native peoples to reserve lands, denying cultural rights and language, etc.), Bill C-31 (affecting Native women's Indian status), the residential schooling system, and forced adoption through the '60s Scoop, have resulted in a marginalization of Indigenous peoples within Canada (Moffitt, 2004). Colonization has been referred to as a *soul wound* (Duran, 2006) to Indigenous peoples as well as a physical and cultural genocide (Moffitt, 2004), and these social issues have resulted in high rates of alcohol abuse, family violence, underemployment, and mental health issues in many Indigenous communities (Smye & Browne, 2002; Stewart, 2008).

In order to address the complex mental health needs of Indigenous peoples facing challenges related to these intergenerational traumas, the political, historical, and social contexts around these health outcomes must be considered within the framework of colonization. In addition, responses to the mental health needs of Indigenous peoples affected by these social, family, inter- and intrapersonal issues must be culturally appropriate and sustainable.

This chapter explores the history of traditional Indigenous healing practices, as well as the contemporary use of these practices, as a culturally appropriate and sustainable approach to care for Indigenous peoples in Canada. This chapter will also consider divergences from Western healing paradigms and the need for multiple understandings of healing to provide integrative care for Indigenous peoples in a contemporary setting.

Indigenous Healing: Theory and Methods

When discussing Native or Indigenous health, it is worth noting specific cultural and geographical groups (Bucko & Iron Cloud, 2008). There are likely some inherent misunderstandings in any discussion on Indigenous healing within North America, as this term implies uniformity in culture and healing practices (Cohen, 1998). Since healing practices have been ongoing for tens of thousands of years in North America, during which hundreds of different cultural groups have evolved, diversity of culture and healing practices is the rule, rather than the exception (Bear Hawk Cohen, 2003). This diversity also makes it difficult to know the extent to which traditional healing is practiced today, although it is clear from many writings that it continues to be practiced widely (Murillo, 2004). Nevertheless, although there is no single source on traditional healing, there are numerous Indigenous teachings on commonly shared beliefs about the fundamental nature of the world and how health and healing are a part of that world (Bear Hawk Cohen, 2003). Keeping in mind regional and ideological differences among North American Indigenous cultures, the following sections will review commonly shared beliefs, values, and healing practices.

Traditionally, a spiritual interpretation of the human condition (Bear Hawk Cohen, 2003) included health and medicine. All things evolved through this cultural and spiritual way of life, rooted in the natural cosmic order; this concept of wholeness is fundamentally part of the consciousness of many—if not all—Indigenous cultures (Begay & Maryboy, 2000). Six Nations Ontario author and healer, Wendy Hill (2009), agrees that all Indigenous peoples of the world share a particular commonality: the connection with the Earth and Spirits. All peoples were spiritual beings, who respected life, nature, and other animals, the ancestors, and our older relatives, such as the sun and moon (Hill, 2009). Shaman healers of Indigenous cultures focused on these natural and spiritual relationships in their work, which served not only to help those who were ill but also to connect spiritually with the sacredness of all things in the universe, fulfilling an existential need to make meaning of our existence here in the cosmos (Begay & Maryboy, 2000; Koss-Chioino, 2003).

It is estimated that the healing traditions of Native Americans have been practiced for at least 12,000 years and possibly as long as 40,000 years (Cohen, 1998). Hultkrantz (1992), a professor of comparative religions, lived among many Native American groups and wrote at length about Indigenous cultures in North America. His writings speak of traditional Anishnawbe peoples as having lived in relative good health, keeping up high standards of hygiene, using sweats to prevent illness, calling on shamans and healers when required, and caring for the infirmed and Elderly until the end of life, even painstakingly carrying them on sleds during migratory periods. Anishnawbe peoples understood disease etiology as rooted in natural and supernatural causes; *Gitchi Manitou* (Lyon, 1996) was the "Great

Mystery," to whom they pledged ethical behaviour (including, for instance, solidarity, generosity, and helpfulness), respectful hunting, and other rules of conduct (Hultkrantz, 1992). Cree peoples too, believed in manitous (spirits) everywhere in nature and often interacted with animal spirits who acted as guardians and helped the hunt. The Cree, too, were charged with following ethical ways of life in keeping with nature's balance (Hultkrantz, 1992). Similar trends can be found in other Native American groups: for instance, the Kashaya peoples of northern California prayed to Coyote (the Creator) and the Redwood trees (the Grandfathers), and they believed all should live in balance with our natural world (Parrish, 2004). The Lakota peoples continue to practice the Sacred Pipe ceremony, which recognizes the spiritual phases of life and offers guidance for walking *the good road* (Bad Hand, 2002). The Navajo peoples healed by walking in balance and harmony with creation (Burkhardt, 2000). Finally, the Pueblo peoples enjoyed collectivist agricultural communities where egalitarian ideals prevailed. Among other traditions, they held ceremonies for rain and fertility out of respect for nature's power (Hultkrantz, 1992).

If we look outside of North American groups to Indigenous peoples in the wider global sphere, we see many interesting similarities between the belief structures of these communities, in terms of their relationship with the earth and the sacredness of existence. For instance, shamanistic practices are common not only to Indigenous cultures in North America but also within South American Indigenous traditions, Qabalah traditions, Anglo-Saxon traditions (Wolf, 1991), and traditional European faith healing (Hultkrantz, 1992), among others. Also, Peruvian shamans use, as one component of their practice, the ayahuasca plant as a healing ritual that allows its followers the perspective of bringing the subconscious into awareness and experiencing a oneness with the earth (Wolf, 2004). The practice induces a timeless state that many spiritual traditions understand as being the key to our sense of harmony with all that is around us (Wolf, 2004). Other ancient spiritual traditions agree; for instance, the Bhagavad Gita, the sacred Hindu text, has at its philosophical core the notion that there exists an infinite, unchanging reality behind the illusions around us and that our life's goal is to connect to this infinite Source (Wolf, 2004). Many other similarities related to notions of time, the egoless self, the energetic, and vibrational harmonies of the planet and universe have been noted in Indian and Chinese societies, among the Aboriginal peoples of Australia, and within Hindu, Sufism, Buddhist, and Taoist practices.

These are but a few similarities of the traditional peoples who, in many corners of the planet, are still seeking a life which is in balance with nature and creation. That many of these groups still enjoy these traditions in the face of an ever-expanding technological globalization speaks to the resilience of all Indigenous peoples around the world. As Paula Gunn-Allen (1986) argues, the presence of survivors is a testament to Indigenous resilience and the human will to survive. She writes, "Tribal systems have been operating in the 'new world' for several hundred thousand years. It is unlikely that a few hundred years of colonization will see their undoing" (p. 2).

Concepts in Indigenous Healing

Healing can be conceptualized as the process of bringing the sacred aspects of the self (physical, emotional, mental, and spiritual) into focus in order to integrate and balance these aspects, with each bearing an equal importance (Hodge, Limb, & Cross, 2009; Hunter, Logan, Goulet, & Barton, 2006). Therefore, the task of the healer becomes to treat the balance, rather than treating the person. Figure 9.1 considers balance and harmony in the Indigenous concept of wellness, as noted by Hodge et al. (2009, p. 215).

While Western medicine reviews disease etiology to treat physical symptoms of illness, traditional healing takes a holistic approach by looking at the four quadrants as well as emotional and environmental contexts (Murillo, 2004).

The notion of "healing"—establishing harmony and well-being—is a lifelong commitment (Bear Hawk Cohen, 2003; Cohen, 1998). Healing connects people to nature and spirit and is not based solely on personal care (Bear Hawk Cohen, 2003). For this reason, healing might also involve ceremonies with the client and can also include relatives and community members; for this reason, healing can also call on social networks and group practices (Murillo, 2004). For instance, if a community member is ill, relatives and

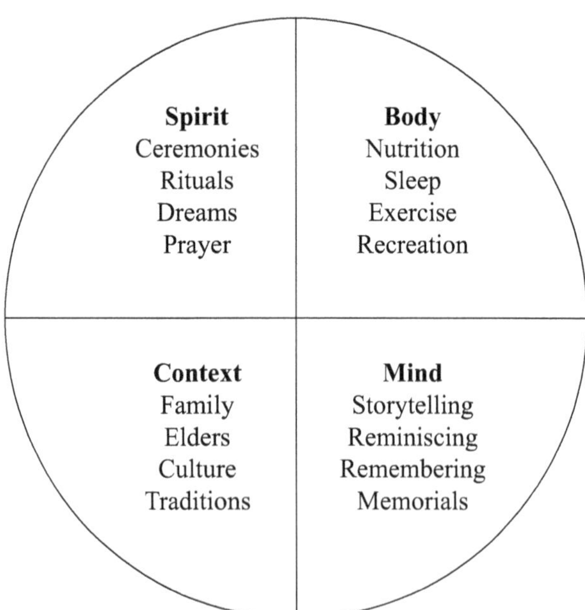

Figure 9.1 Balance and harmony as the pathway to wellness.

friends may gather in prayerful support. Healing extends beyond physical illness, and practices might seek to heal social disruptions and the health of the entire ecosystem (Bucko & Iron Cloud, 2008).

Different healers and groups use a diverse range of formulations and practices for healing (Hultkrantz, 1992). Diversity in healing traditions was likely influenced by the migrations of communities over the years and cultural exchanges along trade routes (Cohen, 1998). Within most healing traditions, diagnostic ability depends on the intuition, sensitivity, and spiritual power of the healer, involves sensing disturbances in energy, and may include seeking information about the illness from spiritual forces (for instance, through dream interpretation, waking visions, spirit guides, and other tools) (Bear Hawk Cohen, 2003; Wolf, 2004). In terms of disease etiology, healers might perceive illness to be caused by spirits, or as a sort of disturbance with the supernatural (Bear Hawk Cohen, 2003; Hultkrantz, 1992). Etiologies also include other external causes, including pathogenic forces that come into the mind, body, and/or spirit (including negative thoughts by others, environmental poisons, and physical or emotional trauma) (Bear Hawk Cohen, 2003; Hultkrantz, 1992).

The usage of the term "medicine man" (Lyon, 1996, p. 168) dates back at least to French Jesuit missionaries during the 17th century; however, this term overlooks the fact that many healers were and are women. Although this term is often used interchangeably with shaman, they are not entirely the same (Lyon, 1996). Hultkrantz (1992) differentiates between groups of traditional healers in his writings. For instance, an *herbalist* is one who cures diseases using herbal medicines and works through natural means. A *medicine person* is a seer who receives healing abilities during vision quests and uses the power of guardian spirits in his or her practice, often including music in the healing experience. Finally, a *shaman* is an individual who is able to harness the power of spirits for healing, as do medicine people; however, a shaman is also a conjurer of sorts, able to take on new forms and transform. Cures in this latter case are typically of supernatural origin. From a general conceptual standpoint, Yeh, Hunter, Madan-Bahel, Chiang, and Arora (2004) suggest that healers are individuals recognized by their communities as possessing special insight and helping skills. They are the keepers of traditional wisdom and use this knowledge and insight to address issues in the community. They also enter into the spirit realm and act as conduits of positive energy from this source (Yeh et al., 2004). As noted earlier, these helpers can be men, women, or two-spirit people (Gunn Allen, 1986; Hultkrantz, 1992; Wolf, 2004).

Indigenous healers do not missionize their practices or coerce patients into accepting their services (Bear Hawk Cohen, 2003). In fact, some illnesses are not treated at all by healers if they are seen as a necessary aspect of the patient's journey (Bear Hawk Cohen, 2003). Also, whereas a Western physician may prescribe standard medicines for particular symptoms, traditional healing often depends on the time, the place, the healer, and the patient, as all must be in harmony to achieve the desired outcome (Bear Hawk Cohen, 2003). The healer does not necessarily see himself or herself as responsible for delivering a cure; rather, she or he is the healing instrument through which healing power flows (Hammerschlag, 2009); in this sense, she or he does not operate as a detached, clinical observer but is emotionally, intellectually, and spiritually attached at all times (Hammerschlag, 2009). Finally, healers themselves are expected to model healthy behaviour for the community (Bear Hawk Cohen, 2003).

Healing Modalities

Traditional healing for many groups involves a combination of spiritual, pharmacological, and physical treatments to aid the sick (Bucko & Iron Cloud, 2008). Healing typically begins with a prayer to help focus the mind on healing and to affirm positive values such as love, thankfulness, and acceptance (Bear Hawk Cohen, 2003). Among the multitude of healing practices, this section will touch briefly on herbal, ceremonial, physical, and counselling medicines.

Smudging is the practice of burning herbs to illicit smoke in order to communicate with, and to honour, the Great Spirit. Its purpose is to cleanse and balance the self and brings about a feeling of being refreshed and rejuvenated (Moondance, 1997). Typically, tobacco, sage, cedar, sweet grass, white spruce, juniper, osha root, and bitter root can be used, among others (Bear Hawk Cohen, 2003; Moondance, 1997). Smudging can also purify a space of toxic energy, negative feelings, or thoughts and create a healing space (Bear Hawk Cohen, 2003).

Plants have also been used widely in herbal remedies, and plants are considered to have strong healing powers (Parrish, 2004). Animals and humans alike have always used plants for food and healing purposes; currently, as much as 80 percent of the world's population relies on herbs for their primary health needs (Burkhardt, 2000). Medicines can be found everywhere in nature, and each healer who works with plants must learn to find, gather, and prepare healing plants. Healers are known to have an astounding knowledge of hundreds of varieties of plants as well as precise methods of preparation (Lyon, 1996). They are taught to listen to the plants for healing instructions, to not pick plants unnecessarily, and to ask permission of a plant for its use in medicine (Burkhardt, 2000). Cedar teas have been used for coughs and cedar twigs to warn off bad dreams; salmon is often baked on cedar wood planks (Bear Hawk Cohen, 2003). Essential oils found in nature are also used for their calming and rejuvenating properties, and natural crystals and stones (such as amber, amethyst, and silver) are considered to have particular energies that bring the human body into balance (Bear Hawk Cohen, 2003; Burkhardt, 2000). Western scholars have often differentiated between plant-based healing (which they consider to be a "rational" treatment) and mystical shamanistic healing (which has been considered "irrational") (Lyon,

1996). The following paragraphs will explore some facets of healing involving this second category.

Within most Indigenous traditions, ceremonies are a natural part of life and serve to bring communities of people together to connect to the Great Mystery (Bad Hand, 2002). The ceremonial circle offers the opportunity for people who share common views to join together for a common focus in harmony with one another and affirms shared cultural identity and values (Bad Hand, 2002; Bear Hawk Cohen, 2003). In ceremony, the ego is laid aside and individuals become one with the larger group, disarming aggression and conflict and offering mutual support (Bad Hand, 2002). Ceremonial experiences also allow mental quiet and focus, which has a secondary effect of decreasing blood pressure and stress hormones, as well as elevating endorphins to bring about positive feelings (Bear Hawk Cohen, 2003). Often during ceremony, the spirit helpers are summoned to join, and participants may use music, drumming, dance, and song to bring past, present and future into alignment (Bad Hand, 2002).

A sweat lodge ceremony is an opportunity to purify the self and to commune with ancestors, animal spirits, and the Great Spirit (Bear Hawk Cohen, 2003). A sweat lodge is a small, low, and round dome-shaped hut with a door facing east, in the sacred direction (Hultkrantz, 1992). Stones are heated over a fire for many hours and are carried into the lodge where water is poured onto them, and they release large amounts of steam (Hultkrantz, 1992). During the ceremony, singing and chanting rituals are enacted in order to bring about spiritual and physical healing and may involve interactions with the spirit world (Smith, 2005). The ceremony itself may bring about stress and frustration, as it takes place in a cramped and extremely hot place. In this sense, the ritual also allows individuals to experience perseverance (Smith, 2005).

Practices to heal the sick body include curing ceremonies, bone-setting, massage, and the removal of the diseased objects (Parrish, 2004). For instance, the sucking shamans typically use hollow bones or reeds to remove intruded objects by sucking. Edwin Denig, a settler who married an Assiniboin woman (Lyon, 1996), recorded an account of this procedure in 1830. Sceptical of the practice, Denig searched the healer for hidden tools and objects but found nothing on him. The healer then continued his practice of drawing and spitting out large objects, including clots of blood and hair from the body of the sick individual. These objects were too large to be easily secreted, and the removal process left no marks on the patient's body (Lyon, 1996, p. 424). The practice of removing diseased objects through sucking remains common today in many places in North America (Hultkrantz, 1992).

With respect to mental well-being specifically, all healing modalities mentioned here are thought to also heal the mind, given that all health matters are seen from a holistic (body/mind/spirit/emotions) perspective (Cohen, 1998). Traditional healing within a mental health sphere represents a wide array of approaches to care, depending on the expertise of the helper. (Some healers lead sweat lodge ceremonies, some helpers utilize the Seven Grandfather teachings, and others converse with spirit ancestors, for example.) What these traditional mental health and healing approaches share in common is the focus on spirit as central to healing and the fact that embedded within the culture are traditional teachings offering guidance for dealing with life's stressors. For instance, traditional customs also provide resources for making sense of the stages of growth and development in life. Spiritual practices and teachings offer a sense of meaning in people's lives and improve mental health outcomes, enhancing well-being, optimism, and acceptance, as well as minimizing stressors. Traditional mental health and healing practices also promote communion with nature, which also has been linked to lasting mental health benefits, including "wilderness rapture," wherein feelings of wonder and humility promote a sense of connectedness. Approaching care with a respect for traditional healing and spirituality helps to close the "secular-sacred divergence" (Gone, 2010, p. 204) present between many mainstream and traditional therapies.

Indigenous mental health and healing practices also recognize the importance of positive identity construction among Indigenous clients, as colonization has disrupted cultural integrity for many communities and individuals. Informing clients about the colonial history and how it may have impacted their communities intergenerationally can offer an explanation of potentially unseen factors influencing their well-being. Gaining an understanding of harmful colonial tactics, as well as community resilience, can offer a deep sense of cultural pride and purpose. This experience of renewal or reawakening (Adelson, 2001) relates to a sense of self-esteem, coping, and sense of "place" in society. Understanding the impacts of racism, oppression, and discrimination on the lives of each client (Shepard, O'Neil, & Guenette, 2006) relates directly to skills needed to provide culturally safe care, as techniques in therapy are largely ineffective without an understanding of individual context (McCormick, 2000).

Western Counselling to Address Trauma

Western counselling services vary considerably in theoretical orientation, framework, and technique (Howard, Riger, Campbell, & Wasco, 2003); for instance, therapies may focus on cognitive restructuring, unearthing social oppressions, improving communication, solving problems, building self-esteem, managing trauma and grief, and gaining self-awareness of thoughts, feelings, and the body, among others. This section briefly outlines a few approaches to psychotherapy when working with individuals who have experienced trauma,[1] including cognitive behavioural therapies which address cognitive schemas and encourage exposure to fearful stimuli, emotion-focused approaches which restructure emotional schemas, feminist approaches which include psychoeducation around oppression and societal power structures, and group counselling. Generally speaking, cognitive-based therapies for survivors of trauma involve identifying maladaptive thoughts, meanings, and effects and replacing them with more adaptive thoughts (Orchowski, Uhlin, Probst, Edwards, & Anderson, 2009). For instance, an assimilation model of cognitive work in therapy includes drawing the client from an avoidant state, or a vague or confused state about the traumatic experience, to a state where he or she can define his or her psychological issues and reach a place of understanding or insight (Orchowski et al., 2009). Once the client has accessed his or her problematic experiences, the client can work through the issues and integrate experience of trauma into his or her cognitive schema in a less fractured way (Orchowski et al., 2009). Cognitive-based work can also look to exposure therapy for post-traumatic stress disorder (PTSD) symptom reduction. For instance, exposure to traumatic memories in a safe environment can alter the feared memories and diminish threat cues (Foa, Rothbaum, Riggs, & Murdock, 1991). This method emphasizes confronting maladaptive beliefs and rehearsing new coping skills while practicing emotional regulation and self-soothing (Resick & Schnicke, 1992). Other cognitive therapies work with belief systems that negatively affect the client's sense of self as well as disruptive interactional patterns that many individuals who are victimized experience (Barnes, 1995).

Emotion focused therapy (EFT) seeks to address not only maladaptive cognitive schemas but also the complex issues stemming from trauma, including affect regulation, self-esteem issues, and interpersonal challenges (Paivio & Nieuwenhuis, 2001). The EFT model emphasizes the central functioning of emotions in therapeutic change, and therefore the emotional content of traumatic feelings and memories need to be accessed in order to be modified and adapted (Paivio & Nieuwenhuis, 2001). For individuals who react to trauma by minimizing or controlling their affective experience, accessing and feeling these emotions may prove therapeutic; for instance, anger helps with empowerment, setting personal boundaries, and assertiveness and sadness permits grieving and acceptance of loss (Paivio & Nieuwenhuis, 2001). Finally, EFT allows the opportunity for the therapist and client to model secure attachment within a safe environment that highlights unconditional positive regard for the client (Baima & Feldhousen, 2007).

Feminist therapy in particular seeks to recognize and problematize social justice issues and power imbalances within society as a whole in order to make sense of the challenges faced by clients on a sociological as well as psychological level (Orchowski et al., 2009). This type of therapy work would seem relevant when working with individuals who have experienced historical oppression and marginalization. Work of this nature with Indigenous peoples who have experienced oppression may involve challenging sociocultural themes around dominant cultural norms that perpetuate a subordinate role among Indigenous groups (Shepard et al., 2006). In this case, this could involve identifying and describing the harmful impacts of colonial policies on Indigenous peoples and fostering internal pride through positive identity work (Adelson, 2001).

Group therapy has also been described as a positive opportunity for individuals who have shared similar trauma experiences to practice socializing techniques, to act as witnesses to one another, to promote collective empowerment and compassion, and to have the sense of not being alone in their grief (Yalom, 1995). Support groups as well as process-oriented psychotherapy groups exist for survivors of trauma and use various modalities, including EFT, solution focused therapy, feminist therapy, and others (Vandeusen & Carr, 2003). For instance, group therapy has been reported to be successful in addressing the outcomes of sexual abuse against women. A group therapy study by Vandeusen and Carr (2003) with university-aged female survivors of sexual assault began with establishing safety within the group prior to taking on deeper, more emotionally vulnerable work; later the group explored the traumatic experience and mourned the abuse. These phases of group work connected the participants to one another through the group process. Results from this study found that the participants felt less isolated, expanded social supports, and increased knowledge about common symptoms and symptom management following sexual assault. They were also able to validate their negative feelings of guilt, shame, and anger. Finally, symptoms related to a fear of being alone, intrusive thoughts, and emotional numbing decreased, while well-being, sense of personal safety and control, and trust in others increased.

Overall, no matter the specific modality used in therapy, efforts to counsel those managing mental health issues have certain commonalities: first, they attempt to minimize negative psychological sequelae associated with various psychological diagnoses (e.g., depression, anxiety, PTSD); second, they assist clients in making healthy decisions; third, they facilitate the rebuilding of clients' lives; fourth, they seek to decrease self-blame and increase self-esteem among clients; and finally, they assist in fostering appropriate coping skills (Howard et al., 2003). The following section will consider some gaps in these therapy modalities when counsellors work with Indigenous clients specifically.

Gaps in Services for Indigenous Clients

Studies have observed lower rates of mental health service use among Indigenous community members as compared to the non-Indigenous population (Harris, Edlund, & Larson, 2005; Oetzel et al., 2006; Shah, 2005). Some authors have suggested that lower rates of mental health service utilization is due to the scarcity of public funding and personnel resources available to meet the higher rates of mental health issues within Indigenous populations (Hodge et al., 2009). While this may indeed be the case, another barrier for Indigenous peoples in accessing mental health services may be the inappropriateness of the services themselves (Hodge et al., 2009). Kirmayer, Brass, and Tait (2000) note that most mental health services in many urban areas have not been adapted to meet the needs of Indigenous clients; this lack of cultural appropriateness of services has resulted in lower rates of mental health service use as well as higher dropout rates from counselling among Indigenous peoples (Harris et al., 2005; Oetzel et al., 2006; Shah, 2005). Counsellors working with those who have experienced trauma must appreciate the specific value systems and unique culture of the client in order to assist in the healing work; in this sense, the most appropriate ways of dealing with intimate partner violence in a European Canadian context, for instance, might not be entirely appropriate or ideal for members of other cultures (Phiri-Alleman & Alleman, 2008). Since the dominant paradigm in Western psychology lacks an Indigenous worldview, services may be inappropriate or irrelevant to the Indigenous clients who use these types of services (Stewart, 2008; Vicary & Bishop, 2005). And individuals are less likely to use health services that are not adapted culturally to their understandings of healing (Blue, 1977; McCormick, 1996).

For instance, the field of psychiatry, from which the *Diagnostic and Statistical Manual of Mental Disorders (DSM)* emanated, is rooted in implicit values of the dominant culture (Kirmayer et al., 2000) and therefore risks over-pathologizing Indigenous clients (Duran, 2006). The field of psychology also draws immensely from the DSM and therefore carries similar risks. Some authors argue that using Western therapy with Indigenous peoples is a continued form of colonization, as some modalities, such as cognitive behaviour therapy, emphasize questioning values in a given framework (Hodge et al., 2009). The questioning of values, however, is rooted in the principle that certain values are correct and others are incorrect. What this theory overlooks is that these so-called implicit values are culture-bound. Even basic assumptions in the Western paradigm of individualism and self-efficacy may be inappropriate for Indigenous clients who may have more community-based values, where the self is defined relationally (Hodge et al., 2009). Finally, many Indigenous people have also noted that the health system remains culturally unsafe for them, as many people have experienced institutionalized discrimination, stereotyping, and racism from their healthcare providers (Shah, 2005). Ironically, this system results in a cycle wherein Indigenous peoples report both the highest rates of mental health issues as well as the highest rate of unmet mental health needs (Harris et al., 2005).

Like all Indigenous groups, Western medicine also had a spiritual ancestry historically (Wolf, 1991). However, it departed from a spirit-based understanding of the world with the advent of scientific advances such as Sir Isaac Newton's laws of mechanics and Descartes's notion of mind-body dualism. By the 19th and 20th centuries, a view of rigid materialism had developed throughout the West. In Western allopathic medicine, the body came to be viewed as a machine and scientific reductionism moved spiritual and other holistic practices out of the realm of medicine (Sulmasy, 1999). While for many Indigenous groups medicine and spirituality are two sides of the same coin (Hultkrantz, 1992), a Western view lacks a holistic framework and overvalues the physical aspects of the self, while defining health as the absence of disease, confirmed through lab tests (Bear Hawk Cohen, 2003; Cohen, 1998). Other criticisms of this system suggest that its scientific methods focus on theory and cures, rather than on helping individuals find meaning in their suffering (Schneider & DeHaven, 2003). In this sense, the Western practitioner is not trained to guide sufferers, to hear stories, and to understand wider contexts—in short, Western health care has no model of what it means to be a whole person and promotes no operational definition of "holistic healing" (Egnew, 2005). Despite the technologically sophisticated medical practices and forward movements in health care, many patients have reported feeling alienated from their healthcare professionals, who now appear simply as technicians, rather than healers (Schneider & DeHaven, 2003). While many Western-trained healthcare practitioners accept the values of this larger scientific framework without question (Hodge et al., 2009), this type of helping lacks a fundamental consideration for the whole person and thus individuals often do not experience the holism of traditional healing practices, which can address physical, emotional, and spiritual dimensions (Egnew, 2005). For this reason, many people turn elsewhere for healing (Schneider & DeHaven, 2003).

Some specific comparisons between Indigenous healing and Western medical paradigms are highlighted by Bear Hawk Cohen (2003): Western medicine focuses on pathology and curing the disease, whereas Indigenous methods focus on client health, healing, and the community; Western medicine sees illness as fundamentally biological in nature, whereas Indigenous healing views diseases as complex and relating to the physical, emotional, social, and environmental realms; Western treatment methods seek to produce measurable outcomes, while Indigenous methods do not always have outcomes which are measurable; Western methods seek to destroy the disease, while Indigenous healing is teleological and asks, what are we to learn from this experience?; Western medicine values intellect, credentialing, and theory, whereas Indigenous medicine values intuition and learning from Elders, nature, and spiritual visions; Western methods focus on dependence on medication and technology and sees the practitioner as a central authority, whereas Indigenous helpers are counsellors and advisors who empower their clients through awareness and involvement of family and community; and Western practices promote standards and uniformity, whereas Indigenous helping is diverse, situational, and individualized.

Due to these historical differences in ways of understanding illness and healing, some Western health practitioners in recent years have begun to recognize their lack of training and ability in addressing the needs of diverse patients, and the movement toward developing culturally relevant psychological practices has expanded dramatically (Gone, 2010). The hope for increasing understanding and respect between Western and Indigenous care services in order to move forward toward providing allied care is expanded on in the following concluding section.

Moving Forward: Integrative Care

From earliest times, all cultures developed their own explanations of abnormal and distressing behaviours, as well as unique culture-specific ways of dealing with these types of issues (Yeh et al., 2004). The Western psychological literature has demonstrated higher rates of mental health issues among Indigenous peoples; however, there is little formal research on the treatment of intergenerational traumas through a lens that considers culture, Indigenous healing, and historical contexts. If Western practitioners working with Indigenous clients intend to move toward a more culturally competent practice in psychology, the acceptance of traditional Indigenous healing, as well as the integration of these traditional methods with contemporary Western practices (where appropriate), is necessary (Gone, 2010).

Western practitioners should first accept the use of traditional helpers among their clients (Murillo, 2004) and allow the clients themselves to determine if and how they will engage in using these services (Bucko & Iron Cloud, 2008). Western practitioners can also request to learn from local Indigenous healers and helpers in order to broaden their understandings of alternative ways of healing. In this sense, they can support their clients by embarking on a similar journey toward learning the history of the local Indigenous community of which their client is a member. Western practitioners can consult with Indigenous healers to ask how the two may work in tandem in supporting the client, and they can be open to hearing an alternate perspective on directions for healing (perhaps even taking direction in their work).

Additionally, a movement within psychology toward holistic healing would involve a consideration of the life systems and social systems of their clients, as individuals do not live apart from the history, culture, and geography of their communities (Nelson, 2004). In order to respond to Indigenous historical trauma specifically, socio-historical factors affecting Indigenous community members need to be acknowledged in the course of therapy treatment and addressed where possible (Cesario, 2001; Kirmayer et al., 2000; Murillo, 2004). As more of the Indigenous population migrates into urban centres, the need for culturally appropriate care increases. All of these arguments lend support for an improvement in practitioner awareness of cultural variations and histories of Indigenous clients and of the need for multiple approaches to healing.

Note

1. Focusing on therapies to address trauma was included purposefully in this section, given the extent to which Indigenous peoples have experienced historical and intergenerational traumas in the wake of colonization.

References

Adelson, N. (2001). Towards a recuperation of souls and bodies: Community healing and the complex interplay of faith and history. In L. Kirmayer, M. MacDonald, &

G. Bass (Eds.), *The mental health of indigenous peoples* (pp. 120–134). Montreal, QB: McGill University.

Bad Hand, H. P. (2002). *Native American healing*. New York, NY: Keats Publishing.

Baima, T. R., & Feldhousen, E. B. (2007). The heart of sexual trauma: Patriarchy as a centrally organizing principle for couple therapy. *Journal of Feminist Family Therapy, 19*(3), 13–36.

Barnes, M. F. (1995). Sex therapy in the couples context: Therapy issues of victims of sexual trauma. *The American Journal of Family Therapy, 23*(4), 351–360.

Bear Hawk Cohen, K. (2003). *Honoring the medicine: The essential guide to Native American healing*. New York, NY: One World Ballantine Books.

Begay, D. H., & Maryboy, N. C. (2000). The whole universe is my cathedral: A contemporary Navajo spiritual synthesis. *Medical Anthropology Quarterly, 14*(4), 498–520.

Blue, A. W. (1977). A study of Native elders and student needs. *United States Bureau of Indian Affairs Education and Research Bulletin, 5*, 15–24.

Bucko, R. A., & Iron Cloud, S. (2008). Lakota health and healing. *Southern Medical Journal, 101*(6), 596–598.

Burkhardt, M. A. (2000). Healing relationships with nature. *Complementary Therapies in Nursing & Midwifery, 6*(1), 35–40.

Cesario, S. K. (2001). Care of the Native American Woman: Strategies for practice, education, and research. *The Journal of Obstetric, Gynecologic, & Neonatal Nursing, 30*(1), 13–19.

Cohen, K. (1998). Native American medicine. *Alternative Therapies in Health and Medicine, 4*(6), 45–57.

Duran, E. (2006). *Healing the soul wound: Counseling with American Indians and other Native peoples*. New York, NY: Teachers College Press.

Egnew, T. R. (2005). The meaning of healing: Transcending suffering. *Annals of Family Medicine, 3*(3), 255–262.

Foa, E., Rothbaum, B., Riggs, D., & Murdock, T. (1991). Treatment of posttraumatic stress disorder in rape victims: A comparison between cognitive-behavioural procedures and counseling. *Journal of Counseling and Clinical Psychology, 59*(5), 715–723.

Gone, J. (2010). Psychotherapy and traditional healing for American Indians: Exploring the prospects for therapeutic integration. *The Counseling Psychologist, 38*(2), 166–235.

Gunn Allen, P. (1986). *The sacred hoop: Recovering the feminine in American Indian traditions*. Boston, MA: Beacon Press.

Hammerschlag, C. A. (2009). The Huichol offering: A shamanic healing journey. *Journal of Religion and Health, 48*(2), 246–258.

Harris, K. M., Edlund, M. J., & Larson, S. (2005). Racial and ethnic differences in the mental health problems and use of mental health care. *Medical Care, 43*(8), 775–784.

Hill, W. (2009). *Understanding life . . . what my ancestors taught me through dreams*. Pittsburgh, PA: Red Lead Press.

Hodge, D. R., Limb, G. E., & Cross, T. L. (2009). Moving from colonization toward balance and harmony: A Native American perspective. *Social Work, 54*(3), 211–219.

Howard, A., Riger, S., Campbell, R., & Wasco, S. (2003). Counseling services for battered women: A Comparison of outcomes for physical and sexual assault survivors. *Journal of Interpersonal Violence, 18*(7), 717–734.

Hultkrantz, A. (1992). *Shamanic healing and ritual drama: Health and medicine in Native North American religious traditions*. New York, NY: The Crossroad Publishing Company.

Hunter, L. A., Logan, J., Goulet, J., & Barton, S. (2006). Aboriginal healing: Regaining balance and culture. *Journal of Transcultural Nursing, 17*(1), 13–22.

Kirmayer, L. J., Brass, G. M., & Tait, C. L. (2000). The mental health of Aboriginal peoples: Transformations of identity and community. *The Canadian Journal of Psychiatry, 45*(7), 607–616.

Koss-Chioino, J. D. (2003). Jung, spirits and madness: Lessons for cultural psychiatry. *Transcultural Psychiatry, 40*(2), 164–180.

Lyon, S. (1996). *Encyclopedia of Native American healing*. New York, NY: W.W. Norton & Company.

McCormick, R. D. (1996). Culturally appropriate means and ends of counselling as described by the First Nations of British Columbia. *International Journal for the Advancement of Counseling, 18*(3), 163–172.

McCormick, R. D. (2000). Aboriginal traditions in the treatment of substance abuse. *Canadian Journal of Counselling, 34*(1), 25–32.

Moffitt, P. M. (2004). Colonialization: A health determinant for pregnant Dogrib women. *Journal of Transcultural Nursing, 15*(4), 323–330.

Moondance, W. (1997). *Star medicine: Native American path to emotional healing*. New York, NY: Sterling Publishing.

Murillo, L. (2004). Perspectives on traditional health practices. In E. Nebelkopf, & M. Phillips (Eds.), *Healing and mental health for Native Americans: Speaking in red* (pp. 109–115). Lanha, MD: Altamira Press.

Nelson, J. (2004). The morning god comes dancing: Culturally competent mental health and HIV services. In E. Nebelkopf, & M. Phillips (Eds.), *Healing and mental health for Native Americans: Speaking in red* (pp. 139–148). Lanha, MD: Altamira Press.

Oetzel, J., Duran, B., Lucero, J., Jiang, Y., Novins, D. K., Manson, S., Beals, J., & the AI-SUPERPFP Team. (2006). Rural American Indians' perspectives of obstacles in the mental health treatment process in three treatment sectors. *Psychological Services, 3*(2), 117–128.

Orchowski, L. M., Uhlin, B. D., Probst, D. R., Edwards, K. M., & Anderson, T. (2009). An assimilation analysis of clinician-assisted emotional disclosure therapy with survivors of intimate partner sexual assault. *Psychotherapy Research, 19*(3), 293–311.

Paivio, S., & Nieuwenhuis, J. (2001). Efficacy of emotion focused therapy for adult survivors of child abuse: A preliminary study. *Journal of Traumatic Stress, 14*(1), 115–133.

Parrish, O. (2004). Healing the kashaya way. In E. Nebelkopf, & M. Phillips (Eds.), *Healing and mental health for Native Americans: Speaking in red* (pp. 117–126). Lanha, MD: Altamira Press.

Paul, D. N. (2000). *We were not the savages*. Halifax, NS: Fernwood Publishing.

Phiri-Alleman, W., & Alleman, J. (2008). Sexual violence in relationships: Implications for multicultural counseling. *The Family Journal: Counseling and Therapy for Couples and Families, 16*(2), 155–158.

Resick, P., & Schnicke, M. (1992). Cognitive processing therapy for sexual assault victims. *Journal of Consulting and Clinical Psychology, 60*(5), 748–756.

Schneider, G. W., & DeHaven, M. J. (2003). Revisiting the Navajo way: Lessons for contemporary healing. *Perspectives in Biology and Medicine, 46*(3), 413–427.

Shah, C. P. (2005). *Health status report of Aboriginal people in Ontario*. Retrieved from http://www.aht.ca/webfm_send/25

Shepard, B., O'Neil, L., & Guenette, F. (2006). Counselling with First Nations women: Considerations of oppression and renewal. *International Journal for the Advancement of Counselling, 28*(3), 227–240.

Smith, D. P. (2005). The sweat lodge as psychotherapy. In R. Moodley, & W. Westerners (Eds.), *Integrating traditional healing practices into counselling and psychotherapy* (pp. 196–209). Thousand Oaks, CA: Sage Publications Ltd.

Smye, V., & Browne, A. (2002). Cultural safety and the analysis of health policy affecting Aboriginal people. *Nurse Researcher, 9*(3), 42–56.

Stewart, S. L. (2008). Promoting indigenous mental health: Cultural perspectives on healing from Native counsellors in Canada. *International Journal of Health Promotion and Education, 46*(2), 49–56.

Sulmasy, D. P. (1999). Is medicine a spiritual practice? *Academic Medicine, 74*(9), 1002–1005.

Vandeusen, K. M., & Carr, J. L. (2003). Recovery from sexual assault: An innovative two- stage group therapy model. *International Journal of Group Psychotherapy, 53*(2), 201–223.

Vicary, D. A., & Bishop, B. J. (2005). Western psychotherapeutic practice: Engaging Aboriginal people in culturally appropriate and respectful ways. *Australian Psychologist, 40*(1), 8–19.

Wolf, F. A. (1991). *The eagle's quest: A physicist's search for truth in the heart of the shamanic world*. New York, NY: Summit Books.

Wolf, F. A. (2004). *The yoga of time travel*. Wheaton, IL: Quest Books.

Yalom, I. D. (1995). *The theory and practice of group psychotherapy*, 4th ed. New York, NY: Basic Books.

Yeh, C., Hunter, C., Madan-Bahel, A., Chiang, L., & Arora, A. (2004). Indigenous and interdependent perspectives of healing: Implications for counselling and research. *Journal of Counseling & Development, 82*(4), 410–419.

10 Colonial Trauma and Political Pathways to Healing

Terry Mitchell

In this chapter, the unacceptable burden of psycho-social-physical-health inequalities borne by Indigenous peoples are identified as a signifier of social injustice with political pathways to resolution. Historical and contemporary forms of colonial violence and related colonial trauma are social issues that settler societies need to increase awareness of, sensitivity to, and accountability for. This chapter provides an overview of the social constructs of Indigeneity, colonialism, and colonial trauma. These constructs provide a foundation for the introduction of six political pathways to advancing social justice as a mental health strategy for promoting the health and wellness of Aboriginal peoples in Canada within a larger framework of reconciliation.

Indigeneity as a Social Construct

First Nations, Métis, and Inuit peoples in Canada are traditionally land-based peoples who are linked to specific territories as political and cultural collectivities with values and lifestyles that are intrinsically linked to their relationship to the land (Blaikie, 2000; Blondin, 1997; Fry & Mitchell, 2015 in press). Indigenous peoples share in common both a deep connectedness to their land and often the loss of territorial homes due to the takeover or displacement of their land (Cohen, 1999; Minister of Supply and Services Canada, 1996a). The land on and with which Indigenous peoples live encompasses their individual and collective physical and spiritual relationship to the land (Kipuri, 2009). Barker's (2009) definition of Indigenous identifies First Peoples as inhabitants of a territory before colonization, stating "Indigenous people in the context of Turtle Island (North America) are those people whose societies predated colonization, who exist in a complex relationship to the land and who have been and continue to be primary targets of active colonization" (p. 328). Alfred and Corntassel (2005), in contrast, view Indigeneity as a political construct arising out of colonialism and as a social process of resistance and struggle against the oppression of settler populations, stating,

> Indigenousness is an identity constructed, shaped and lived in the politicized context of contemporary colonialism . . . It is this oppositional,

> place-based existence, along with the consciousness of being in struggle against the dispossessing and demeaning facts of colonization by foreign people, that fundamentally distinguishes Indigenous peoples from other people in the world.
>
> (p. 597)

The 1983 definition from Cobo's final report for the United Nations on the *Study of the Problem of Discrimination against Indigenous Populations: Conclusions, proposals, and recommendations*, identifies Indigenous communities as contemporary populations "having a historical continuity with pre-invasion and pre-colonial societies that developed on their territories" (chap. xxi–xxii, para. 379). The final report (1983) bridges the pre-colonial perspective with the response to colonization viewpoint by discussing Indigenous peoples globally as pre-colonial societies and as a distinctive population that has resisted assimilation through attention to the preservation and dissemination of their land base and cultures "in accordance with their own cultural patterns, social institutions and legal systems . . ." (chap. xxi–xxii, para. 379).

The social-political definition of Indigeneity is therefore framed in terms of both a primary relationship to traditional lands and cultural practices, as well as confrontation with the colonial forces of land appropriation and cultural interference. Despite huge variances in cultures and geographic location, Indigenous peoples are constituted as a politically created world population through the shared experience of being subjected to historical and current colonial practices which profoundly disrupt and interfere with their diverse cultures and complex social, cultural, and spiritual connectedness to the land. Significantly, Indigeneity is also characterized by a third factor of resistance to genocide and assimilation with enduring persistence in the practices of cultural preservation and renewal (McGregor, 2004; Thomas, Mitchell, & Arseneau, 2015 in press). As McGregor (2004) stated,

> We have learned to resist and thus have survived. Understanding colonialism and its devastating impacts upon us, as well as learning how to resist various forms of colonialism (including internalized forms), constitute an important part of our traditional teachings today.
>
> (p. 77)

Colonialism

The concepts of Indigeneity, trauma, resistance, and renewal must be considered in terms of their relationship to both historical and contemporary forms of colonization. Colonialism has been defined as "the takeover of territory, appropriation of material resources, exploitation of labour and interference with political and cultural structures of another territory or nation" (Loomba, 2005, p. 11). Indigenous peoples worldwide have been subjected to land seizure without being conquered through war (Asch, 1997) as well as the takeover of natural resources and cultural and political interference (Cohen, 1999). Indigenous peoples have been "legally infantilized and politically patronized" (Miller, 2004, p. 102), and their cultures, communities, families, and selves battered by an unrelenting "vicious assimilative assault" (p. 251). This colonial violence, which is politically legitimated by state governments and upheld by majority populations, persists in various forms today, including resource extractive industries where Indigenous peoples are often characterized as "standing in the way of development" (Cohen, 1999, p. 7).

Miller (2004) defines assimilation as "ideology and policy that seeks to eradicate a people's identity and cultural practices in favour of another group's way of doing things" (p. 225). In keeping with this definition, central to Canada's assimilation policy, the Indian residential school system involved forcibly removing very young children from their homes, often relocating them to distant communities. These residential schools, which lasted for over a century from the 1870s until the1990s, have been identified as one of the most devastating expressions of the assimilative policy thrust of the federal government (Archibald, 2006; BBC News, 2008; Indian and Northern Affairs, 2008; Truth and Reconciliation Commission, 2015). On June 11, 2008, the prime minister of Canada, Mr. Stephen Harper, offered an apology to Aboriginal peoples for the nation's regressive and harmful social policy that affected 150,000 students and their families for generations (Harper, 2008). The prime minister's apology reveals the mechanisms of the colonial assimilation project, and the source of the colonial trauma resulted in intergenerational impacts, which have been described as cumulative "becoming more severe as it is passed onto subsequent generations" (Duran, 2006, p. 16). The government apology is a political and social record of wrongdoing and a moral awakening to the devastating long-term impacts of cultural interference and colonial violence.

Colonial Trauma

Indigenous peoples continue to be colonized by having their land and resources appropriated as they experience ongoing cultural interference. The continual conflict and interference of Indigenous land and cultures have imposed high degrees of long-term stress on Indigenous peoples around the world. However, despite the global practice of colonialism, land seizure and vicious assimilative assaults, non-Indigenous settler institutions generally fail to identify and assess the impact of systemic racism, displacement, assimilation, and cultural genocide as explanatory factors in relation to the extremely deleterious health status of the world's Indigenous peoples (Mitchell & Maracle, 2005). Furthermore, there is a general dearth of research on Indigenous mental health within Canada and around the world (Cohen, 1999). The limited available data regarding Indigenous mental health indicates Indigenous peoples are experiencing high rates of depression, alcoholism, suicide, and violence, which have been linked to cultural discontinuity and oppression (Kirmayer, 2000). The enduring impact of persistent and pervasive acts of colonial violence have been described as colonial trauma characterized as complex, continuous, cumulative, and collective with long-term intergenerational effects (Mitchell, 2011; Mitchell, 2015 in press).

Colonial trauma requires that mental health professionals place their work within the wider scope of social justice (Cohen, 1999) to identify and address the traumagenic forces that have impacted Indigenous communities (Mitchell & Maracle, 2005). "The state of Indigenous people's health, including addictions and mental health, cannot in Canada be extricated from colonial projects" (de Leeuw, Greenwood, & Cameron, 2010, p. 292). The mental, physical, social, and spiritual health of Indigenous populations in Canada and across the world have been impacted by the shared phenomenon of historical and contemporary colonialism. There has been a comprehensive and relentless assault on the spiritual, emotional, intellectual, and socio-ecological nature of Indigenous peoples and their cultures (Duran, 2006; Mitchell, 1996). Trauma is therefore experienced not just by individuals but also by the collective. This collective trauma signifies an external agent and the political nature of the crimes against Indigenous people, supporting the thesis that Indigenous mental health is a social justice issue with political pathways to healing.

Identifying Agency

There are many terms used to characterize the enduring collective trauma of Indigenous peoples: post-traumatic stress (Manson et al., 1996), historical trauma (Brave Heart, 1999), intergenerational trauma (Brave Heart & DeBruyn, 1998), Native Holocaust (Stannard, 1992), soul wound (Duran, 2006), and colonial trauma (Evans-Campbell, 2008). I support the use of colonial trauma, as it names the external nature and political source of the trauma and allows for an awareness of current colonial expressions while respecting the historical wounds of Elders and ancestors. Colonial trauma is defined by Evans-Campbell (2008) as "both historical and contemporary events that reflect colonial practices to colonize, subjugate, and perpetrate ethnocide and genocide" (p. 335). The mental, spiritual, social, and physical health of Indigenous individuals and communities has been impacted by the systematic and enduring exposure to colonial violence. Colonial trauma reflects the pervasive nature of the crimes committed against Indigenous peoples and signifies the systematic and institutionalized violence that is legitimized by policy, law, and other institutions of government. Colonial trauma has been inflicted on Indigenous peoples for hundreds of years due to the ravages of political interference through dislocation, depopulation, and the systematic repression and interference of culture (Brave Heart, 1998; Brave Heart & DeBruyn, 1998; Brave Heart-Jordan & DeBruyn, 1995; Cohen, 1999; Duran & Duran, 1995; Jilek, 1981; Townsley & Goldstein, 1977).

Colonial trauma persists into the present with a strong historical context. Colonial trauma reflects the long-term nature of the crimes against Indigenous peoples that are neither a brief human aberration, nor a specific historical event. Colonial violence and colonial trauma frame a traumatic era—an era of over five centuries of political assaults against Indigenous peoples (Whitbeck, Adams, Hoyt, & Chen, 2004). To conceptualize Indigenous trauma as colonial trauma as a psychologist or mental health professional is to do two significant things: first to externalize the trauma and second to identify a traumagenic agent.

The focus of this chapter is to look upstream to see what is contributing to the phenomenon of the psycho-social-physical health crisis of the world's Indigenous peoples. In externalizing the trauma and identifying traumagenic agents, we begin to assign social and political agency for the trauma. Colonial trauma is neither natural nor inevitable but rather a socially constructed and politically maintained phenomena in which the sources of trauma are in large part external to the individual, the community, and the culture. The health status of Indigenous peoples should, therefore, no longer be viewed simply as an individual or population health issue but rather as a complex social justice issue with political origins and political and policy solutions (Mitchell & MacLeod, 2014).

Political Pathways

The International Covenant on Economic, Social and Cultural Rights, widely considered as the central instrument of protection for the right to health, recognizes "the right of everyone to the enjoyment of the highest attainable standard of physical and mental health" (art. 12, para. 1). The World Health Organization maintains that most health disparities are avoidable and health disparities representing significant inequalities are unacceptable. Since colonial trauma, as argued here, is a key political determinant of health and a political reality that serves as an explanatory factor for the health inequities borne by Indigenous peoples, then colonialism itself needs to be addressed and taken up within society as a whole and addressed within mental health services. Working toward improving population health and reducing social disparities requires a serious focus on both the social and political determinants of health as well as application of social policy tools and human rights laws available both nationally and internationally.

Shifting the focus and dialogue on Indigenous mental health from the individual to the collective, and from the personal to the political, calls for the development of political pathways to healing. While Canadians as a whole enjoy the benefits and relative security of a social democracy, not all Canadians benefit equally from the social arrangements within Canada. In fact, Canadian Aboriginal peoples experience social, economic, and health conditions comparable to developing nations (Anaya, 2013; Minister of Supply and Services Canada, 1996b; Mitchell & Maracle, 2005; Waldram, Herring, & Young, 2006; Young, 2003).

Increasingly, we need to understand the historical, political, and policy processes that have created the enormous and unacceptable gap between the mental and physical health of Indigenous peoples and settler populations as a social justice issue. There is a growing consensus that we must move beyond an understanding of population health rooted in an analysis of the biological antecedents of health, lifestyle, behaviour choices, and health systems as the primary determinants of health (Loppie Reading & Wien, 2009; Mikkonen & Raphael, 2010). There is an increasing need to adopt a critical social determinant of health perspective to assist in addressing the gross disparities in health status endured by Indigenous communities. The Public Health Agency of Canada has identified a Social Determinants of Health Framework for all populations, which includes twelve determining factors: income and social status, social support networks, education and literacy, employment/working conditions, social environments, physical environments, personal health practices and coping skills, healthy child development, biology and genetic endowment, health services, gender, and culture (Public Health Agency of Canada, 2003). However, issues of systemic racism, policies of assimilation, ongoing land and resource struggles, cultural genocide, and colonial trauma are rarely identified within the dominant culture as explanatory factors in relation to the contemporary Indigenous health crisis. The Public Health Agency's framework falls short of adequately addressing the social-political factors that contribute to the poor health outcomes for Indigenous peoples. Historical and contemporary practices of colonization, land issues, and social policy need to be identified as factors contributing to health status. The social determinants of health need to be significantly modified to include political dimensions, such as globalization, cultural imperialism, government policy, and environmental protection, all of which are critical to protecting and improving the health status of Indigenous populations. There is a need to extend the determinants of the health framework to both social and political determinants as seen in Australian health innovations (Auditor-General, 2010). To address the pervasive impacts of colonial trauma, I propose six political pathways to Indigenous health and wellness: 1) self-determination and decolonization, 2) social policy, 3) protection of territory and environmental protection, 4) resilience and resurgence, 5) reconciliation and reparation, and 6) revitalization.

1. *Self-Determination and Decolonization*

Strongly linked to the mental and physical health of Indigenous peoples is the right to self-determination, which is a fundamental principle of human rights law embodied in the Charter of the United Nations; the International Covenant on Civil and Political Rights; and the International Covenant on Economic, Social and Cultural Rights. Common Article 1, paragraph 1 of these Covenants provides that "all peoples have the rights of self-determination.

By virtue of that right they freely determine their political status and freely pursue their economic, social and cultural development." The issue of sovereignty acknowledges the collective nature of Indigenous health and wellness and privileges Indigenous perspectives on moving from resilience, to reconciliation, and to revitalization.

Canadian Indigenous scholars Alfred and Corntassel (2005) view the path to healing of individuals and collectives as integrally connected to Indigenous engagement with culture, language, and land. They caution against privileging colonialism as the only or most important narrative of Indigenous peoples and urge Indigenous people to focus on reclaiming and engaging in Indigenous culture. They write of four interlocking concepts, "sacred history, ceremonial cycles, language and ancestral homelands," as important for healing (p. 609). They urge people to seek healing in the strengths of their cultures, not waiting for resources, consent, or participation from the colonizer. Significantly, they speak of "zones of refuge that are immune to the reaches of imperialism and globalization" (p. 605) and the importance of decolonization.

> We begin to realize decolonization in a real way when we begin to achieve the re-strengthening of our people as individuals so that these spaces can be occupied by decolonized people living authentic lives . . . true power as Indigenous people ultimately lies in our relationships with our land, relatives, language, and ceremonial life.
>
> (p. 605)

2. *Social Policy*

Access to social and economically supportive living conditions and the protection of environments that promote and sustain individual and community health are issues that are governed by social policy. Social policy is an important avenue for addressing health disparities endured by Indigenous peoples. While "zones of refuge" are critical and Indigenous leadership is essential for political pathways to healing, settler populations also have a responsibility in achieving historical redress, reparation, and reconciliation. As stated in the *Highlights from the Report of the Royal Commission on Aboriginal Peoples* (Minister of Supply and Services Canada, 1996d), redress of the harms of the past and the social and political structures that currently sustain them should not be left to Indigenous people to address alone:

> Just as social problems spring in part from collective experience, so solutions require change at the collective level. Aboriginal people acting alone cannot shift the weight of disadvantage and discrimination. But solutions that lift the weight for Aboriginal people collectively shift it for everyone.
>
> (Minister of Supply and Services Canada, 1996d)

Social policy must be developed to address the social and political origins of community- and population-level health problems rather than solely focusing on and allocating resources to the symptoms of distress and disease (Mitchell & MacLeod, 2014). The improvement of social, economic, and environmental living conditions is a critical vehicle for reducing social stress and improving population health (Loppie Reading & Wien, 2009; Mikkonen & Raphael, 2010). Political engagement and sound social policy, developed in collaboration with the populations they affect, are powerful pathways to addressing colonial trauma and to fostering community conditions for social, emotional, spiritual, and political wellness.

The 1996 Royal Commission on Aboriginal Peoples (RCAP) (Minister of Supply and Services Canada, 1996c) made a number of policy recommendations that were developed through an intensive process of engagement. Participatory policy development is a strategy for culturally relevant redress to a multitude of interlocking social and environmental factors that determine the health status of Indigenous communities. The RCAP participatory process provided important, specific, and powerful policy recommendations to advance the health, well-being, and security of Indigenous peoples in Canada. Recommendations emerging from the *Highlights from the Report of the Royal Commission on Aboriginal Peoples* addressed issues of sovereignty and self-governance, as well as many critical social determinants of health: education, housing, capacity building, and leadership (Minister of Supply and Services Canada, 1996c).

3. Protection of Territory and Environmental Protection

Critical to the process of decolonization is the recognition of the essential importance of land and territory to Indigenous peoples to their very identity and existence. Treaty issues, restitution, and reparation, as well as protection from further displacement through development, expansionism, or environmental degradation and industrial pollution must be addressed through all available political avenues domestically and internationally. It is critical, therefore, to consider the concept of Indigeneity, the unity of Indigenous peoples and their collective rights to their ancestral lands (National Aboriginal Health Organization, 2011). Indigenous societies are culturally, spirituality, and historically connected to their lands in complex ways that non-Indigenous peoples have failed to understand, or simply cannot understand.

> Our knowledge comes from the land, and the destruction of the environment is a colonial manifestation and a direct attack on Indigenous knowledge and Indigenous nationhood . . . In present times environmental destruction of Indigenous territories facilitated by state governments and instituted by large multinational corporations continues to remove Indigenous peoples from the land and prevent Indigenous peoples from living our knowledge.
>
> (Simpson, 2004, pp. 4–5)

To address colonial trauma, to promote the healing of individuals and collectives, the collective relationship to land and territory must be addressed through decolonizing processes that respect the significant cultural relationship to land. Historical treaties and modern-day land claim agreements, environmental protections, and the right to free prior and informed consent regarding development on traditional territories must be honoured in order to protect, preserve, and restore Indigenous lands, resources, cultures, and community wellness.

4. Resilience and Resurgence

Decade after decade, century after century, Indigenous peoples have resisted colonial aggression and colonial interference (Thomas et al., 2015 in press). The initial development of Canada resulted in the decimation of the Indigenous population from approximately two million people at contact to a low of one hundred and fifty thousand. In the past decade, there has been resurgence in the Indigenous population that has now surpassed a population of over one million (Employment and Social Development Canada, 2015). The Aboriginal population currently represents 4.3 percent of the total Canadian population of 34 million (Employment and Social Development Canada, 2015). To discuss the Aboriginal population as 4 percent of the Canadian population minimizes and misrepresents the important presence of First Nation, Inuit, and Métis peoples within the Canadian population, not only because they are the descendants of the First Peoples, but because they represent 23 to 86 percent of the population of the three territories and 15 percent to 16 percent of the population in the provinces of Manitoba and Saskatchewan (Statistics Canada, 2011). This population distribution represents a very strong political force. One of the political opportunities in exercising the identity politics of Indigeneity is to develop national and international partnerships between Indigenous populations to share data collection and tracking systems of social-political determinants of health and outcome data (Smylie & Anderson, 2006) and to lobby collectively for the implementation of the United Nations declaration on the Rights of Indigenous Peoples (Association, I.B. et al., 2011; Mitchell, 2014).

5. Reconciliation and Reparation

In order to heal the wounds of colonial trauma, it will be necessary to acknowledge the nature and impact of colonial relations of the past and the present. The Canadian Truth and Reconciliation Commission (2015) was established to create a record of the residential school experience, to commemorate former residential school students, and to repair relations between Aboriginal and non-Aboriginal peoples. One of the principle tasks was to promote awareness and public education about the Indian residential school system and its impact. As asserted by de Leeuw et al. (2010), "Comprehensive and meaningful decolonization of both Indigenous and settler communities is required in order to heal the deeper 'causes of causes' of health disparities in Canada" (p. 295).

6. Revitalization

Decolonization has been identified as a critical strategy for Indigenous wellness. Indigenous scholars have identified cultural renewal, decolonizing of the mind, and reclaiming languages and Indigenous concepts as critical pathways to cultural revitalization (Anderson et al., 2003; King, Smith, & Gracey, 2009; Kirmayer, Simpson, & Cargo, 2003). The United Nations Declaration of Indigenous Rights is an international document that provides an opportunity for increased political action on addressing colonial trauma and revitalizing Indigenous communities. *Through parallel processes of zones of refuge, public education, and participatory social policy, we may strive to approach the national goal of respectful coexistence and Aboriginal wellness* (Minister of Supply and Services **Canada, 1996c;** Truth and Reconciliation Commission, 2015).

Conclusion

The social and health inequalities borne by Indigenous peoples were identified as a gross social injustice with political pathways to resolution. Acknowledging and addressing both historical and contemporary forms of colonial trauma is a critical mental health strategy to advance the strength and sovereignty of Indigenous peoples. Indigeneity, defined as an essential connection to territorial homelands and to the resistance to and survival of various forms of colonialism and imperialism, was presented as a useful construct to both understand and address colonial trauma. A commitment to culturally appropriate, just, and effective social policies developed in collaboration with affected populations was proposed. Six strategies—1) self-determination and decolonization, 2) social policy, 3) protection of territory and environmental protection, 4) resilience and resurgence, 5) reconciliation and reparation, and 6) revitalization—were identified as political pathways to individual and collective wellness within a larger framework of reconciliation.

References

Alfred, T., & Corntassel, J. (2005). Being indigenous: Resurgences against contemporary colonialism. *Government and Opposition, 40*(4), 597–614.

Anaya, J. (2013). *Report of the Special Rapporteur on the rights of Indigenous peoples, James Anaya* (No. A/HRC/24/41). United Nations Human Rights Council. Retrieved from http://unsr.jamesanaya.org/docs/annual/2013-hrc-annual-report-en.pdf

Anderson, J., Perry, J., Blue, C., Browne, A., Henderson, A., Khan, K., & Smye, V. (2003). "Rewriting" cultural safety within the postcolonial and postnational feminist project. *Advances in Nursing Science, 26*(3), 196–214.

Archibald, L. (2006). *Decolonization and healing: Indigenous experiences in the United States, New Zealand, Australia and Greenland.* Ottawa, ON, Canada: Aboriginal Healing Foundation.

Asch, M. (Ed.) (1997). *Aboriginal and treaty rights in Canada: Essays on law, equity, and respect for difference.* Vancouver, BC: UBC Press.

Association, I. B., et al. (2011). *Understanding and implementing the UN declaration on the rights of indigenous peoples: An introductory handbook.* Winnipeg: Indigenous Bar Association.

Auditor-General, North Coast area health service. (2010). *North Coast area health service: Notes to and forming part of the financial statements for the year ended 30 June 2010.* Retrieved from www.health.nsw.gov.au/publications/Publications/Annual-Report-2009–10 /Financial-Statements-North-Coast-AHS.pdf

Barker, A. J. (2009). The contemporary reality of Canadian imperialism: Settler colonialism and the hybrid colonial state. *The American Indian Quarterly, 33*(3), 325–351.

BBC news online. (2008). Canada apology for Native schools. *British Broadcasting Corporation.*

Blaikie, N. W. H. (2000). *Designing social research: The logic of anticipation.* Cambridge, UK: Polity.

Blondin, G. (1997). *Yamoria the lawmaker: Stories of the dene* (p. 18). Edmonton: NeWest Press.

Brave Heart, M. Y. H. (1998). The return to the sacred path: Healing the historical trauma and historical unresolved grief response among the Lakota through a psychoeducational group intervention. *Smith College Studies in Social Work, 68*(3), 287–305.

Brave Heart, M. Y. H. (1999). Oyate ptayela: Rebuilding the Lakota nation through addressing historical trauma among Lakota parents. *Journal of Human Behaviour and the Social Environment,* 2(1/2), 109–126.

Brave Heart, M. Y. H., & DeBruyn, L. M. (1998). The American Indian holocaust: Healing historical unresolved grief. *American Indian and Alaska Native Mental Health Research, 8*(2), 60–82.

Brave Heart-Jordan, M., & DeBruyn, L. M. (1995). So she may walk in balance: Integrating the impact of historical trauma in the treatment of Native American Indian women. In J. Adleman, & G. Enguidanos (Eds.), *Racism in the lives of women: Testimony, theory, and guides to anti-racist practice* (pp. 345–368). New York, NY: Haworth Press.

Cohen, A. (1999). *The mental health of Indigenous peoples: An international overview.* Retrieved from http://www.who.int.remote.libproxy.wlu.ca/mental_health/media/en/72.pdf (p.7)

de Leeuw, S., Greenwood, M., & Cameron, E. (2010). Deviant constructions: How governments preserve colonial narratives of addictions and poor mental health to intervene into the lives of indigenous children and families in Canada. *International Journal of Mental Health and Addiction, 8*(2), 282–295.

Duran, E. (2006). *Healing the soul wound: Counseling with American Indians and other Native peoples.* New York, NY, US: Teachers College Press.

Duran, E., & Duran, B. (1995). *Native American postcolonial psychology.* New York, NY: New York Press.

Employment and Social Development Canada. (2015). *Indicators of well-being in Canada: Canadians in context—Aboriginal population.* Retrieved from http://well-being.esdc.gc.ca/misme-iowb/.3ndic.1t.4r@-eng.jsp?iid=36

Evans-Campbell, T. (2008). Historical trauma in American Indian/Native Alaska communities: A multilevel framework for exploring impacts on individuals, families, and communities. *Journal of Interpersonal Violence, 23*(3), 316–338.
Fry, B., & Mitchell, T. (2015, in press). Towards coexistence: Exploring the differences between indigenous and non-indigenous perspectives on land. *Native Studies Review.*
Harper, S. (2008, 11 June). *Prime Minister Harper offers full apology on behalf of Canadians for the Indian Residential Schools system.* Office of the Prime Minister, Ottawa, Ontario. Retrieved from http://pm/gc.ca/eng/media.asp?id=2149
Indian and Northern Affairs. (2008). Statement of apology to former students of Indian Residential Schools. Retrieved from https://www.aadnc-aandc.gc.ca/eng/1100100015644/1100100015649
International Covenant on Civil and Political Rights. Adopted and opened for signature, ratification and accession by General Assembly. (16 December 1966) Retrieved from http://www.ohchr.org/en/professionalinterest/pages/ccpr.aspx
International Covenant on Economic, Social, and Cultural Rights. Adopted and opened for signature, ratification and accession by General Assembly. (3 January 1967) Retrieved from http://www.ohchr.org/EN/ProfessionalInterest/Pages/CESCR.aspx
Jilek, W. G. (1981). Anomic depression, alcoholism and a culture-congenial Indian response. *Journal of Studies on Alcohol, 9*, 159–170.
King, M., Smith, A., & Gracey, M. (2009). Indigenous health part 2: The underlying causes of the health gap. *The Lancet, 374*(9683), 76–85. doi: 10.1016/S0140-6736(09)60827-8.
Kipuri, N. (2009). Chapter II: Culture. In *State of the world's indigenous peoples* (pp. 51–81). New York: United Nations publication. Retrieved from http://www.un.org/esa/socdev/unpfii/documents/SOWIP/en/SOWIP_web.pdf
Kirmayer, L. J. (2000). Rethinking psychiatry with indigenous peoples. *Australian and New Zealand Journal of Psychiatry, 34*(S1), A37.
Kirmayer, L., Simpson, C., & Cargo, M. (2003). Healing traditions: Culture, community and mental health promotion with Canadian Aboriginal peoples. *Australasian Psychiatry, 11*, 15–23.
Loomba, A. (2005). *Colonialism/postcolonialism.* New York, NY: Routledge.
Loppie Reading, C., & Wien, F. (2009). *Health inequities and social determinants of Aboriginal peoples' health.* Prince George: National Collaborating Centre for Aboriginal Health.
Manson, S., Beals, J., O'Nell, T., Piasecki, J., Bechtold, D., Keane, E., & Jones, M. (Eds.). (1996). *Wounded spirits, ailing hearts: PTSD and related disorders among American Indians* Washington, DC: American Psychological Association.
McGregor, D. (2004). Traditional ecological knowledge and sustainable development: Towards coexistence. In M. Blaser, H. A. Feit, & G. McRae (Eds.), *The way of development: Indigenous peoples, life projects and globalization* (pp. 72–91). London, UK: Zed Books Ltd.
Mikkonen, J., & Raphael, D. (2010). *Social determinants of health: The Canadian facts.* Toronto, ON, Canada: York University School of Health Policy and Management.
Miller, J. R. (2004). *Lethal legacy: Current Native controversies in Canada.* Toronto, ON, Canada: McClelland & Stewart Ltd.
Minister of Supply and Services Canada, Highlights from the Report of the Royal Commission on Aboriginal Peoples. (1996a). *People to people, nation to nation,*

Chapter 1: Looking Forward, Looking Back (Cat no. Z1–1991/1–6E). Retrieved from http://www.aadnc-aandc.gc.ca/eng/1100100014597/1100100014637

Minister of Supply and Services Canada, Highlights from the Report of the Royal Commission on Aboriginal Peoples. (1996b). *People to people, nation to nation, Chapter 2: Restructuring the Relationship* (Cat no. Z1–1991/1–6E). Retrieved from http://www.aadnc-aandc.gc.ca/eng/1100100014597/1100100014637

Minister of Supply and Services Canada, Highlights from the Report of the Royal Commission on Aboriginal Peoples. (1996c). *People to people, nation to nation, Chapter 3: Gathering Strength* (Cat no. Z1–1991/1–6E). Retrieved from http://www.aadnc-aandc.gc.ca/eng/1100100014597/1100100014637

Minister of Supply and Services Canada, Highlights from the Report of the Royal Commission on Aboriginal Peoples. (1996d). *People to people, nation to nation, Chapter 4: Perspectives and realities* (Cat no. Z1–1991/1–6E). Retrieved from http://www.aadnc-aandc.gc.ca/eng/1100100014597/1100100014637

Mitchell, T. (2011). *Colonial trauma and pathways to healing, Canadian psychological association convention*, June 2–4, 2011, Toronto, ON, Ontario.

Mitchell, T. (2014). *International gaze brings critical focus to questions about indigenous rights and governance in Canada.* CIGI Special Report The Internationalization of Indigenous Rights: UNDRIP in the Canadian Context, 43–47.

Mitchell, T. (2015 in press). Colonial Trauma: Complex, continuous, collective, cumulative and Compounding. In J. Stone, & T. Wise (Eds.), *Intergenerational trauma in Indian country*. Arizona, US: University of Arizona Press.

Mitchell, T., & MacLeod, T. (2014). Aboriginal Social Policy: A critical community mental health issue. *Canadian Journal of Community Mental Health, 33*(1), 109–122.

Mitchell, T. L. (1996). *Old wounds, new beginnings: Challenging the missionary paradigm in Native-White relations, a cross-cultural perspective on sexual abuse service development in a Yukon community* (Doctoral dissertation). Retrieved from Scholar's Portal.

Mitchell, T. L., & Maracle, D. T. (2005). Healing the generations: Post-traumatic stress and the health status of Aboriginal populations in Canada. *Journal of Aboriginal Health, 2*(1), 14–24.

National Aboriginal Health Organization. (2011, July 25). *Holistic health and traditional knowledge.* Retrieved from http://www.naho.ca/blog/2011/07/25/holistic-health-and-traditional-knowledge/

Public Health Agency of Canada. (2003). What Makes Canadians Healthy or Unhealthy. Retrieved from http://www.phac-aspc.gc.ca/ph-sp/determinants/determinants-eng.php. (Retrieved, June 6th, 2011).

Simpson, L. R. (2004). Anticolonial strategies for the recovery and maintenance of indigenous knowledge. *American Indian Quarterly, 28*(3–4), 373–384. Retrieved from http://www.nebraskapress.unl.edu.remote.libproxy.wlu.ca/product/American-Indian-Quarterly,673174.aspx

Smylie, J., & Anderson, M. (2006). Understanding the health of indigenous peoples in Canada: Key methodological and conceptual challenges. *Canadian Medical Association Journal, 175*(6), 602–605.

Stannard, D. E. (1992). *American holocaust: Columbus and the conquest of the new world*. New York, NY, US: Oxford University Press.

Statistics Canada, National Household Survey. (2011). *Aboriginal peoples in Canada: First Nations People, Métis and Inuit* (catalogue no. 99–011-X2011001).

Retrieved from Statistics Canada website: http://www12.statcan.gc.ca/nhs-enm/2011/as-sa/99–011-x/99–011-x2011001-eng.cfm#a2

Study of the problem of discrimination against indigenous populations, 21 Chapter: Conclusions, proposals and recommendations. Final report submitted by the Special Rapporteur, Mr. José Martínez Cobo UN Doc. No. E/CN.4/Sub.2/1983/21/Add.8 (30 September 1983)

Thomas, D., Mitchell, T., & Arseneau, C. (2016). Re-evaluating "resilience": From individual vulnerabilities to the strength of cultures and collectivities among indigenous communities. *Resilience: International policies, practices and discourses, 4*(2), 116–129.

Townsley, H. C., & Goldstein, G. S. (1977). One view of the etiology of depression in the American Indian. *Public Health Reports, 92*(5), 458–461.

Truth and Reconciliation Commission. (2015). *Honouring the truth, reconciling for the future: Summary of the final report of the Truth and Reconciliation Commission of Canada*. Retrieved from www.trc.ca/websites/ . . . /**2015**/ . . . /Exec_Summary_**2015**_05_31_web_o.pdf

Waldram, J. B., Herring, D. A., & Young, T. K. (2006). *Aboriginal health in Canada: Historical, cultural, and epidemiological perspectives*, 2nd ed. Toronto, ON, Canada: University of Toronto Press Incorporated.

Whitbeck, L. B., Adams, G. W., Hoyt, D. R., & Chen, X. (2004). Conceptualizing and measuring historical trauma among American Indian people. *American Journal of Community Psychology, 33*(3), 119–130.

Young, T. K. (2003). Review of research on Aboriginal populations in Canada: Relevance to their health needs. *British Medical Journal, 327*(7412), 419–423.

Part 4

North

Healing Through Western and Indigenous Knowledges

11 Cultures in Collision

"Higher" Education and the Clash Between Indigenous and Non-Indigenous "Ways of Knowing"

Michael Chandler

This chapter is all about the "worldviews" and "epistemic practices" common to many Indigenous learners, as well as how such distinct "ways of knowing" likely shape the ongoing educational prospects of Canada's contemporary First Nations, Métis, and Inuit students. Although such culturally driven "beliefs about belief" will be argued to contribute to many of the academic missteps that stymie Indigenous learners on every rung of the usual educational ladder, special attention will be focused here on the common difficulties faced by those who, against the odds, have succeeded in gaining admission to institutions of "higher" learning.

The broad thesis to be explored here is that, rather than being counted as fair commentary on the competencies of individual students, the whole panoply of academic difficulties encountered by Indigenous learners is better understood as the aftermath of a drive-by shooting—a collective wound inflicted in the course of that ongoing cultural war still being waged against those whose "ways of knowing" are foreign to, and regularly at odds with, what Rorty (1987) has called the dominant "Judeo-Graeco-Roman-Christian-Renaissance-Enlightenment-Romanticist" (p. 57) framework of understanding that, over centuries, has dominated mainstream Eurocentric educational practice.

Any serious attempt to defend the possible merits of this thesis—the idea that the educational inequities suffered by Indigenous learners are part and parcel of an across-the-board effort to discount the very possibility of bona fide Indigenous ways of knowing—requires persuading you of a minimum of at least *three* things.

The *first* of these arguments is easily, if painfully, won, and only requires rehearsing that familiar litany of defamatory statistics regularly used to demonstrate that, in comparison to their culturally mainstream counterparts, Indigenous learners too often prove to be academic underachievers, too frequently leave school at a tender age, and are sorely underrepresented among those who graduate from high school, or succeed at various levels of postsecondary training. If there are any remaining surprises in these well-rehearsed educational woes, it is, perhaps, that something like half of those Indigenous students who do make it all the way to some institution of "higher" learning regularly end up leaving empty handed, without the "degree" that they and their communities had so much hoped for (DeGagné, 2002). In short, the common plight of far too many Indigenous learners is a recurrent story of lost opportunities and failed prospects—failures that, if anything, increase in volume and volubility in the ideologically driven world of postsecondary education. In what follows, only a short and beginning space will be allotted to rehearse these grim statistics.

The *second* and more expansive of the arguments to be detailed here takes the form of a synopsis of those emerging lines of argument meant to persuade you that Indigenous persons, in Canada and around the world, actually do subscribe to distinctive ways of knowing, or folk epistemologies that set them apart from, and put them at a serious educational disadvantage relative to, their non-Indigenous counterparts. Unfortunately, the state of the available evidence required to substantiate these claims continues to be too anecdotal, too loosely observational, too casually ethnographic, too dependent upon the reports of one-off knowledge stewards, and, otherwise, too reliant upon introspective accounts to successfully persuade the "tougher minded" empiricists among us. At the same time, however, the full body of this newly emerging literature—all given over to supporting the proposition that Indigenous persons commonly hold to paradigmatic frameworks, worldviews, tacit epistemologies, and, more loosely, distinctive "ways of knowing"—is, nevertheless, too detailed, too internally consistent, and too convergent to be casually set aside for the sake of some narrow allegiance to any otherwise tighter-lipped species of scientific rigor. For such reasons, a substantial part of this chapter will be given over to a rough accounting of the multiple claims currently being made in favour of the existence of such distinctively Indigenous ways of knowing.

In the *third* and concluding part of this chapter, an attempt will be made to "connect the dots" by arguing that responsibility for many of the educational shortfalls that defeat some, but of course not all, Indigenous learners can be legitimately laid at the door of all those who insist that anything short of a full, root-and-branch conversion to classic Eurocentric beliefs about belief is equivalent to a stubborn refusal to take advantage of what *bona fide* Westernized knowledge is widely imagined to be. The chapter will end with a gesture in the direction of the sort of research program that would seem to be required if existing claims about Indigenous ways of knowing are to be taken with new seriousness by the usual guardians of Western scientific respectability.

On Falling Short of Eurocentric Standards of Academic Success

As is generally known, major disparities between the health and general well-being of Indigenous and non-Indigenous groups are commonly found across the whole of the postcolonial world (cf. Battiste, 2002; Durie, 2006).

Canada, despite its privileged social and economic status, offers no exception. Just about every bad thing one might imagine happening has been shown to happen more often and more vengefully within Indigenous communities. So much so, in fact, that there is suspect merit in repeating, even one more time, this or that litany of woes. Increasingly, among those most opposed to the constant rehearsing of such shortcomings are Indigenous persons themselves, many of whom are rightly concerned that the relentless tallying up of such miseries threatens to become part of the problem, rather than its solution.

What is not, however, repeated nearly enough is that, notwithstanding generic disparities commonly known to count against Indigenous communities (including the educational disparities to be featured here), available evidence already makes it plain that the educational and sundry other social ills routinely regarded as "epidemic" throughout much of the Indigenous world are not uniformly distributed across Canada's (or anyone else's) many Indigenous communities (cf. Chandler & Lalonde, 1998, 2009; Chandler, Lalonde, Sokol, & Hallett, 2003). When viewed at the band level, for example, the rates of school failures, accidents, and youth suicides for more than half of the communities studied prove to be equal to, and sometimes lower than, those found in the general population (Chandler & Lalonde, 2009; Hallett et al., 2008). Because more generic numbers aggregated at the level of whole provinces or whole countries only partially lie, the opposite is, of course, also true. In many Indigenous communities, health and social problems really are present in epidemic proportions—rates so high that, when added to the running average, the resulting summary statistics often prove to be as alarming as they are misleading. To take only a brace of examples from British Columbia (BC), province-wide rates of youth suicide (said to be five to twenty times the national average), or school dropout rates (widely reported to exceed 60 percent), although arithmetically real enough, actually describe only a small handful of communities, while many others have no suicides and produce a proportionate number of high school graduates (Chandler et al., 2003; Hallett et al., 2008). All of this evidence of radical variability in the health and well-being of various Indigenous communities makes it plain that easy generalizations about the world's, or Canada's, or BC's Indigenous groups amount to little more than "actuarial fictions"—synthetic numbers that obscure the fact that, whatever else may be going on, the various ills in question are clearly not features of indignity as such, but merely serve instead to characterize some communities and not others.

All such cautionary tales about the dangers of generalizing across the whole of any Indigenous world notwithstanding, it nevertheless continues to be true that the prospects—including the educational prospects—of an unacceptably large number of Indigenous persons remain unacceptably bleak. Across Canada, embarrassingly few First Nations, Métis, and Inuit students enjoy a fair measure of educational parity or success at any grade level. Notwithstanding the unsatisfactory and obscurant ways in which "Aboriginal" status is officially determined, the continuing failures of

Canada's educational systems to adequately address the training and educational needs of the Indigenous population are, on balance, so profound and so unconscionable as to be beyond all serious dispute (Castellano, Davis, & Lahache, 2000).

Across the country's more than six hundred First Nations bands, generic differences continue to be present at effectively every level of educational achievement (Applied Research Branch, HRDC, 2000). Although, as hinted at earlier, there do exist scattered communities in which Indigenous students are known to outperform their non-Aboriginal counterparts (cf. Hallett et al., 2008), the more generic picture is one of chronically inequitable treatment, academic failure, and lost educational opportunities. In BC, for example, First Nations learners of all ages regularly underperform on standardized achievement measures, dropout of school at surprisingly tender ages, graduate from high school at a rate less than half of that of their non-Indigenous counterparts, and are dramatically underrepresented in the province's more than fifty institutions of "higher" learning (DeGagné, 2002).

Evidence for these discrepancies can be found at every rung in the educational ladder. Again, in BC, the 2003 dropout rate for "Aboriginal" youth was 57 percent—compared to a counterpart rate for non-Aboriginals of only 2 percent (BC Ministry of Education, 2003) and, according to the *Report of the Royal Commission on Aboriginal Peoples. Vol.1* (1996), those Indigenous students that do drop out tend to do so early—typically between grades seven and ten. Although there has been modest improvement in these figures—only five years earlier the BC provincial Aboriginal dropout rate was 66.2 percent—the gap between these two cultural groups continues to widen (DeGagné, 2002), especially for those youth living on reservations.

Similarly, the overall rate of high school graduation among First Nations youth across Canada is commonly reported to be less than 30 percent (Council of Ministers of Education, 2002), compared to approximately 70 percent for the general population. In BC, for example, First Nations' learners again graduate from high school at rates less than half that of their culturally mainstream counterparts (British Columbia Ministry of Education, 2003).

The transition from high school graduation to college admission is equally problematic. Recent evidence compiled by the University of Victoria indicates that of the approximately three thousand college-age First Nations students currently in BC, less than three hundred will actually gain admission to some sort of postsecondary training, and fewer still will emerge with a degree. By all of these measures, then, the unmet training and educational needs of Indigenous learners are beyond dispute.

Although all of these lost opportunities obviously need to be redressed, the problems associated with the low numbers of Indigenous persons who successfully gain admission to and eventually graduate from institutions of higher learning are, perhaps, the most sorely felt. Over and above all of the familiar reasons that go along with squandering this resource, there is a broad consensus, within both Indigenous communities and the larger society, that "building capacity" through the successful professional training of Indigenous learners is a key requirement for hurrying the day when Indigenous groups regain real control over their own lives. Consequently, every Indigenous learner who fails to gain entry to some postsecondary educational program, or is otherwise left stranded along the educational wayside, is a serious brake upon all agreed upon wheels of progress.

The actual magnitude of the problem of producing a fair proportion of Indigenous college graduates is widely recognized (Council of Ministers of Education, 2002), but poorly documented. Although the number of First Nations learners enrolled in any sort of postsecondary educational program has, for example, increased dramatically (from only 60 in 1961 to 27,100 in 1997–1998), it continues to be the case that Indigenous persons remain among the least successful postsecondary students in North America (DeGagné, 2002). According to DeGagné (2002), while the percentage of the Canadian Indigenous population holding a university degree increased between 1988 and 2003 from 2.6 percent to 4.5 percent, the counterpart numbers for the non-Aboriginal population are almost four times higher. More broadly still, as of 2006 (Statistics Canada), of all Indigenous persons of working age (between twenty-five and sixty-four years), only 8 percent held university degrees, compared to 23 percent for the rest of the Canadian population. Similar comparison of the proportions of the same populations completing community and technical college diplomas also shows the same increasing disparity (Castellano et al., 2000). These unconscionable gaps are even larger for the postgraduate and professional educational levels.

Considerably less well known than data concerned with the low admissions and graduation rates among Indigenous learners is the fact that, of all those who do successfully apply to institutions of "higher" learning, less than half actually stay the course and obtain the degrees for which they, and their communities, have held out so much hope (DeGagné, 2002). Doing the math, every Indigenous learner with a degree in hand stands on the shoulders of twenty-five or more others whose early academic aspirations were defeated somewhere along the hard road to postsecondary graduation.

Although responsibility for these educational disparities is, no doubt, broadly shared, credible explanations that do not "blame the victim" by assigning such failures to some imagined shortcoming on the part of Indigenous learners themselves, remain thin on the ground. Setting such racist accounts to the side, any shortlist of alternative explanations would, according to DeGagné (2002), need to include efforts to erase existing a) funding barriers, b) ambivalent attitudes towards formal education on the part of many Indigenous groups owed to the legacy of residential schools, c) inadequate preparation from kindergarten to grade 12, and d) lack of appropriate role models or family support.

Beyond all of these sometimes reasonable prospects, a further and little explored possibility is that some important part of all of the educational difficulties faced by Indigenous learners can be usefully understood as a direct consequence of an intolerance for what is thought to be distinctive about the tacit epistemologies or culturally sanctioned ways of knowing common to many Indigenous groups. On such accounts, there are, to quote the contemporary philosopher Steven Stich (1990), "no intrinsic epistemic virtues," (p. 01) only historically informed differences in the distinctive ways that diverse cultural groups have come to understand the knowing process—differences that become increasingly problematic when control over the whole architecture of education is determined unilaterally by practitioners of only one of these warring worldviews.

If, on this view, Indigenous learners routinely subscribe to "epistemological frameworks" or *ways of knowing* that are importantly different from those commonly practiced within the cultural mainstream, and *if* the forms of pedagogy to which such students are routinely exposed are typically set within knowledge frameworks that Indigenous learners experience as foreign and hostile, *then* trouble is automatically afoot, and school failures and lost educational opportunities are sure to follow.

In light of this open prospect, it becomes a matter of first importance to become as clear as contemporary scholarship allows about what it could possibly mean to hold to any one of potentially many "Indigenous ways of knowing." Part Two, to follow, explores the existing literature concerning such proposed "Indigenous epistemologies."

Epistemologies in General and Indigenous Epistemologies in Particular

Epistemic Violence

Given the chronically subjugated status of Indigenous peoples, and the long history of epistemic violence directed against their ways of being, it should come as no great surprise that such groups often show themselves to be mistrustful and less than welcoming of whatever appears next in the ongoing train of government initiatives meant to improve their lot—initiatives, all of which are alleged, in their turn, to be just what the doctor ordered. Alternatively, as postcolonial and colonial discourse analysts would have it (cf. Duran & Duran, 1995; Fanon, 1965; Gandhi, 1998; Said, 1978), knowledge invented in London or New York City or Ottawa and rudely transplanted root and branch into someone else's back yard is often and rightly understood to be just another flexing of the dominant culture's "technologies of power" (Foucault, 1980)—another weapon wielded by those who have such power against those who must suffer it.

A usual key plank in the platform of such critical accounts is that conquering cultures routinely work to brand "indigenes" as childlike, to label their knowledge systems as mere superstitions, and to reframe their own attempts to colonize the life-worlds of conquered peoples as well intended educative or civilizing missions (Gandhi, 1998), all generously aimed at dragging some otherwise "stone-aged" peoples (often kicking and screaming) into the "modern" world. Such acts of "epistemic violence," whatever else they may do, guarantee the positional inferiority of Indigenous people, further marginalize their voices, and undermine any possibility that they might be seen to know how to best manage their own affairs and educate their own children. Instead, such fundamentally elitist views especially promote the idea that serious thoughts about how education ought best to proceed, and what is to account as true knowledge, all ends up being regarded as the exclusive province of culturally mainstream experts.

Not surprisingly, objections to such assimilatory practices are growing in volume and volubility. Owed in important part to what has become an international renaissance in Indigenous scholarship, Aboriginal philosophers, ethnologists, and social historians have as part of this resistance movement recently mounted ambitious efforts to document and give equal pride of place to their own non-Western systems of knowledge (cf. Del, 2009; Ermine, 1995; Foley, 2003; Gegeo, 2001; Meyer, 2001; Ogbor, 2000; Quanchi, 2004; Rigney, 1999; Smith, 2005; West, 1998; and many others). In particular, an international cadre of First Nations, Maori, Pacific Islander, and Australian Aboriginal scholars have collectively sparked a recent explosion of new interest in the distinctive ways in which Indigenous groups think about the process of knowledge acquisition.

As one might expect, these far-flung accounts, often fail to speak with a single voice. The relevant literature is, for example, replete with regular talk of "foundational epistemologies," "empirical epistemologies," "natural epistemologies," and "subjectivist research epistemologies," not to mention "anti-colonial epistemologies" (Foley, 2003), "emancipatory epistemologies" (Rigney, 1997), and "Kaupapa Maori epistemologies" (Smith, 2005).

All of these and sundry other candidate possibilities aside it, nevertheless, appears to be generally agreed upon that Indigenous and non-Indigenous epistemologies of every stripe necessarily represent accounts that, as the "Native" Hawaiian scholar Gegeo points out, are concerned

> with who can be a knower, what can be known, what constitutes knowledge, sources of evidence for constructing knowledge, what constitutes truth, how truth is verified, how evidence becomes true, how valid inferences are to be drawn, and the role of belief in evidence, and related issues.
>
> (1998, p. 290)

As thus understood, the several foundational epistemologies that have dominated the more analytic branches of 20th century Anglo-American philosophy and science turn out to have played to extremely poor reviews among many Indigenous scholars. Such criticisms are owed primarily to the complex relations that are assumed to obtain between spirituality, land, power, and knowledge—relations that give talk of epistemology as an almost inescapable political character. According to Rigney (1997, p. 113), for example, epistemologies found to operate within the mainstream of Euro-American thought have all "been constructed essentially for and by non-Indigenous persons," and, as a result, are widely deemed to be discriminatory, gender-biased, ethnocentrically determined, and ideologically controlled (cf. Ogbor, 2000).

Because it "barters [well] within the currency of mainstream academia" (Meyer, 2001, p. 146), however, many contemporary Indigenous scholars have chosen not to abandon the widely suspect study of epistemology, but instead to "decolonize" and re-"color" such efforts by taking up the task of "rediscovering and reaffirming" (Rigney, 1999, p. 113) what are held out to be Indigenous ways of knowing. Reclaimed in these ways, the study of Indigenous epistemologies is, according to Meyer (2001, p. 125), widely regarded, not only as a "sword against anthropological arrogance and [a] shield against philosophical universalisms," but as a key plank in the shared platform of Indigenous studies programs.

Despite this growing concert of opinion, with rare exceptions, the great bulk of contemporary Indigenous scholarship has relied, up to the present, almost exclusively upon introspection, informal observations, and key informants or traditional knowledge stewards as sources for such insights. What is largely missing from this burgeoning literature are programs of *empirical* research that might serve to help test or further elaborate existing claims concerning such distinctive Indigenous ways of knowing. Beginning thoughts about how such more dedicated empirical efforts might be undertaken will be briefly hinted out in Part Three. Before any of this, however, more attention still needs to be focused on what are most commonly held out to be the defining differences that set Indigenous *epistemologies* apart from other aspects of Indigenous *knowledge systems*.

Demarcation Criteria

Notwithstanding certain obvious differences between the claims of often widely scattered Indigenous scholars, there, nevertheless, appears to be a subset of common *demarcation criteria* most often said to differentiate Indigenous epistemologies from other concepts. Key among these are that Indigenous epistemologies—in contrast to those deemed to characterize the Anglo, Judeo-Christian, post-Enlightenment, Eurocentric West—are said to "stand in binary opposition to 'scientific,' 'western,' 'Eurocentric,' or 'modern' systems of knowing" (Battiste, 2002); to be *holistic* rather than *analytic* (Ermine, 1995; West, 1998); to be *context-sensitive* and especially moved by immediate circumstance and lived experiences (Rigney, 1999); to describe physical geography as a foundational stone of Indigenous knowledge building (Quanchi, 2004); to make room for the *sacred* as opposed to only the physical and human worlds (Whitt, 2009); to view prayers, rituals, and ceremonies as links to this spiritual world providing relevant guidance to sacred knowledge; to consider "the people of the animal and plant world

[as] stewards to certain doors of knowledge" (Ermine, 1995, p. 106); to regard knowledge as ecologically situated and unique to specific knowledge systems and settings (Gegeo, 2001); and to count among the "epistemological agents," whole *communities* rather than only *individuals*, and true knowledge as the result of a process that can only be validated by cultural groups (Gegeo, 2001).

Although certain of these claimants would appear to have been, perhaps, injudiciously "lured" (Foley, 2003) by the liberationary agendas of various critical sociologies and post-positivist philosophies (Battiste, 2002) and so run the risk of recreating the "other" by mistakenly rough sorting everyone into opposing halves of the same false Indigenous versus non-Indigenous dichotomy (or by wrongly imagining that "indigenes," wherever one finds them, all occupy the same quasi-universalistic, pan-Indian horizon), it nevertheless remains the case that several common and testable themes run through these deeply felt either-or accounts. Over and above the claims that Indigenous worldviews are somehow more normative or "spiritual," such broadly shared assumptions also include the more readily testable convictions that Indigenous epistemologies subscribe to a) an *"incremental"* as opposed to an *"entity*-based" view of learning (Dweck, 2006); b) tend to be *holistic* rather than *analytic* (Masuda & Nisbett, 2001; Nisbett, Peng, Choi, & Norenzayan, 2001); c) *particularistic* versus *universalistic*, or more *context-dependent* than *independen*t (Nisbett, 2003); d) more *subjective*, as opposed to *objective* (Norenzayan, Choi, & Peng, 2007); and e) more *narrative-like* than *essentialistic* in their usual patterns of thought (Chandler et al., 2003).

Connecting the Dots

What the proceeding section was meant to make clear is that, while much that has been said about Indigenous epistemologies, or ways of knowing, may not yet satisfy the "tough minded" standards of proof demanded by the *academy*, it nevertheless continues to be true that there is a surprising concert of opinion about what it might and might not mean to view the world through such Indigenous lenses. If any half of these recurrent insights can be shown to stand up to more rigorous scrutiny, then those charged with shaping the future course of existing educational practices would be obliged to introduce real change. That is, *if* it were the case that the particulars of various Indigenous knowledge systems were already well understood and documented, and otherwise shown to be as distinct as the scholars cited earlier regularly claim, and *if*, in some imagined spirit of intercultural sharing and mutual respect, there was a sufficient public appetite for real educational change, *then* everyone's marching orders would be reasonably straightforward. As Marlene Brant-Castellano made clear in the 1996 Report of the *Royal Commission on Aboriginal Peoples*:

> For Aboriginal people the challenge [would be] to go beyond the deconstruction of oppressive ideologies and practices [and], to give expression

> to aboriginal philosophies, world-views, and social relations. For non-Aboriginal people the challenge [would be] to open up space for Aboriginal initiatives in schools and colleges, work sites and organizations so that Indigenous ways of knowing can flourish.
>
> (p. 23)

Unhappily, this appears not to be the world in which we currently live. Even where openness to change and mutual respect does exist in sufficient supply, it still remains the case, according to Battiste (2002), that "when educators encounter [such] cultural differences, they have very little theory, scholarship, research, or tested practice to engage Aboriginal education in a way that is not [strictly] assimilative" (p. 9). As a consequence, contemporary education practices—especially "higher" education practices—are too often reduced to a form of proselytizing aimed at converting Indigenous learners to a way of thinking that is not their own. The result is that, for far too many such students, the available options are seen to reduce to a "Hobson's choice" between reluctantly abandoning their hopes for academic success or committing to a form of intellectual assimilation that threatens both their personal identity and the persistence of their culture. Many (roughly half) would appear to count the obligation to renounce their Indigenous ways of knowing as too high a price to pay and choose to end their struggles for a postsecondary degree as simply the lesser of two evils. If we are to free Indigenous learners from the horns of this dilemma, then what seems required is some repair for what Battiste describes as our still missing body of required theory, scholarship, and research. The open questions are, of course, what theory, what sorts of research, and scholarship barking up what sort of tree?

At present, there is, of course, more than a little ongoing research given over to studying the utilities of Indigenous "head start" programs, the efficacy of "Indigenizing" middle school and high school curricula, and the problem of early school leaving. Similarly, as DeGagné (2002) has suggested, still others are currently focusing research attention on the existing shortage of appropriate role models, or the corrosive effects of institutional racism. While all of these things are of critical importance and obviously need to be done, they are not, I suggest, the only or perhaps even the best first place to concentrate our scarce resources.

Among the reasons for suggesting that this is true are the facts that arranging for a minimally acceptable K–12 educational experience, eliminating racism, or otherwise supplying appropriate numbers of appropriate role models are all necessary, but amount to slow work at best. Rather, and in the short run, I would propose that the most efficacious and best theory-guided point of entry into the "capacity building" problem facing Indigenous communities lies along a path that directs special attention on that roughly 50 percent of Indigenous learners who have already succeeded in gaining entry to some institution of higher learning, but who, nevertheless, end up leaving empty handed, without the degree or certificate they sought. Any measure of success with these "earlier college leavers"—these students that have somehow managed, against odds, to overcome whatever handicaps might have otherwise undermined their earlier educational efforts, and who have already earned their way into colleges and universities—are role models in waiting and offer the quickest possible "fix" to the common "lack of capacity" that hamstrings the efforts of Indigenous communities to lift themselves up by their own bootstraps.

Despite their other unique qualifications, it is these same students who also face the most challenging of confrontations between their own Indigenous ways of knowing and the Eurocentric epistemologies that especially govern the inner workings of many or most institutions of higher learning. There is no doubt that the differences between the tacit epistemologies of students and their teachers also operate at every other rung of the educational ladder, but nowhere are such differences likely to count as much as they do in the inner sanctum of the "academy"—ground zero of what Battiste (2002) has called the natural home of the "classic Eurocentric order of life" (p. 2). In short, it is, I propose, postsecondary learners who need to be counted as the worst casualties of the ongoing collision between contrasting beliefs about belief and the best prospects for telling researchers what they need to know in order to make a difference.

This hypothesis—the proposition that the "failure to launch" common to so many Indigenous postsecondary students is not the result of some contest between the more and less able, but is better understood as symptomatic of an ongoing clash between combatants in a paradigm struggle between those who do and do not subscribe to the Eurocentric assumptions that drive Western conceptions of knowledge—is increasingly open to test.

An important part of such optimism about the timeliness of undertaking serious research into possible differences between the "folk" epistemologies of Indigenous and non-Indigenous learners is owed to the fact that of late, and largely behind the backs of contributors to literature outlined in Part Two, other armies of more culturally mainstream researchers have been hard at work honing a variety of measurement tools meant to cut through more casual observations and to rigorously document differences in the tacit epistemologies of various age and cultural groups. To date, almost all of these investigators have focused their attention on possible differences between North American and Asian college-age students. While none of these investigators has made Indigenous epistemologies the focus of their research efforts, they have developed a large cache of well-oiled measurement tools that, with proper attention to matters of "cultural safety," could well be brought to bear in carrying out a close-hauled program of empirical research meant to explore those distinctive "ways of knowing" thought to divide Indigenous and non-Indigenous postsecondary learners.

This is not the place to expand upon such a possible research undertaking. What has, however, hopefully been made clearer than it was at the outset of this chapter are the serious prospects a) that some important part of the ills currently facing First Nations, Métis, and Inuit communities is owed to an ongoing culture war in which many of the worst casualties are Indigenous learners; b) that among the several campaigns still being waged against the world's Indigenous populations, perhaps the most hard fought are those between the many who wish to champion and others intent upon eradicating what are being increasingly held up as distinctive Indigenous ways of knowing; c) that a promising and convergent account, due to a recent renaissance in Indigenous scholarship, is beginning to emerge that gives substance to what talk of Indigenous epistemologies may be talk about; and, finally, d) that current circumstance afoot in the world of contemporary cross-cultural research conspires to make programmatic research into the particulars of Indigenous ways of knowing and their relations to Indigenous education newly possible.

References

Applied Research Branch, Strategic Policy, Human Resources Development Canada (HRDC). (2000). *Dropping out of high school: Definitions and costs.* Available Online: http://www11.sdc.gc.ca/en/cs/sp/hrsdc/arb/publications/research/2000–000063/r-01–01e.pdf

Battiste, M. (2002). *Indigenous knowledge and pedagogy in First Nations Education-A literature review with recommendations.* Report prepared for the National Working Group on Education, Indian and Northern Affairs Canada, Ottawa, ON.

British Columbia Ministry of Education. (2003). *How are we doing? Demographics and performance of Aboriginal students in B.C. public schools.* Available Online: http://www.bced.gov.bc.ca/abed/performance.htm

Castellano, M. B., Davis, L., & Lahache, L. (Eds.) (2000). *Aboriginal education: Fulfilling the promise.* Vancouver: UBC Press.

Chandler, M. J., & Lalonde, C. E. (1998). Cultural continuity as a hedge against suicide in Canada's First Nations. *Transcultural Psychiatry, 35*(2), 191–219.

Chandler, M. J., & Lalonde, C. E. (2009). Cultural continuity as a moderator of suicide risk among Canada's First Nations. In L. J. Kirmayer, & G. G. Valaskakis (Eds.), *Healing traditions: The mental health of Aboriginal peoples in Canada* (pp. 221–248). Vancouver, BC: UBC Press.

Chandler, M. J., Lalonde, C. E., Sokol, B. W., & Hallett, D. (2003). Personal persistence, identity, and suicide: A study of Native and non-Native North American adolescents. *Monographs for the Society for Research in Child Development, 68*(2), 1–138.

Council of Ministers of Education. (2002). *Best practices in increasing Aboriginal postsecondary enrolment rates.* Victoria: The Council of Ministers of Education.

DeGagné, M. (2002). Of Successful First Nations Students in Canadian Post Secondary Education. Doctoral dissertation, Michigan State University.

Dei, G. J. S., & Simmons, M. (2009). The indigenous As a Site of decolonizing knowledge about conventional development and the link with education: The case of ghana. In Jonathan Langdon (Ed.), *Indigenous knowledge, development and education* (pp. 15–36). Rotterdam: Sense Publishers.

Duran, E., & Duran, B. (1995). *Native American Postcolonial Psychology.* Albany: State University of New York Press.

Durie, M. (2006). Indigenous resilience: *From disease and disadvantage to the realization of potential.* [CONGRESS PAPER]. Rapu Oranga Pacific Region Indigenous Doctors Congress.

Dweck, C. (2006). *Mindset.* New York: Randomhouse Inc.

Ermine, W. J. (1995). Aboriginal epistemology. In M. Battiste, & J. Barman (Eds.), *First Nations Education in Canada: The circle unfolds* (pp. 101–112). Vancouver, Canada: University of British Columbia Press.

Fanon, F. (1965). *A dying colonialism* (H. Chevaliar, Trans.). New York: Grove Press.

Foley, D. (2003). Indigenous epistemology and indigenous standpoint theory. *Social Alternatives, 22*(1), 44–52.

Foucault, M. (1980). George canguilhem: Philosopher of error. *Ideology and Consciousness, 7*, 53–54.

Gandhi, L. (1998). *Postcolonial theory: A critical introduction.* New York: Columbia University Press.

Gegeo, D. W. (1998). Indigenous knowledge and empowerment: Rural development examined from within. *The Contemporary Pacific, 10*(2), 289–316.

Gegeo, D. W. (2001). (Re)visioning knowledge transformation in the Pacific: A response to subramani's "The Oceanic Imaginary". *The Contemporary Pacific, 13*(1), 178–183.

Hallett, D., Want, S. C., Chandler, M. J., Koopman, L. K., Flores, J. P., & Gehrke, E. C. (2008). Identity in flux: Ethnic self-identification, and school attrition in Canadian Aboriginal youth. *Journal of Applied Developmental Psychology, 29*(1), 62–75.

Masuda, T., & Nisbett, R. E. (2001). Attending holistically versus analytically: Comparing the context sensitivity of Japanese and Americans. *Journal of Personality and Social Psychology, 81*, 992–934.

Meyer, A, M. (2001). Our own liberation: Reflections on hawaiian epistemology. *The Contemporary Pacific, 13*(1), 124–148.

Nisbett, R. E. (2003). *The geography of thought: How Asians and Westerners think differently . . . and why.* New York: The Free Press.

Nisbett, R. E., Peng, K., Choi, I., & Norenzayan, A. (2001). Culture and systems of thought: Holistic versus analytic cognition. *Psychological Review, 108*, 291–310.

Norenzayan, A., Choi, I., & Peng, K. (2007). Cognition and perception. In S. K. D. Cohen (Eds.), *Handbook of cultural psychology* (pp. 569–94). New York: The Guilford Press.

Ogbor, J. O. (2000). Mythicizing and reification in entrepreneurial discourse: Ideology-critique of entrepreneurial studies. *Journal of Management Studies, 37*(5), 605–630.

Quanchi, M. (2004). *Indigenous epistemology, wisdom, and tradition: Changing and challenging dominant paradigms in Oceania.* Paper presented to the Social Change in the 21st Century Conference, Centre for Social Change Research, Queensland University of Technology.

Rigney, L. I. (1997). Internationalisation of an indigenous anti-colonial critique of research methodologies: A guide to Indigenist research methodology and its principles. *The Journal for Native American Studies, WICAZO as Review, University of Minnesota Press, 14*(2), 109–121.

Rigney, L. (1999). Internationalization of an Indigenous anticolonial cultural critique of research methodology and its principles. *Wicazo Sa Review, 14*(2), 109–121.

Rorty, A. O. (1987). Persons as rhetorical categories. *Social Research, 54*(1), 55–72.

Royal Commission on Aboriginal Peoples (RCAP). (1996). *Report of the Royal Commission on Aboriginal Peoples*, Canada Communications Group—Publications, Ottawa.

Said, E. (1978). *Orientalism*. New York: Pantheon Books.
Smith, L. T. (2005). Building a research agenda for indigenous epistemologies and education. *Anthropology and Education Quarterl, 36*, p. 93.
Stich, S. (1990). *The fragmentation of reason*. Cambridge, MA: MIT Press.
West, Japanangka Errol. (1998). *Speaking towards an Aboriginal philosophy*. Indigenous Philosophy Conference, Linga Longa, April 1998.
Whitt, L. (2009). *Science, colonialism, and indigenous peoples: The cultural politics of law and knowledge*. Cambridge: Cambridge University Press.

12 An Ally in Northern Community Health

Respectful Engagement in Healing Relationships

Linda O'Neill

Ally in Mental Health

He wears sadness on this day; his usual humour is missing, and his head is down. "I need the waterfall today. Can we go?" he quietly asks. We climb into the vehicle and drive up the road. Car therapy in the north appears to be his favourite intervention, and this is not an unusual request. We slide down to the rocks above the waterfall and sit side by side on the moss, feeling the mist from the pounding water on our faces. We are silent for a long time, as the water seems to inform him. In that moment, I suddenly understand that the elements of this place are an essential part of the therapeutic relationship we are developing, a relationship between this youth and the land and me.

From twenty-five years of living in a remote northern community, I have been guided by community members in my development as an ally for the First Nations people living there and elsewhere in the world. Through my therapeutic alliance work with community members' children and youth, I have come to understand aspects of the unique issues faced by First Nations people living in that context. Those issues are different from the issues faced by any other racial or ethnic group personally, politically, and socially (France, McCormick, & Rodriguez, 2004). Issues of racism, colonization, and residential school legacies, as well as the Indian Act and collectivism ideals present challenges to non-First Nations counsellors, and I hold experience stories reflecting aspects of all these issues in my role as helper.

The question of whether non-Aboriginal counsellors can be effective for Aboriginal clients has been asked in very general terms, particularly in the context of Native Americans (Morrisette, 2008). It is a question I have asked myself hundreds of times as I sought personal and professional balance between my own culture and the culture of my clients. Aboriginal and Western worldviews in the knowledge realm have been described as being diametric trajectories (Poonwassie & Charter, 2001). As a further challenge, Indigenous knowledge acquired by community members through enculturation is not a universal concept, resulting in the essential need for various researchers, practitioners, and institutions to accept diversity within Indigenous knowledges (Battiste & Youngblood, 2000). Overgeneralizing cultural groups' traits can lead to limiting stereotyping notions regarding psychological traits. The learning piece that comes out of the variety of realities for Aboriginal people is to avoid the overgeneralization of First Nations, Métis, and Inuit clients and respecting instead the diversity within the culture. As an ally within the helping profession, I have learned that both diversity and universality need to be understood within each counselling relationship and within relationship to community.

Culture: Walking the Bridge

He is tall and very thin, stretched by a recent growth spur. He is working to get a sense of his new body, and his movements might be described as awkward. He is frustrated with the stillness required of him in the classroom and his seeming difficulty in working with the material and required tasks. On this day, Elders come to the school to teach a traditional stick handling game. As the drum begins, I watch, and he begins to move his upper body, following the rhythm. I have never seen him move like this, with deliberation and grace, with a surety and an inner knowledge. I am aware that I am in the presence of something sacred, a transmission of ancient movement that words can never do justice to.

Christopher (1996) conceptualizes culture as moral visions—constellations of values and assumptions that shape our life experience. He describes culture as preceding us, permeating our lives. Lives can be viewed as structures of care, indicating what each cultural group cares for and values. Different cultures provide different moral visions.

The goal in counselling education and practice appears to be finding ways to bridge the gap between various Aboriginal groups' and Western beliefs on mental health and healing. The space between these cultural beliefs might be viewed as a tyrannical space (Berman, 2006) or as an "experiential domain that relates entities to one another in terms of position and movement" (Gone, 2008, pp. 371–372). Perhaps the analogy of alliance in understanding and negotiating this space is one focused on the goal of advancing diverse yet compatible interests of all members (Morrow, 1991). Summerfield (1999) suggests that definitions of health and mental health need to be changed so they reflect Indigenous conceptualizations and can then be socialized. One of the most critical aspects of worldview to understand are beliefs about the nature of human suffering and distress, problems related to behaviour, their cause, and how healing occurs: what helps and what is standard practice (Christopher, 1996). Throughout history, all cultures have developed explanations for abnormal or unhealthy behaviours and have created culture-specific, Indigenous methods for dealing with resulting problems (Yeh, Hunter, Madan-Bahel, Chiang, & Arora, 2004). Dana (2000) describes how assessment of culturally diverse people can be competently accomplished only by clearly understanding the contribution of culture to presenting problems.

Emic Lens in an Etic World

The need for change and consideration of how counselling is taught and practiced rests with the suggestion that psychological counselling services are underutilized by minority groups due to "mistrust, perceived irrelevance, and insensitivity to their cultural norms and personal meanings" (Nelson-Jones, 2002, p. 133). Culture-specific, or emic, conceptualizations exist for a variety of psychological problems. Western-based practitioners are advised to validate the client's cultural conception of mental health problems because this conception of mental illness affects help-seeking action, the expectations of treatment outcome, and the manifestation of symptoms (Dana, 1998). An emic approach views the counselling process as being informed by culturally specific knowledge, with a basic understanding of the client's cultural context as essential. Geertz (1973) views culture as webs of significance, and an emic approach values that significance by understanding the uniqueness of each web while at the same time recognizing the threads of connection.

An etic approach tends to present all counselling as being multicultural due to significant differences present in every client/counsellor relationship based on unique cultural backgrounds and worldviews (Dana, 1998). In counsellor education, we inform students that our task is to meet each client's needs, including aspects of cultural identity. The risk in this approach is that the counsellor may perceive significant cultural diversity as basic individual differences, resulting in a superficial understanding of the deeper context. Western educators sometimes use an etic approach when the traditional theories of counselling are not presented as Western in origin, leading some new counsellors to assume that these theories can be applied universally. Our Western theories are reflections of the dominate beliefs of our society, including a focus on individualism and autonomy (Gysbers, Heppner, & Johnston, 2003). It is suggested that three-quarters of the world's population use some form of Indigenous (non-Western) or alternate methods of healing, including the healing of mental health issues (Bemak & Chung, 2002), and this fact alone should stimulate the need to present alternative methods in counselling education.

Practitioner Culture

Pettifor (2001) describes professionals who lack awareness of diversity and their own cultural bias as being unintentionally racist, a difficult stance to address when awareness is lacking and motives are not clear even to the source. Dana (2005) concurs, describing bias among clinicians in cross-cultural interactions as "typically inadvertent, denied (and) below thresholds of awareness" (p. 11). A major factor in developing a culturally congruent manner is the cultural awareness of the practitioner. If professionals are unaware of their own cultural schemas, these schemas may be projected onto the client resulting in improper assessment and intervention (Kress, Eriksen, Rayle, & Ford, 2005). Roysircar (2004) suggests that practitioners work to understand what their cultural heritage is in order to understand what significant beliefs and attitudes from that cultural base define their belief systems—systems that come into each counselling encounter.

As a counsellor educator, I observe how difficult it is for Caucasian student counsellors to define their culture schemas. For many of these students, family and religion define culture, without a strong affiliation to a specific culture. In my development as an ally, I had to put words to my culture and try to articulate my own worldview in order to grasp the lens that I bring to each interaction with my First Nations colleagues and clients. If I cannot identify my own cultural map and the teachings and social interactions that drew that map, I cannot know theirs. Self-reflection and self-awareness are the essential tools for this process.

Counselling Context: Enduring Legacy

From the time I first saw her as a young child, she appeared to be fuelled by anger. This strong emotion was the only thing that kept her in the world, and one night it left and was replaced by overwhelming sadness. As we talk about her survival and her new life, the scar ridges on her arms are growing fainter. She describes her view of life as being transformed through the diagnosis of PTSD and the knowledge that everything she went through should not have happened, especially to a child, and was not done to her because she was a bad person. I begin to adjust my more pessimistic views on the usefulness of diagnosis in a cultural context.

Alliances are often formed to increase security by massing capabilities against a common enemy (Morrow, 1991). In the context of my story, the enemy is historical trauma and continued racism, with security increased through empathic engagement. Wise and gifted colleagues and community members have informed my journey as a helper as they shared the context of their own trauma work and transformation. Implications for cross-cultural counselling related to historical issues are key to the challenge of supporting First Nations clients (Morrissette, 2008). Culturally sensitive engagement demands an understanding of historical trauma—the cumulative complex trauma from psychological, emotional wounding across generations and over the lifespan resulting from massive group trauma experiences inflicted on a group who share an affiliation (Brave Heart, 2003; Evans-Campbell, 2008). In this context, historical trauma refers to intergenerational trauma affecting First Nations people, including trauma from genocide policies, including assimilation attempts through the residential school system.

The definition of trauma characterized by loss of control, connection, and meaning (Herman, 1992) fits the description of profound loss described by residential school survivors (Assembly of First Nations, 1994; Corrado & Cohen, 2003; Glavin, 2002; Kinnon, 2002). Studies focusing on the determinants of mental health with First Nations people suggest the need for extensive analysis of the structure, dynamics, and history of such communities (Kinnon, 2002; Kirmayer, Simpson, & Cargo, 2003). According to many researchers, one cannot address ways to promote mental health for First Nations people without discussing the profound impact both colonization and the residential school system has had on families and communities (Chrisjohn, Young, & Maraun, 1997; Kinnon, 2002; Mussell, Cardiff, & White, 2004; Tafoya & Del Vecchio, 1996).

Moving from the history of colonization and the residential school system to understanding the long-term consequences found in many First Nations clients "requires a model of the transgenerational impact of cultural change, oppression, and structural violence" (Kirmayer et al., 2003, p. 21). An analogy could be made between the residential school experience and the phenomenon of addiction, as the effects go far beyond the addicted individual (Chrisjohn et al., 1997), affecting families, communities, and nations.

Community-based helping practitioners may identify the effects of trauma, or they may continue to work with the effects unacknowledged. Brave Heart (2003) suggests that in order for helpers to be effective, an understanding of the ongoing transmission of trauma across generations in Aboriginal populations in addition to culturally relevant trauma theory is required. When I inquired about a culturally appropriate trauma model for work with First Nations clients, I was gently informed by a First Nations colleague that trauma transcends culture and that trauma takes all of us to a place of commonality. My colleague suggested instead that the basic trauma model presented by Herman (1992) would be appropriate (Ed Anderson, personal communication, July 2007).

First Nations citizens are challenged not only from intergenerational effects but also from racism encountered on a daily basis, sometimes referred to as race-based traumatic stress (Bryant-Davis, 2007; Tafoya & Vecchio, 1996). Race-based trauma includes the psychological consequence of institutional or interpersonal racial discrimination, and consequences may have compounding effects on survivors of other traumatic experiences (Bryant-Davis, 2007). In my community work, I have walked into stores with children and youth and felt the tone of encounters change, and the vigilant eyes of clerks hone in. For Western practitioners, one of the hardest concepts to consider is that "violent acts are not committed, necessarily, by perverted individuals but by ordinary people who are caught up in tragic circumstances . . ." (Papadopoulos, 1998, p. 463). Whether these spontaneous acts of racism are violent or not, the "tragic circumstances" in many small communities appear to include generational lack of understanding and fear.

Ally as Advocate for Change: Counselling Education

She has struggled through the theories class and can find no place for her world in the pages of male, White therapists' and theorists' ideas on helping and change. She has come to my office to share the pain and frustration of not finding resonance or representation. Books on the office shelf by Roland Chrisjohn, Duran and Duran, Rubert Ross, Marie Battiste, Peter Cole, Linda Tuhiwa-Smith, and the shared stories from the north seem to ease the frustration. She works to articulate her theory, and I quietly thank again all those people from my community who have informed me and allowed me once again to work as an ally by bridging the cultural space with resources.

My journey as a helper working in two cultures has led me, with a few twists and turns, to become a counsellor educator. The task now is how to facilitate the development of additional allies with the intent of assuring that new counsellors become effective for First Nations clients and to facilitate a place for First Nations students and Aboriginal theories of mental health in this heavily Westernized profession.

The role of an alliance is sometimes defined in the pursuit of changes to the status quo (Morrow, 1991); one area of change sought in my story includes changes in counsellor education in terms of how we present cross-cultural work. The culture and diversity component of counselling that Pedersen (2001) referred to as the fourth force, multicultural counselling training, continues to grow, with counselling programs using various models for implementation. Offering one or two multicultural counselling and diversity classes in the separate course model is common, but an integrated, infused model throughout the entire counselling programs is recommended (Abreu, Chung, & Atkinson, 2000). In the context of northern work where the Aboriginal population is much larger than other areas of the country, a focus on appropriate counselling and support for First Nations, Métis, and Inuit should be a priority in counsellor education.

The challenges in counselling education in presenting respectful, sensitive, and effective support to members of Aboriginal cultures are many. The need for balance between Western and Aboriginal approaches is required in practice and in counsellor education. In trying to address the psychological needs of clients from other minority cultures, Bemak and Chung (2002) suggest that psychotherapy has tended to focus on a Westernized view of mental health. This view contains individualistic ideologies used to help find coping strategies and improve client functioning—a philosophical approach that does not fit the cultural background of many clients, where culture is based on family and community connections. One person's trauma experience and resulting problems are often considered to be those of their family and community, with mental well-being dependent on and not to be separated from community (France & McCormick, 1997). Clients from minority groups, such as First Nations populations, and Western practitioners often have very different perceptions of what "good" mental health looks like, as well as what constitutes effective intervention strategies (Bemak & Chung, 2002). I have experienced this phenomenon first-hand with helping practitioners who come from "outside" a community without the benefit of cultural awareness.

Mental Health Inequalities

Health practitioners and counsellors have often judged First Nations clients' high attrition rate as lack of commitment rather than practitioners' lack of cultural sensitivity in their approach and to the context of client issues (Duran & Duran, 1995). Poor housing, poverty, political alienation, and the resulting despair are some of the root causes for many of the traumatic mental health problems found in Aboriginal communities (Bryant-Davis, 2007; Smye & Browne, 2002). Smye and Browne (2002) suggest that current policies, practices, and research may recreate traumas inflicted on Aboriginal people. Approaches and practices need to be viewed through the lens of cultural safety in order to identify and critique issues of institutional racism and discrimination. A focus on the meaning of mental health and illness for Aboriginal people and appropriate responses is required. Cultural safety may not exist in counselling relationships if holistic Aboriginal approaches, or the historical context of Aboriginal mental health, are not acknowledged.

Holistic approaches are difficult to convey to those with a more linear, process-oriented worldview. In counsellor education, we often use beginning skills texts that rely heavily on a progressive stage model, or we discuss stages of change and stages of grief and loss. These stages models appear to be much more relevant for many First Nations clients when used in a circle or web model and given context through lived experience stories.

Community Wisdom: Traditional Education

She brought her community out of a destructive cycle of addiction that she herself had struggled with for so many years by going door-to-door, checking on family and others, and speaking of alternatives. The community and many of the people all bore visible scars from that cycle, yet as the years went by and more people were converted to a different life by her hope and spiritual strength, those scars became less visible, and it was harder to remember that time. This one small woman had restoried her community with her own transformation, her energy, and her spiritual belief that people could be healthy and find a different meaning in their lives. We have shared clients and a long work history, but she is aging now, and her health is not staying true to her spirit. On this day, I sit on the floor beside her couch as she tells me stories of times before residential school—stories that transform my understanding of who she is.

In very general terms, the well-being of individuals in Aboriginal communities cannot be separated from the context of community, leading traditional healing to focus on the person within the context of his or her community, considering the individual to be embedded in the community (France et al., 2004). The support of local practitioners and the use of local resources are essential to community work. Community resources include traditional healers and Elders, parents and influential family members who provide networks of support (Wessells, 1999). A concern for some of my First Nations colleagues is that the expertise, knowledge, and ideas of front-line workers are not heard and respected. They struggle with how to get the information that they hold out to all practitioners working with First Nations clients.

In recent conversations with adult children of respected Elders living in northern communities, stories were used to illustrate what Elders did and continue to do in their helping work. These stories are not mine to present, but I realized after these conversations that language, the English language in particular, is inadequate when trying to define the complex subtleties of how Elders help. A question that several First Nations colleagues ponder is if Elders' ways of helping and providing counsel will be sustained in future generations and how these ways can be taught in this evolving world of culture and acculturation.

There is a recent movement advocating for the therapeutic integration of traditional and conventional Western models of helping (Gone, 2008; Trimble, 2010). There is such hope inherent in this approach, but great care needs to be taken to prevent the disrespectful and inappropriate use of Aboriginal traditional activities and rituals by non-Aboriginal practitioners (Trimble, 2010), a particular concern of mine based on the spiritual aspect and resulting reverence surrounding such activities and ceremonies. Wessells (1999) cautions that local resources be used critically, as some local practices and traditions go against the practitioner's own cultural ethics and may even cause harm when used by inexperienced practitioners. He suggests that traditional approaches and local practices be neither romanticized nor too quickly rejected and that practitioners keep in mind that cultures, and therefore practice, continually evolve. In my work, I refer clients in need of more traditional approaches to First Nations counsellors, helpers, and Elders who have the expertise and context.

Conclusion

She has taken a long time to decide who I am and if I can be of use to her. She exudes a depth of reflection and quiet as she watches me work with other youth, and slowly she begins to have short interactions with me. Her parents have a difficult relationship after a painful divorce that occurred many years ago. She has aligned herself with her father this particular year, and he lets me know that he is concerned. She gives words out carefully, but her non-verbals provide clarity as to her emotional state. I find her one afternoon softly crying in the corner of a room. I slide down to the floor by her and . . . I wait. I have had to learn to wait, quieting my cultural tendency to fill the air with many empty words, while using gentle coercion of empathic sounds. I now know to let her be. I am attuned to the sound of her breathing and her weeping and a sense of what she is working through. Several hours later, she clarifies her pain for me. I have met her criteria for trustworthiness and understanding by waiting and . . . being.

The ability of a practitioner to accommodate another's reality and to take an empathic understanding of worldview has been proposed as the essence of cross-cultural counselling (Bojuwoye, 2001). Due to the space between the cultures in this type of work and advocacy, a question asked is how much cultural knowledge is required for competent cross-cultural practice (Trimble, 2010). Cultural knowledge is directly tied to community and understanding community. Learning about the reality of the First Nations people I have worked with has resulted in a long relationship with community, echoing Trimble's (2010) point that the only way for true partnerships to form between First Nations and non-First Nations is in collaboration with community and the establishment of long-term relationships. Reciprocity, which is the norm in First Nations communities (Salois, Holkup, Tripp-Reimer, & Weinert, 2006), is the interaction that sustains these relationships.

In looking at the cultural imperatives listed by Morrisette (2008) as being essential for relationship development with First Nations clients, including interconnectiveness, empowerment, spirituality, non-intervention, and the personal qualities of respect, honesty, and love, it is the quality of respect that is the foundational element for the work that I have done and the relationships I have formed. Through my emergence and development as ally and helper, I have learned to respect and honour connection to land; the ancient transmission of culture; resistance and resilience in the face of trauma; the deep need for connection, diversity within culture; Elder wisdom and spirituality; and the mindful importance of being. I continue to spread the word while holding close the stories and experiences that have informed me.

References

Abreu, J. M., Chung, R. H. G., & Atkinson, D. R. (2000). Multicultural counseling training: Past, present, and future directions. *The Counselling Psychologist, 28*, 641. doi: 10.1177/0011000000285003.

Assembly of First Nations. (1994). *Breaking the silence: An interpretive study of residential school impact and healing as illustrated by the stories of First Nations individuals*. Ottawa, ON: First Nations Health Commission.

Battiste, M., & Youngblood, J. (2000). What is indigenous knowledge? In M. Battiste, & J. Youngblood (Eds.), *Protecting indigenous language and heritage: A global challenge* (pp. 35–56). Saskatoon, SK: Purich Publishing Ltd.

Bemak, F., & Chung, R. C. (2002). Refugees and terrorism: Cultural innovations in clinical practice. In C. E. Stout (Ed.), *Psychology of terrorism: Clinical aspects and responses* (Vol. 2, pp. 1–26). Westport, CT: Praeger Publishers/Greenwood Publishing Group, Inc.

Berman, G. S. (2006). Social services and indigenous populations in remote areas: Alaska Natives and Negev Bedouin. *International Social Work, 49*(1), 97–106.

Bojuwoye, O. (2001). Crossing cultural boundaries in counselling. *International Journal for the Advancement of Counselling, 23*, 31–50.

Brave Heart, M. Y. H. (2003). The historical trauma response among Natives and its relationship with substance abuse: A Lakota illustration. *Journal of Psychoactive Drugs, 35*(1), 7–13.

Bryant-Davis, T. (2007). Healing requires recognition: The case for race-based traumatic stress. *The Counselling Psychologist, 35*(1), 135–143.

Chrisjohn, R., Young, S., & Maraun, M. (1997). *The circle game*. Penticton, BC: Theytus Books Ltd.

Christopher, J. C. (1996). Counseling's inescapable moral visions. *Journal of Counseling & Development, 75*, 26–34.

Corrado & Cohen. (2003). *Mental health profiles for a sample of British Columbia's Aboriginal survivors of the Canadian residential school system*. Ottawa, ON: The Aboriginal Healing Foundation.

Dana, R. H. (1998). Personality assessment and the cultural self: Emic and etic contexts as learning resources. In L. Handler, & M. J. Hilsenroth (Eds.), *Teaching and learning personality assessment* (pp. 325–346). Mahwah, NJ: Lawrence Erlbaum Associates.

Dana, R. H. (2000). Handbook of cross-cultural and multicultural personality assessment. In A. L. Comunian & U. P. Gielen (Eds.), *International perspectives on human development* (pp. 233–258). Lengerich, Germany: Pabst Science Publishers.

Dana, R. H. (2005). *Multicultural assessment: Principles, applications, and examples*. Mahwah, NJ: Lawrence Erlbaum Associates.

Duran, E., & Duran, B. (1995). *Native American postcolonial psychology*. Albany, NY: State University of New York Press.

Evans-Campbell, T. (2008). Historical trauma in American Indian/Native Alaska communities. *Journal of Interpersonal Violence, 23*(3), 316–338. doi: 10.177/088 6260507312290.

France, M. H., & McCormick, R. (1997). The helping circle: Theoretical and practical considerations of using a First Nations peer support network. *Guidance & Counselling, 12*(2), 27–32.

France, M. H., McCormick, R., & Rodriguez, M. (2004). Issues in counselling in the First Nations community. In M. H. France, C. Rodriguez, & G. Hett (Eds.), *Diversity culture and counselling: A Canadian perspective* (pp. 65–91). Calgary, AB: Temeron Press.

Geertz, C. (1973). *The interpretation of cultures*. New York, New York: Perseus.

Glavin, T. (2002). *Amongst god's own: The enduring legacy of St. Mary's Mission*. Mission, BC: Mission Indian Friendship Centre, Longhouse Publishing.

Gone, J. P. (2008). So i can be like a whiteman: The cultural psychology of space and Place in American Indian mental health. *Culture Psychology, 14*(3), 369–399. doi: 10.1177/ 1354067X08092639.

Gysbers, N. C., Heppner, M. J., & Johnston, J. A. (2003). *Career counselling: Process, issues, and techniques*, 2nd ed. Boston, MA: Allyn & Bacon.

Herman, J. (1992). *Trauma and recovery*. New York, NY: Basic Books.

Kinnon, D. (2002). *Improving population health, health promotion, disease prevention and health protection services and programs for Aboriginal people*. Ottawa, ON: National Aboriginal Health Organization.

Kirmayer, L., Simpson, C., & Cargo, M. (2003). Healing traditions: Culture, community and mental health promotion with Canadian Aboriginal peoples. *Australasian Psychiatry, 11*, 15–23.

Kress, K., Eriksen, K., Rayle, A., & Ford, S. (2005). The DSM-IV-TR and culture: Considerations for counsellors. *Journal of Counselling & Development, 83*(1), 97–104.

Morrissette, P. J. (2008). Clinical engagement of Canadian First Nations couples. *Journal of Family Therapy, 30*(1), 60–77.

Morrow, J. D. (1991). Alliances and asymmetry: An alternative to the capability aggregation model of alliances. *American Journal of Political Science, 35*(4), 904–933.

Mussell, B., Cardiff, K., & White, J. (2004). *The mental health and well-being of Aboriginal children and youth: Guidance for new approaches and services*. Chilliwack, BC: Sal'i'shan Institute.

Nelson-Jones, R. (2002). Diverse goals for multicultural counselling and therapy. *Counselling Psychology Quarterly, 15*(2), 133–143. doi: 10.1080/095150701101 00965.

Papadopoulos, R. K. (1998). Destructiveness, atrocities and healing: Epistemological and clinical reflections. *Journal of Analytical Psychology, 43*(4), 455–477.

Pedersen, P. B. (2001). Multiculturalism and the paradigm shift in counselling: Controversies and alternative futures. *Canadian Journal of Counselling, 35*(1), 15–25.

Pettifor, J. (2001). Are professional codes of ethics relevant for multicultural counselling? *Canadian Journal of Counselling, 35*(1), 26–35.

Poonwassie, A., & Charter, A. (2001). An Aboriginal worldview of helping: Empowering approaches. *Canadian Journal of Counselling, 35*(1), 63–73.

Roysircar, G. (2004). Cultural self-awareness assessment: Practice examples from psychology training. *Professional Psychology: Research and Practice, 35*(6), 658–666.

Salois, E. M., Holkup, P., Tripp-Reimer, T., & Weinert, C. (2006). Research as spiritual covenant. *Western Journal of Nursing Research, 28*(5), 505–524. doi: 10:1177/0193945906286809.

Smye, V., & Browne, A. (2002). 'Cultural safety' and the analysis of health policy affecting Aboriginal people. *Nurse Researcher, 9*(3), 42–56.

Summerfield, D. (1999). A critique of seven assumptions behind psychological trauma programs in war-affected areas. *Social Science & Medicine, 48*(10), 1449–1462.

Tafoya, N., & Del Vecchio, A. (1996). Back to the future: An examination of the Native American holocaust experience. In M. McGoldrick, & J. Giordano (Eds.), *Ethnicity and family therapy*, 2nd ed. (pp. 45–54). New York, NY: Guilford Press.

Trimble, J. E. (2010). The virtues of cultural resonance, competence, and relational collaboration with Native American Indian communities: A synthesis of the Counseling and psychotherapy literature. *The Counseling Psychologist, 38*, 243. doi: 10.1177/0011000009344348.

Wessells, M. G. (1999). Culture, power, and community: Intercultural approaches to psychosocial assistance and healing. In K. Nader, & N. Dubrow (Eds.), *Honoring differences: Cultural issues in the treatment of trauma and loss* (pp. 267–282). New York, NY: Brunner/Mazel, Inc.

Yeh, C., Hunter, C., Madan-Bahel, A., Chiang, L., & Arora, A. (2004). Indigenous and interdependent perspectives of healing: Implications for counselling and research. *Journal of Counselling & Development, 82*(4), 410–419.

13 *A'tola'nw*

Indigenous-Centred Learning in a Counselling Graduate Program

Anne Marshall, Larry Emerson, Lorna Williams, Asma Antoine, Colleen MacDougall, and Ruby Peterson

A'tola'nw (SENĆOŦEN) means *"a time of hope and respecting one another."* This is the name gifted to our Indigenous Communities Counselling Psychology (ICCP) graduate program (originally the Aboriginal Communities Counselling Program or ACCP) by Elder John Elliot of the Tsartlip Nation on southern Vancouver Island, British Columbia. Our shared story is one of Aboriginal and non-Aboriginal learners and educators in a graduate counsellor education program. The learners are training to be counsellors and helpers who will return to or take up work in Indigenous communities. However, deep Indigenous-centred and decolonized learning is difficult to negotiate and navigate in the Western academy. In our journey together, we are challenged to find new spaces to learn, think, and feel that are inclusive and authentic—free from oppression and colonial control.

Traditional leaders tell us the answers lie within. Yet there are few maps to follow with little time and few opportunities for the type of learning we desire. To simultaneously engage Western and Indigenous learning is not easy; it is often traumatic and always challenging. We face a host of dichotomies and apparent contradictions. We know and do not know our cultures and languages. We are of mixed ancestry. We have inherited unresolved residential school trauma, whether we know it or not. We understand and do not understand community, kinship, and place. We are connected and disconnected. We feel both joy and pain. We are humanized and dehumanized. We sense beauty and contradictions among ourselves and among those with whom we work.

We have hopes and aspirations for healthy communities and nations. We understand what the Western academy wants from us. However, we must be vigilant and courageous learners or we will be immobilized and discouraged and among ourselves perhaps end up reproducing the very same conditions that have disrupted our communities. We must also take care in this process to remember the promise to our communities, families, and ourselves.

In this chapter, we begin with a brief background of why and how the program came to be, including a description of the values and principles that underpin everything in it. We then share our experiences and insights from the program, written in the first-person plural (we) to signify our collective voice. This format is a conscious and agreed upon choice that is consistent with Indigenous oral traditions. Certain specific observations and quotes from several different students, gathered through reflections and interviews during the first program, are interwoven within our narrative and are indicated *in italics*. Our experiences are organized around what we have found to be recurring themes: Indigenous-centred learning (ICL), ceremony and traditional knowledge, sacredness of dreams and visions, and walking in two worlds. We conclude with lessons learned, the beginnings of the second ICCP graduate student cohort, and our vision for the future.

Background

Postsecondary education is seen as key to closing the social and economic gaps between Aboriginal and non-Aboriginal people (Simpson, 2004; Warner, 2006). As stated in the *Aboriginal Post-Secondary Education Strategy and Action Plan* (2007), the goal of the Ministry of Advanced Education in British Columbia is to increase participation, retention, and success in postsecondary education for Aboriginal people. Some of the barriers related to success include a lack of Aboriginal involvement in decision making regarding postsecondary programs, cultural issues and bias in postsecondary programs and institutions, lack of relevant programming, and geographic distance to most postsecondary sites for Aboriginal learners. The success rate for Aboriginal learners increases significantly when these difficulties are addressed (British Columbia Ministry of Advanced Education, 2007). One suggested strategy to address these barriers is the development and delivery of culturally relevant Aboriginal programming that reflects the goals of Aboriginal learners and leads to meaningful employment. A further goal is to incorporate long-term, self-sustaining Aboriginal community involvement into the planning and implementation of these programs in significant partnerships, while at the same time balancing the university's autonomy in terms of program and service development and delivery—a challenge to be sure. The first ICCP at the University of Victoria adopted these goals and strategies to address the barriers to postsecondary education for Aboriginal learners. This graduate professional program has been designed for adult learners working in counselling and mental health settings within an Aboriginal context.

The ICCP delivery model was created through a collaborative partnership between the Department of Educational Psychology and Leadership Studies and the Office of Aboriginal Education (now the Office of Indigenous Education) in the Faculty of Education at the University of Victoria to develop and deliver a graduate counselling program relevant to and consistent with the values and traditions of Aboriginal communities. The vision for the program model was explored at a 2006 retreat of Aboriginal and non-Aboriginal faculty, educators, students, Elders, and community professionals. The retreat participants stayed together to form the Advisory and Planning Committee that has continued to guide the ideas, issues, and decisions related to the development and implementation of the program. What makes this graduate program different and unique is the integration of Indigenous values and traditions into both the undergraduate prerequisite and graduate courses in the program. In addition, Aboriginal community needs and partnerships are a central focus of every aspect of this initiative; community voices and needs have guided and will continue to guide the direction of the program.

In March 2007, the Advisory and Planning Committee members along with additional community educators and practitioners worked with Indigenous Diné scholar Dr. Larry Emerson to establish the seven key values and principles that guide the vision of the program:

- The Indigenous paradigm is central
- The sacred and the spiritual dimension
- The ancestral dimension
- Stories, ceremony, culture, language, and communal healing
- The earth and our relatives
- The circle
- The vocation and practice of professional helping

These values and principles guided the curricular enhancement and revision of undergraduate prerequisite and graduate courses in the existing University of Victoria Counselling program to make the content and delivery methods more relevant to the needs and traditions of Aboriginal communities. New courses have also been developed specifically for this program, such as a course entitled "Indigenous Development Across Generations." Aboriginal community members and prospective students have long expressed a desire for graduate counsellor training that would enable graduates to become registered professionals with national and provincial accrediting bodies yet also incorporate Aboriginal worldviews and values. Thus the University of Victoria Aboriginal Communities Master's in Counselling program is what Duran (2006) terms a "hybrid" program—one that integrates two paradigms, Indigenous and Western, that complement and contrast each other. Course materials and delivery models incorporate Indigenous ways of knowing. Indigenous philosophy, practices, and counselling methods are used to help students working in Aboriginal contexts where the dimensions of the spiritual, ancestral, and cultural (stories, ceremony, language, and communal healing) play a vital part in how people live (Emerson, 2006). The program follows a "generative model" of curriculum (Ball, 2004) in which courses are structured using an open architecture that leaves room for the voices of students, Elders, and the community to enter into active dialogue with the material. Within the framework of graduate studies regulations and counselling professional registration requirements, the students and communities involved have further shaped the program and curriculum.

The program was launched in September 2008 with nineteen students, beginning with a four-day immersion in Indigenous ways of knowing and relating; instructor Dr. Larry Emerson characterized this approach as "no books, no pens, no papers, no computers."

Recognizing the critical importance of relationships and mentoring in Aboriginal communities, a community mentorship component was established for the program and funded by the Counselling Foundation of Canada (http://www.counselling.net). Ongoing relationships and interactions with Aboriginal community Elders, educators, professionals, and supervisors are consistent with Indigenous community traditions and are seen to be vital to the success of the Aboriginal Communities Counselling graduate program. Organized by a mentorship coordinator, the mentorship project includes Elder participation, an Indigenous Healing Speakers' series, counselling supervision support, resource development, and special events.

As articulated by Dr. Larry Emerson:

> Collectively, we are addressing: How do we learn? How do we know what to know? How can, we as a learning community, successfully understand ourselves? How do we assess our situation without harsh judgment? How do we restore and regenerate our own and others' capacity to articulate our own solutions, using principles of traditional knowledge and cultural self-determination as a guide for healing, decolonization, transformation, and mobilization?

Our Stories of Learning

Welcome to our experiences. We are a cohort of seventeen Indigenous and two non-Indigenous students in the ACCP at the University of Victoria. These are the personal stories of our learning. What brought us together is our common vision from deep within our spirits. Like many others on this journey, we are all finding ways to answer the call or the promise that our spirits made before entering this world. We have been seeking a place to learn that would honour our ancestral teachings. This program has offered that to us, and for this, we are eternally grateful. We are learning how to take our place in the way of our ancestors and look through the lens of our own traditional knowledge. This foundational work of decolonizing our minds, hearts, and spirits has been pivotal in our ability to learn all that we need to while standing with and being accountable to our communities. This journey of integrating traditional knowledge with Western counselling practices is possible. We offer our stories. We have written them collectively, drawing on notes, conversations, videotaped classes, online discussions, and reflections.

Indigenous-Centred Learning (ICL)

From the beginning, we were invited to the sacred circle of learning with our mind, body, and spirit. It began with the statement of values and principles sent prior to our first class. When we first came together, we were offered a voice for what we hoped to experience in this program. The words echoed again and again among the students on the first day of the program were, *we have been waiting and searching a long time for something that would honour our culture and teachings to be present within the learning environment.* This meant a great deal to all of us. ICL has offered us freedom to be all of who we are. ICL is learning within a holistic format. We do this through finding our voice from within and connecting to the sacred, ancestral, spiritual dimension. When we approach critical thinking with traditional knowledge (TKn) and Western knowing, we offer a way to integrate these perspectives within our communities. Figure 13.1 illustrates this process.

Learning/Relearning How to Learn Holistically

In the Western academy and practice, there is great emphasis placed on categorization and the knowledge of Western experts. This is not consistent with Indigenous-centred knowing and has been a source of great tension for us. We needed to trust that our voices and Indigenous knowing would be honoured in the academy. We needed to build trusting relationships with each other. The teachings we received, from our first professor, Dr. Larry Emerson, set the tone for our expectations for the rest of the program. With

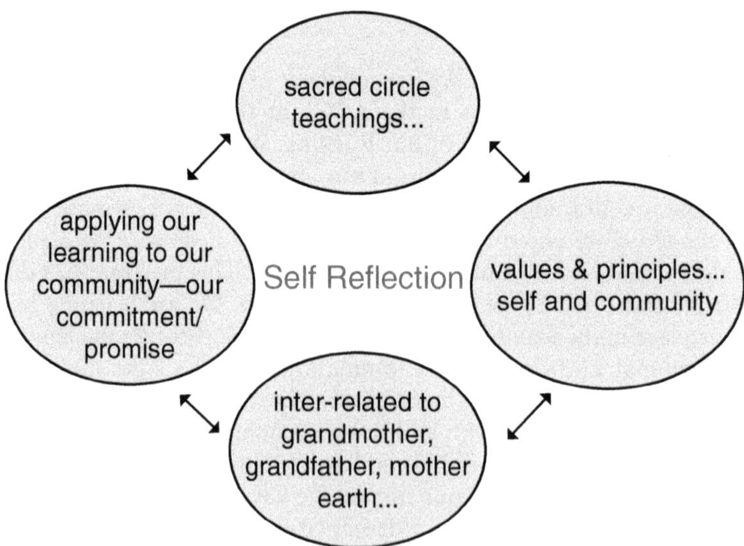

Figure 13.1 Our ICL process.

him we experienced learning how to learn holistically, which took us to the place deep within our teachings that we hoped and ached for. We went far deeper than just our minds—we entered our physical, emotional, and spiritual dimensions of knowing. The effects have been life changing.

> *I feel ten shades of grateful for [the] open discussions . . . where my whole learning takes place. By whole, I am referring to integrating this knowledge with my emotional, mental, spiritual, and physical self. I am thankful to be part of a program that resists the "colonized mind frame" that is soaked into the "modern society." Focusing [instead] on our ancestors, communities, families and identity.*

Through looking within ourselves to find our own values, beliefs, and principles we made many discoveries. Through exercises, ceremonies, and teachings, we were guided to be intentional in looking through this lens of our traditional knowledge. Using the sacred medicines as our filters, we were asked to view our learning through our sacred teachings of medicines. We were put back in touch with our own knowing, which previously had been put away for many of us, so we could endure the Western academic process that normally would not allow us to open up our holistic knowing.

> *I didn't know before that what I know could be called traditional knowledge (TKn). I didn't know the way I look at life is from an Aboriginal perspective; I thought it was from my family and community. For it to be called TKn was a breakthrough—I already had that, I just didn't know it. I allowed myself to remember what I was taught as a young person; youth knowledge was so engrained, I just didn't know . . . this was good to apply to course material.*

Looking through the lens of our sacred medicines to learn the difference between Western and Indigenous ways of knowing and learning was both freeing and exhilarating. This knowledge helped us take ownership of this stepping stone for our journey of ICL.

Finding Our Voice From Within

Exploring how to find our voice from within was an additional gift we received in this program. While most of us have been advocating to have our voice and knowledge honoured in the academy, this program has offered us the sacred space to really become clear and connected to our voices within. The experience of finding voice within this program has empowered, humbled, and inspired us in different times and ways.

> *Voice? What's critical . . . there are 19 ways of doing things, 19 different tools, multiple voices . . . TKn is a key aspect to look at—to be open*

> *and aware of and always acknowledging the history of each individual. We all strive for the same outcome of our relatives; it takes practice to get there. We'll stumble, we don't know it all, we don't have all the answers. We're willing to create the path for others; a true honouring of traditional culture without taking meaning away from it. It's important to acknowledge that. It's like referencing the TKn of our grandmothers, not just other (Western) authors . . . it's our inner voice too.*

In our efforts to decolonize ourselves, we have at times seemed unsure about our voices. Our learning environment was largely without competition with Western ways of knowing, and we did not need to justify our Indigenous knowledge. There seemed to be times when we were not sure if we could trust this new way of being in a learning environment. Sometimes we did not feel sure enough to express ourselves, and other times we voiced our needs and beliefs strongly, as we found balance. What the program has offered us is the experience of bringing our voice and knowing into the academy. Now that we have experience with this decolonized way of learning and bringing our TKn, we know what to expect and want to share it so others can experience freedom from a dependence on mainstream culture. *It has been about finding voice through an inner search as opposed to an externalized search and was based on different principles. It has been about using voice in different ways.*

We are also learning and relearning that voice does not always have words. Voice also presents itself in the presence of our knowing and understanding. *It creates sacred space for us to know that we know.* Understanding voice through the lens of TKn is understanding that sometimes having voice and using it wisely means to be quiet and allow nature and spirit and ancestors to speak to us and through us to our loved ones. Sometimes our most powerful voice is silence.

Ancestral and Spiritual Connection to Knowing

The ancestral dimension comes through the self and through ceremony. Ancestors exist and become part of our journey. To have a Western post-secondary institution make that important is central to our pathway. While some of us grew up with these teachings, it is important to acknowledge that not all of us have. For some, this was fairly new territory, so there is the process of awakening this knowing within each of us again. The learning process is always on a continuum of understanding, and while some understand some things, others have different knowledge. We are all being asked to look deep within.

> *I'm trying to be open to ask questions and be open to say "I don't know." I've never really questioned myself in this way before. I do need the spiritual aspect, doing more ceremonies, in my personal life—not*

just talking about it with clients. Not knowing enough of tools and knowledge is on because there's a big fire inside of me that makes me feel whole and strong. At times, though, I feel empty and lacking in self-confidence.

In our ICL, we are each grappling with what the ancestral and spiritual means for us, and it has certainly led us to explore our sacred teachings further. It is through ceremony that we learn so much.

Connecting ICL to All Our Relations

Building relationships is central to our teachings; we need to carry this into our lives and our work. It is a natural process, and we are continuing to discover that there is not one right way to approach counselling from ICL. There are no easy answers and there are no quick answers, either. However, there are many possibilities rooted in our relationships.

I once worked with a grandma—needed help for young son who didn't attend school for four years and was at grade one level. I talked to grandma, took cookies and tea—made several visits. Her son's problems reminded her of herself when she was a little girl; she was a residential school survivor. Her concern over her grandson was really about her own anxiety—a fear of white man's school that brought up issues for her so that negatively affected her grandson's approach to schooling. Western counsellors might not find out or know these things because of their lack of knowledge and experience regarding Native people and traditional knowledge. My approach was to just drop by for tea and talk. Even if we have our own offices, we will always have those kinds of visits possible.

The possibilities for what we can do are endless! What we are learning from ICL is that the grounding teaching is based in all our relations, physical and spiritual, with other human beings, Mother Earth, and all living things. The goal of Indigenous-centred counselling is to achieve balance, harmony, beauty, and love. We are learning that when our relationship with our physical and spiritual self is in balance, we can use both dimensions in our work.

I have within me the presence of the healing "spirit." I cannot explain it in words. It is a feeling that is swirling around me, an energy that comes to me when I am encountering a relationship when someone is needing to be heard.

All that we are learning is connected to the teaching of interdependence rather than the emphasis on independence in mainstream counselling. When we remember this, we can stay grounded and humble in doing the work we have made a commitment to our communities to do. We are all human beings learning to be the best we can be.

We are on this journey together.

> *[I] realize how busy I already am before class [and] was exhausted in [our] first class. I was quiet and observing and experiencing that uncertainty. But seeing 18 other women where they were at and seeing their spirits and emotions, I recognized this was important . . . [I am] not the only one struggling with time, learning process . . . hearing other frustrations, similar life situations, so I don't feel alone. It feels good to be walking on the same journey everyone else is on. Sitting in circle hearing stories calms the spirit and emotions. Ok, I'm like these others . . . similar journey . . . children, work, family. This awareness resulted in a feeling of togetherness.*

Ceremony and Traditional Knowledge

Entering into our program of ICL felt like we were entering into sacred ceremony. From the beginning of our first course, our respected Elder and teacher Dr. Larry Emerson centred us in holistic learning of TKn through the modality of ceremony. *The process might be called ceremonial learning interspaced with humour, community, emotion, and a process of opening up—not necessarily protecting oneself.* This was a transformational time for each of us as women and intensified and propelled our learning to a depth that would not have otherwise been able to be obtained with such speed in a Western framework of learning.

Ancestral and Spiritual Dimension in Learning

Through traditional ceremonies, we were guided rather than just told about what it means to practice living with the balance of physical and spiritual dimensions. *We learned through ceremonies and their translation and connection to learning and [also] through learning the spirit of things.* We experienced and reflected on our own learning first. Then, as time went on, we received teachings about the intentions behind what we experienced. This form of learning can be very challenging if one is not familiar with working from a TKn format, and we all had to challenge ourselves to shift from the Western academic mental learning process to the more holistic learning we were experiencing. *Medicines, such as cedar, sage and sweet grass, had input into our learning.* From these processes, we came to understand and remember what we knew to be true. *The ancestral dimension comes through the self and through ceremony. Ancestors exist and become part of our journey.*

The ancestral dimension comes through the self and through ceremony. Ancestors are with us on our journey. Having a learning environment in the program that makes this understanding a central part of learning creates so many more possibilities for us to return to our communities with meaningful tools to participate in healing. We came to understand that we already know things intuitively. We are searching for knowledge that we already carry. *It was a powerful day when [a student] was acting, but not acting, when demonstrating traditional counselling*. The student's needs echoed our need for traditional knowledge. *The "welcoming home" learning ceremony using stones was memorable*. The learning from these lessons has been endless.

Although some of us have experienced these teachings previously, we all required the process of awakening this knowing within each of us again. The learning process was always on a continuum of understanding, and each of us held various areas of knowing. We needed to support each other, using the gifts each brought to the circle. All of us had many questions, and we found ourselves searching *within*.

In differing forms and times, we all seemed to be asking ourselves difficult, soul-searching questions. Ceremony offered us the sacred space to look within ourselves for the meaningful learning we were seeking. *Ceremony is the framework and process that pulled us together and helped us create harmony in order to pursue tough issues.*

Using the modality of ceremony for teaching TKn in the Aboriginal Community Counselling program has been very effective. Ceremony connects us with all our relations and with ourselves. It guides us to discover values and ways for developing healthy relationships. As grandmother Clara Shinobu Iura of the Amazon says, "Personal healing is the essential first step toward healing the world" (Schaefer, 2006, p. 140). This counselling program has honoured the teachings that have been passed down from generation to generation, and our counselling work lies within sacred knowledge. Learning this sacred knowledge holds healing for our communities, because we first need to understand what we value. As Lane, Bopp, Bopp, Brown, and Elders (2004) put it,

> values are the way human beings pattern and use their energy. If there is not a balance between our values concerning ourselves and our values concerning others, we cannot continue to develop our true potential as human beings. Indeed, if there is an imbalance, individuals, and whole communities suffer and even die.
>
> (p. 18)

This understanding has been with Indigenous peoples since the beginning of time and is situated in our creation stories. These stories are teachings of how to live in harmony and balance with all our relations: Mother Earth, Father Sky, Grandfather Sun, and Grandmother Moon. It is the teaching of connection. This teaching of connection is the natural response to restoring balance. Regenerating our balance in physical, emotional, mental, and spiritual realms is what our traditional knowledge provides. We can offer Indigenous-centred counselling or guidance to restore wholeness from the fragmentation of mind, body, and spirit, as well as to address the fragmentation that has come from disconnection, isolation, depression, trauma, and abuse.

The Sacredness of Dreams and Visions

Dreaming and visioning are processes that assist Indigenous helpers to find solutions and dig deeply into an issue to present different perspectives (Maracle, 2008; Sefa Dei, 2002). Using messages, dreams, and visions is important to support the *relative* (client or individual) trying to achieve wellness. It is a journey to see the vision and bring it into being. When interpreting the dream, we honour the way to best convey the message in order to be of help. Dreams have shaped our personal and community visions. Learners in this program described personal transformations related to dreams and visions. Indigenous dreams and visions are words from our ancestors, our grandmothers, and our grandfathers—the teachers who came before us. Their words have brought us here, to the present day. One student shared her experience:

> *From a dream, I was guided to create a drum bag for the group. The bag became an essential symbol in my learning process, giving me the teachings to acknowledge my story and inner strength. These teachings have taught me the significance of following my intuition. The meanings behind the drum bag bring forth the need to nurture and protect the drum as it represents our connection with Mother Earth and our communities.*

The tradition of honouring our dreams and visions is a practice we want to bring into our counselling, as a means of healing for our community members. If we have good intentions and a loving spirit, then a guiding symbol will be there. *I believe that when I feel lost or beaten I can call on my intuition. I hope to be able to encourage my community members to uncover their own symbols to empower them on their healing path.* We can help people to create their own intentions and symbolic visions. In Blackfoot language, the words *Mokakit Iiyiikaakimaat* stand for wisdom (knowledge) and the strength to persevere no matter what the journey in life brings forth. These Indigenous terms speak to a counselling vision where we as helpers will guide people in finding their own inner strength to strive and to be courageous in life. It is important that we are open to this wisdom and guidance that comes from our hearts and spirits.

Many of us describe our learning process as one of transformation, self-actualization, and visioning. As we have progressed through the program, we have realized that, along with the faculty, we are in the midst of transformation; we are establishing a program that values the essence of who we are as Aboriginal people. This program considers our own personal foundations along with our family and community fundamental beliefs. It encourages us to delve deep within to understand what these beliefs represent. Another student shares one of her dreams:

> *Before I even entered the First Peoples House [at the University of Victoria] and before it was finished being built, I experienced this dream where I was in my new home sharing it with my friends. Only when classes began did I realize that this was the house in my dreams. It was a vision of what my education is, that it is close to my heart and a part of me because it is about my experience, my growth, my process in life and how I will share that with others. My challenge has been dealing with sharing that vision. As I write I am confident and determined in my journey that I'm where I'm supposed to be and doing the right thing, but at the same time my confidence is also linked to how I feel about the institution that ironically was principal in creating the First Peoples House. I feel as though my dream will be denigrated by the institution, that somehow it won't be understood as I understand it.*

She continues:

> *The dream I had was a vision of the spirit that flows through me and into my work with others. I continue to find value and significance in my process, my experience and my vision. The learning process I have gone through in understanding my educational experience has been an effort in actualization. It is personal, distinguished, and indicative of the elements of who I am. To make the most out of my learning experience I must embrace who I am and understand my relationship with myself, the university, my family, and the community.*

Yet another student speaks of her own humbling learning experience:

> *I have journeyed to a place far deeper and of greater significance for myself, my family, my community—our world—in a way that cannot be described effectively using words. Our lessons are grounded through sacred ceremony into our spirit, mind, and heart knowing.*

We began by being invited to enter into this sacred journey of ceremony to reconnect to the knowing that has always been with us, but we questioned. We have been challenged to review our knowing, including Western counselling values and beliefs, through the lens of TKn. Using ceremony has enhanced the remembering of sacred practice and helped us to find healing for ourselves and for those who seek reconnection, rejuvenation, restoration, and support. Our place of understanding is within our hearts and spirits. *Being intentional of my purpose for learning is central . . . and ensuring my purpose is responsive and accountable to my community.*

Also in this experience is the call to understand the Western counselling philosophies and practices and learn how to honour both. Maintaining this integrity for the good of our communities has been a great challenge, and applying the teaching of inclusion to a way of knowing that has been harmful in the past to our people and nations has required a great deal of humility and faith. *Finding the balance of when and where to stand up to a colonial history and when to embrace the "gifts" within the same system continues to be an ongoing challenge.* There are many challenges, daily challenges, that we face, but we stand united and work with the same intentionality, moving with a clear intention of love. As a cohort, we have learned that we needed to follow this way of keeping our spirits strong, healthy, and balanced. *I have also learned that when I am not working from this place [of love], then I participate in the disconnection, alienation and suffering—physically and spiritually.*

One student describes these teachings as parallel to what she has been taught in the Kwak'wak'ka'wakw (northern Vancouver Island First Nation) big house. *All things are connected, relationship is key, and it all comes back to our connections to our Mother Earth.* This is where our healing will really become significant. When we are in balance with Mother Earth, and all living things, then our soul wounds will be healed on that journey.

Another student writes that her learning has been about the value of trusting her inner knowing and nurturing it. In Shuswap (central British Columbia First Nation), there is a word that has to do with a style of learning, *Etsxe*. Translated, *Etsxe* means "the value of knowing your gifts." This student describes how traditional teachings are a lens for remembering and refreshing knowledge within:

> *Unlike my previous experience with formal education offered through the institution, where learning was structured through gaining knowledge from outside, the learning in this program is also about remembering and refreshing the knowledge from within. From that lens, I have been able to be critical of the external research and academic writings, and have begun to deconstruct from a true, personal, and Aboriginal lens. From learning and growing from the heart and my own intuition, I have been guided toward my own truth and a reassurance of who I am and where I am from. Although I have been questioning much of what I know along my journey, I have been inspired to seek out the answers in an honourable and respectful way, and in a traditional way: by seeking out stories from my family and culture, by prayer, and by dreams.*

Walking in Two Worlds

In this Indigenous community-oriented counselling program, we struggle to articulate this puzzle of *walking in two worlds* and teaching back to what our experiences have been. One classmate has described this journey of bridging these two worlds as *braiding our hair together*. As we are weaving, our intention is for strands of balance, awareness, and truth based in traditional knowledge, while harmoniously incorporating strands of Western thought. Some came to the program firmly grounded in knowledge and practice of helping from an Indigenous centre. Others were unclear about what that meant. In order to practice Indigenous-centred counselling while often working in Western frameworks, we must learn to walk within these two worlds so we can connect with others independently of their worldview. This program has gifted us the time and space to grapple with the complications that come from walking in two worlds. We have learned we must all have a clear vision of what it means for us to work from an Indigenous centre and to be accountable to the people and communities we are helping. Another significant part of our learning has been developing our skills of communicating to others in Western writing, words, and actions what it means to work in a way that respects Indigenous knowledge. Developing an Indigenous lens and learning about helping and healing as a community have brought us to a more holistic understanding of counselling.

From the beginning, Dr. Larry Emerson encouraged us to see that we all have an Indigenous self, one in which we can uncover the layers of modernity that affect us all to varying degrees. Although it was uncomfortable at times, he pushed us to identify and define our Indigenous lens in traditional modalities and in more Western written formats. Our Indigenous lens is essentially the way we see and experience the world that weaves in and respects traditional knowledge. Modalities representing knowledge in our cohort included dreamcatchers, woven bags to carry sacred objects, and traditional drinks. Each modality had a unique meaning connected to our communities, families, experiences, and spirits. Our lenses illuminate the promises we make to our communities, our families, and ourselves and speak to the intentions we have as helpers.

Our teachers, Elders, professors, and community practitioners have showed us how traversing in two worlds is done with honour and respect. They have shared their stories and teachings. The challenges they have overcome are echoes of our own. As one classmate reflects:

> *One challenge is taking the academy's and traditional knowledge and trying to integrate them . . . Traditional knowledge was just there for us to embrace and integrate . . . it becomes a path. It's about finding balance and harmony, trying to walk in that way. We are pushed by program demands to perform to certain "standards," while at times wrestling with beliefs that these requirements are unnatural and part of Western institutionalized practice.*

In this program, we are constantly asked to step outside our comfort zone and take on new activities. At times, we can become so focused on an unfamiliar format that we lose our way. Through this process, I have learned patience! Patience with my own limitations and patience to see that, with practice, I will learn what is being asked of me.

The guidance and support from the community, as well as from non-Aboriginal professors who are allies in helping and healing in Indigenous communities, has been ever present. It was good to have teachers and Elders who have a sense of spirituality and academics who know how to build community and remember that our community is bigger than the classroom. *We celebrated our beginning—not just the end—in the Long House and were embraced by the community.*

The journey this program is taking us on has been described as being about the innate wisdom we carry and use to look at our processes and to understand this with a sense of harmony. Ideally, in the folds of our group, we are gifted the time and space to explore these identities, refine our Indigenous lenses, and honour ceremony such as singing, drumming, and prayer. These are the times when our program nurtures our growth with gentle smiles and guidance with the grace of a grandmother's touch. Ceremony presents a unique opportunity for non-Aboriginal students with limited experience in this realm to witness and understand how ceremony heals and restores. We then learn how an understanding of traditional knowledge can be shared among Aboriginal and non-Aboriginal peoples and practiced harmoniously across cultures. These differences in culture are not only between Aboriginal and non-Aboriginal students but among all of us. The women in the inaugural ACCP program have come from communities across Canada, and the teachings we bring to our group have been an enriching experience for us all. Carrying Indigenous knowledge into the community is integrated into our helping practices. We have expressed our appreciation for practicum field placements that honour a collaborative effort. Regular team meetings, debriefings, and brainstorming strategies are recognized as familiar experiences in practicum placements. We also try to work as much as possible in a circle, with a traditional opening and introduction about why we are meeting, an Aboriginal story or process, and a traditional closing, much like how the ACCP classes operate, but this depends on the situation.

We will continue to navigate through these two worlds with focus, discipline, and intentionality. The challenges we face will no doubt at times feel insurmountable, and that is when we will hopefully rest into the moment and look through to the promises we have made to our communities and in turn to ourselves. This journey is summarized in the words of our professor Larry Emerson, who guided us in finding our Indigenous voice and lens:

> *The walk may not always be pretty, but if we observe carefully along the way, if we are mindful to learn and unlearn, to let go and embrace, we find harmony, beauty and balance hidden in the trail. We just have to look and be confident that our ancestors, our grandmas, and grandpas are watching . . . Periodically, we have to assess our struggles to see the successes, to align the successes to glimpse that dimension of our story.*

Lessons Learned

We are learning to decolonize our minds, to free ourselves from the *expert* mind frame of Western knowing and move into the teachings of how to be a good human being. It also means to walk humbly, with the understanding that we have gifts to receive from others. Our goal then becomes one of walking in harmony, beauty, and balance with all our relations. We believe we have been set on Mother Earth to help restore, rejuvenate, and revitalize the law of nature given to us by our Creator and passed down through our ancestors. We do this through ceremony and through the ways of song, dance, and language. Had we attended a Western-centred graduate counselling program, we would likely still be struggling individually to have our voices heard. Because of our experiences with ICL, we are better equipped to return to our communities and provide our helping gifts in ways that are meaningful and relevant to Indigenous ways of knowing. Furthermore, we are focusing less on justifying our knowledge, thus minimizing Western modes of dichotomous knowing. Instead we have a safe, sacred space to learn how to *braid our [Western and Indigenous knowledge] hair together* (teaching from Kwak'wak'ka'wakw Elder/mentor, Wa'ta [Christine] Joseph).

Today there are a growing number of practitioners and researchers who are demonstrating the value of traditional knowledge in the counselling field and showing how to integrate Indigenous and Western approaches into a harmonious joining of worldviews (Duran, 2006; McCormick, 2009; Stewart, 2007). The University of Victoria Indigenous Communities Counselling Psychology program has embraced this integration so that our communities will experience the benefits of this innovative work. All nineteen students in the first ACCP cohort have graduated and are working in different helping positions. Most are working within Indigenous contexts. A second cohort of thirteen students began their ICCP program in January 2014. Similar to the inaugural ACCP cohort, they are also Indigenous and non-Indigenous, as well as from diverse backgrounds and professional experiences. They, too, are learning to walk in two worlds and to integrate Indigenous and Western knowledge in their own particular ways. As they move through the second year of their program, they echo many of the hopes, fears, and goals of the first cohort yet have new experiences to share that will enrich their classmates' learning and understanding of how to blend the best of both worlds to support individuals, families, and communities. As one ACCP student observed, *As human beings, we all seek this connection and balance and we all once knew these teachings. It is time to return to the ways of helping and healing that feed our spirits.*

References

Ball, J. (2004). As if indigenous knowledge and communities mattered. *American Indian Quarterly, 28*(3–4), 455–479.

British Columbia Ministry of Advanced Education. (2007). *Aboriginal post-secondary education strategy and action plan*. Retrieved Nov. 23, 2007, from http://www.aved.gov.bc.ca/aboriginal/documents/strategy.pdf

Duran, E. (2006). *Healing the soul wound: Counseling with American Indians and other native peoples*. New York, NY: Columbia University Teachers' College Press.

Emerson, L. (2006). Through an indigenous lens: Teacher education program honours Kainai community. *Tribal College Journal of American Indian Higher Education, 18*(2), 18–21.

Lane, Jr., P., Bopp, J., Bopp, M., Brown, L., & Elders. (2004). *The sacred tree: Reflections on Native American spirituality*. USA: Lotus Press.

Maracle, L. (2008). Decolonizing Native women. In B. A. Mann (Ed.), *Make a beautiful way: The wisdom of Native American women* (pp. 29–52). Lincoln: University of Nebraska Press.

McCormick, R. (2009). Aboriginal approaches to Counselling. In L. J. Kirmayer, & Gabor G. Valaskakis (Eds.), *Healing traditions: The mental health of Aboriginal peoples in Canada* (pp. 337–354). Vancouver: UBC Press.

Schaefer, C. (2006). *Grandmothers counsel the world: Women elders offer their vision for our planet*. Boston: Trumpeter Books.

Sefa Dei, G. J. (2002). Rethinking the role of indigenous knowledge in the academy. *NALL Working Paper, 58*, 1–25.

Simpson, L. (2004). Anticolonial strategies for the recovery and maintenance of indigenous knowledge. *American Indian Quarterly, 28*(3–4), 373–384.

Stewart, S. (2007). *Indigenous Mental Health: Canadian Native Counsellors' Stories* (Unpublished doctoral dissertation). University of Victoria, Victoria, British Columbia.

Warner, L. (2006). Native ways of knowing: Let me count the ways. *The Canadian Journal of Native Education, 29*(2), 149–164.

Acknowledgements

We are grateful for Lorna Williams's vision and tenacity; for Anne Marshall's trust, support, and perseverance, and her desire to keep seeing that there is something more; the Advisory Committee's commitment and dedication to bring this vision to reality; and to all the instructors and Elders for guiding us with their own teachings and honouring our knowing—giving sacred space for us to unfold our gifts. Many thanks to our Elder and teacher, Larry Emerson, who has guided us and this program into the light and vision of our own traditional knowledge through ICL with the use of sacred ceremony. Larry's teachings and role modeling have been our grounding and for this we cannot give enough thanks. And to all our mentors within our communities, thank you for keeping us connected to what is important—the reason we are doing this work. With offer much respect to all who have paved the way for the new trailblazing we are taking on!

14 A Partnership With the People

Skilful Navigation of Culture and Ethics

Melinda A. García, Gayle S. Morse, Joseph E. Trimble, Denise M. Casillas, Beth Boyd, and Jeff King

> Politics (the "social and collective") does not begin where ethics ("the behavior of individuals") ends. . . . there must be a commonness, a humanity, to make ethics possible.
>
> (Grosz, 1989, p. xvii. Further,

> Every question that is political is also moral. Every question. And you have to answer morally. Moreover, issues of power in ethics, especially in the ethics of science, are rarely, if ever, absent. They continue to be played out vividly and resolutely in ongoing struggles over biocolonialism.
>
> (Lyons, 1993)

The words of the distinguished Haudenosaunee (Iroquois) leader, Oren Lyon (Juagquisho), point to the need for field-based researchers to establish ethical behaviour as defined by communities built on respect for different life ways and thought ways. Community voices all over the world are demanding ethical research and challenging the way research has been conducted and the way that respondents were treated during the research process. Ethnocultural communities are no longer interested in scientists who conduct research *on* research subjects. Increasingly, communities are requiring that researchers demonstrate they have the dialogic capacity that will allow them to develop critical knowledge with and alongside community members (ATFE, 1996; Ho-Chunk Legislature, 2005; Navajo Human Research Review Board, 2007a; Navajo Human Research Review Board, 2007b; Trimble & Fisher, 2006; Watkins & Shulman, 2008).

The recent increase in research conducted among ethnocultural groups around the world has been accompanied by mounting community concerns and negative reactions to the Western-based models of research in which the researcher is the expert and is not accountable to the community. These concerns have resulted in active efforts by communities to set standards for respect and accountability and have often been accompanied by the emergence of community-based research review committees. The expectations of communities for respect, trust, equity, and ethical research, as defined by those communities, present unplanned and unusual challenges for many researchers who have not been trained in methodologies that encourage relatedness, interdependence, and transparency with the community. One of the most important challenges is the ethical conduct, as defined by the community, of researchers while they are in the field. What the community defines as ethical may not coincide with the time and productivity demands of Western universities and granting agencies. Another important challenge is the co-development of research goals and research methodology with the community as opposed to the researcher being the expert who sets the research agenda. Finally, the question of who owns the data and interprets the outcomes has become highlighted in recent years. Though controversial in Western universities, most communities now consider the data collected to be community owned, and they require input into the interpretation of the data (Santiago-Rivera, Morse, Hunt, & Lickers, 1998; Navajo Human Research Review Board, 2007a; Navajo Human Research Review Board, 2007b). Communities now require that the process of the research, as well as its fruits, benefit the community (American Indian Law Center, 1999; Rivkin et al., 2011; Watkins & Shulman, 2008).

Community research that is conducted with a lack of cultural sensitivity and ethical clarity has frequently lead to field-based research that has been harmful to the participants. Yet research can be beneficial to these communities if appropriate measures are taken to ensure cultural responsiveness and solid grounding in the cultural worldviews of communities.

Ethnocultural Research and Complaints From North American/Alaskan Indian Communities

Psychology has a long history of cultural ignorance and bias when conducting research with Native communities (Capriccioso, 2010; Foulks, 1989; García & Tehee, 2014; Norton & Manson, 1996; Trimble & Fisher, 2006). As such, tribes have come to view psychological research with the same critical eye that they use with anthropological and medical research. Researchers from each of these disciplines have failed to follow the principles of informed consent, reporting their findings back to the communities, and sharing the data with communities. There have been systematic failures to engage either individuals or the community in order to come to a consensus of the nature of "the problem" being studied (Foulks, 1989). Deception regarding the purpose of the research has been common. In the United States, surveys of ethnocultural populations reveal suspicion with individual and community surveys, intervention studies, informant reports, blood sampling, and genetic research (Corbie-Smith, Thomas, & St. George, 2002; Fisher & Wallace, 2000). Susan Reverby also exposed the U.S. Public Health Service's syphilis and gonorrhea experimentation in Guatemala from 1946 to 1948, in which hundreds of people, including institutionalized mental patients, were intentionally infected with gonorrhea and syphilis (Reverby, 2011). Lest one should be tempted to think of these as the most egregious examples of research hubris and abuse of institutional power, Harriet Washington's groundbreaking history, *Medical Apartheid* (2006), provides evidence of almost four hundred years of medical experimentation on Black Americans from colonial times to the present. Recent highly publicized complaints from Native communities include the Barrow Alaska Study (Davis et al., 2002; Norton & Manson, 1996), the lawsuit brought by the Havasupai tribe against Arizona State University (Hendricks, 2004), and the Human Genome Diversity Project (Whitt, 2009).

In the Barrow Alaska Alcohol Study (Foulks, 1989), Intersect (a consulting firm based in Seattle, whose director had previously worked in Barrow) developed a study to examine alcohol abuse and the local treatment detoxification program among the Inupiat tribal members. The research design team included people from the Alaska Department of Health as well as outside consultants. The research design and initial publications did not consider ethnocultural factors. The resulting publications reinforced Native stereotypes and created a firestorm of controversy between the local community, the local researchers, and outside research team. The subsequent damage to the community eclipsed any opportunity to better understand the scientific merit or utility of the study (Foulks, 1989; Norton & Manson, 1996; Trimble & Fisher, 2006).

In the early 1990s, Arizona State University (ASU) researchers collected blood samples from Havasupai tribal members to search for genetic links for diabetes risk (Trimble, Scharron-del Rio, & Casillas, 2013). An unsuccessful attempt to find a genetic link to type 2 diabetes led the ASU researchers to reorganize their study to use the blood samples to study schizophrenia and inbreeding, as well as to potentially uncover factors that could explain human migration patterns. Tribal members learned in a public lecture at ASU that the blood samples had been used for purposes other than those they agreed to when signing the human subjects consent forms. The tribe filed a lawsuit in 2004. In 2010, the Arizona Board of Regents settled the lawsuit, agreeing to pay $700,000 to the tribe, provide funds for a clinic and a school, and to return the blood samples (Capriccioso, 2010; Hendricks, 2004).

In yet another example, requests for confidentiality from tribal authorities were ignored by researchers when they published the results of a series of studies on the hantavirus pulmonary syndrome that appeared in journal articles in 1993 and 1994; authors named the Diné (Navajo) location in their articles, even after the tribe had specifically asked investigators to keep the information confidential. Thus, as a direct consequence of the recurring abuse of trust by researchers, many American Indian tribes' interest in participating in research has diminished; in this case, the Diné did not approve of any further research for over a year after these publications, although the hantavirus continued to spread throughout the area (Childs et al., 1994; Davis & Reid, 1999; Nichol et al., 1993).

Indigenous communities across the world led in part by U.S. American Indians have uniformly condemned the Human Genome Diversity Project that has also been called the Vampire Project (LaDuke, 2005). This project attempts to define groups of Indigenous people with genetic material and has been condemned by Indigenous populations and the United Nations Educational, Scientific and Cultural Organization's International Bioethics Committee. Yet the project continues with external funding because, as the scientists argue, they were merely trying to document *all* people and not leave anyone out. Further, they suggested that those opposed (primarily Indigenous groups) simply misunderstood their project (LaDuke, 2005; Whitt, 2009). This echoes the colonial view that outsiders know what is best for the Indigenous people. At this time, more American Indian groups, such as the Society of Indian Psychologists, are speaking out with examples of this harmful colonial view and possible solutions to the problem specifically related to research and publication (García & Tehee, 2014).

The Society of Indian Psychologists Commentary on the APA Ethics Code (García & Tehee, 2014) includes over a dozen recent examples of pervasive and consistent ethical violations on the part of researchers. In this document, Native psychologists provided examples of current problems with every part of Standard 8: Research and Publication in the APA Ethics Code (APA, 2010). A Native psychologist described racist comments on the part of an anonymous reviewer during the peer-review process for a publication. Although the editor of the publication told the psychologist to ignore the comments, there was no recourse regarding this reviewer or the inappropriate comments (García & Tehee, 2014, p. 76). This incident suggests that psychologists may be allowed to make racist comments under the cover of anonymous review without any fear of exposure or censure.

Further, Native psychologists have a much more challenging burden when describing their proposed research for grants because the reviewers have little or no cultural knowledge in order to understand the quality and potential impact of the proposal (García & Tehee, 2014, pp. 79–80). The Native psychologist then has to add additional explanatory material, which uses precious and extremely limited space, to their grant applications because they must educate the potential reviewers. This short-changes the discussion of the research design and its implications for the community. Equal space to describe the research in the grant proposal does not lead to equity in access to research resources. A level playing field assumes that the reviewers will be culturally competent to review all research designs with all populations. This level playing field does not exist at this time. The result is that grants do not get funded because the reviewers are not culturally competent to assess whether the proposal is scientifically necessary.

Western-based psychology continues to maintain that a "no treatment" control condition is the gold standard for determining empirically relevant interventions. Withholding treatment or intervention for a number of participants is completely unacceptable in many Native communities. It is incompatible with the cultural view of caring for each other equally and is seen as cruel (García & Tehee, 2014, p. 77). It is likely that informed consent is culturally informed in ways unknown to an outside researcher and that this may not include a "no treatment control" condition. Although the researcher is the expert in Western methodology, the community members are the experts in their community beliefs and processes through which they interpret research methodology. In order to respect the reciprocal relationship, the process and utility of research must be explained before the specific issue needing consent can be presented (Watkins & Shulman, 2008, p. 303). Researchers should not assume that the community is too naive or uneducated to understand the research. It is incumbent upon ethical researchers to clearly explain their methodology in language understood by the community. This requires researchers to use language and communication methods that are not in common use in academia. For example, in one study, before the project was submitted for review, not only was the method for participant engagement reviewed with the community but also the proposed measures were evaluated by focus groups to determine their potential reliability, validity, and acceptability to the community (Santiago-Rivera, Morse, Haase, & McCaffrey, 2007). As Foulks (1989) argued, it is not the method that causes problems but rather the participants' naiveté that is responsible for a lack of understanding. Researchers must understand their own cultural naiveté with respect to the intersection of research methodology and cultural context so they do not miss important cultural taboos specific to each group. Examples of this include recording voices or taking pictures for research (García & Tehee, 2014, p. 77).

Regarding the reporting of research results, a Native psychologist noted, "There is such a strong mainstream Western ideology of what research is, that there is virtually no room to put any Indigenous context to publications arising from research with Native populations" (García & Tehee, 2014, p. 78). Another added, "Respecting the dignity and sovereignty of the community dictates that a community member should be included in the writing process and subsequent publication as a community expert in interpreting research outcomes" (García & Tehee, 2014, p. 78). This is important so both emic and etic perspectives can be utilized in interpreting the data that allows the cultural context to become an important part of the narrative and frame the outcomes.

Professional Ethical Guidelines and Standards of Conduct

In response to widespread grievances from ethnocultural communities as a result of culturally incompetent and unethical research practices, many tribal groups have developed guidelines to improve the quality of the research process and collection and use of research data, as well as interpretation of results. This movement began with the American Anthropological Association (AAA) in 1967 as a response to continued abuses in research with ethnocultural populations. Subsequently, the AAA released a special publication on research ethics (Cassell & Jacobs, 1987) designed to improve and advance the ethical considerations in anthropological research and practice.

Other professional organizations followed. The American Psychological Association issued the *Guidelines for Research in Ethnic Minority Communities* (APA, 2000) and *Guidelines on Multicultural Education, Training, Research, Practice, and Organizational Change for Psychologists* (APA, 2002). The Canadian Institutes of Health Research published their *Guidelines for Health Research Involving Aboriginal People* (2007) as a result of an interdisciplinary and multicultural multiyear effort in developing them.

In 2009, the International Union of Psychological Science, the International Association of Applied Psychology, and the International Association for Cross-Cultural Psychology issued the *Universal Declaration of Ethical Principles for Psychologists* (2009), which acknowledged that a single way of defining respect and ethics is not appropriate.

> Respect for the dignity and worth of human beings is expressed in different ways in different communities and cultures. It is important to acknowledge and respect such differences. On the other hand, it also is important that all communities and cultures adhere to moral values that respect and protect their members both individually and collectively.

More recently, a consortium of researchers from New Mexico tribal communities and researchers from the University of New Mexico issued the *Guiding Principles for Engaging in Research with Native American Communities* (Straits et al., 2012). All of these guidelines are thoughtful and sincere attempts to provide a structure for responsible research with ethnocultural populations. Unfortunately, all of them are voluntary, and none of them address the deep-seated bias that characterizes the training and practice of psychology in the United States today.

Most psychologists in the United States follow the APA Ethics Code (APA, 2010) without understanding the cultural values, or automatic attitudes, embedded in the code. For example, Principle B states, "Psychologists consult with, refer to, or cooperate with other professionals and institutions to the extent needed to serve the best interests of those with whom they work." This principle ignores the cultural views or needs of a community and suggests an automatic colonial and patriarchal view that the researcher will know what is best for the community. Similar automatic or implicit attitudes consist of associative knowledge for which we may lack awareness, while reflective or explicit attitudes are those that we are aware of having (Banaji & Greenwald, 2013). There is a large body of research that indicates that everyone has automatic attitudes, also known as hidden biases, even psychologists. Those automatic attitudes about social groups can influence our behaviour and decisions towards those groups while we remain oblivious to their presence. Most people, including psychologists, are often unaware of disagreement between the explicit and the automatic, or hidden, forms of their own attitudes and stereotypes (Banaji & Greenwald, 2013; Kahneman, 2011).

Researchers have also attempted to analyze the factors that have contributed to problems in doing studies with various ethnocultural groups

(Bengsten, Grigsby, Corry, & Hruby, 1977; Burhansstipanov, Christopher, & Schumacher, 2005; Cassell & Jacobs, 1987; Foulks, 1989; Hillabrant, 2002; Ibrahim & Cameron, 2005; Malgady, 1996; Rogler, 1999; Tierney, 2001; Trimble, 1977). Many have also suggested positive ways to address research with ethnocultural populations (Blume, 2014; Casillas, 2006; Castellano, 2004; Fisher et al., 2002; Goodenough, 1980; Letiecq & Bailey, 2004; Santiago-Rivera et al., 1998; Smith, 1999; Straits et al., 2012; Trimble & Fisher, 2006; Trimble & Mohatt, 2006).

After decades of struggling with researchers to practice in a respectful and competent way with Indigenous communities, the Society of Indian Psychologists (SIP) decided to write and publish a commentary on the APA Ethics Code (APA, 2010) in order to expose the continuous difficulties arising from dealing with the consequences of hidden biases and ongoing cultural ignorance (García & Tehee, 2014). According to the SIP Commentary, the biases embedded in the APA Code of Ethics, but never made explicit, are

a) Behaviour can be best studied as discrete units to understand the whole
b) Compartmentalism is helpful in promoting the understanding of how humans function
c) It is best for individuals to be autonomous and self-reliant (p. 13).

In contrast, Indigenous people of the Americas as well as other parts of the world have defined health as complex, holistic, and interrelational for thousands of years. A person cannot be understood outside of the context of his/her family, group, and community. A person seeks intervention because his/her life is out of balance. The restoration of balance (physically, emotionally, mentally, spiritually, and contextually) is often the goal of intervention, not individual efficacy or individual understanding. The community, whether tribal or urban, is considered an entity in addition to individuals. There are many stories throughout the Commentary that illustrate the tension between the competing values of American individualism and Indigenous community engagement (García & Tehee, 2014).

Most of the stories in the Commentary refer to a lack of competence (Standard 2, APA, 2010) in all areas of psychology, including training, delivery of services, and research. These stories illustrate that it is not possible to be competent as a psychologist without cultural competence. The process of recalling and writing the stories in the SIP Commentary was painful for many of the participants. Some occurred last year, which felt like yesterday and not so long ago, while some occurred thirty years ago. The overall lack of cultural competence or cultural humility in the field of psychology, including in research, remains a constant flaw. In response to Standard 3: Human Relations (APA, 2010), which addresses avoiding discrimination and harm, the SIP Commentary states:

> This Standard may be the least enforced Standard in the Ethics Code. Which types of discrimination are fair? Discrimination by psychologists

> often comes from implicit and unacknowledged biases that are expressed as micro-aggressions. While the term is called "micro," the effect on the receiving party is profound. This Standard only represents lip service or window dressing towards the idea that psychologists should seek out and demonstrate multicultural competence skills.
>
> (p. 42)

Through the Commentary, SIP maintains that it is not possible to understand ethics as separate from culture. Culture is the frame through which behaviour is considered to be ethical or unethical. The abuse of power through the privilege of ignoring culture or by assuming that White values are universal plays a major role in the harm experienced by Indigenous people as well as other marginalized and stigmatized people from researchers. While the APA Ethics Code encourages psychologists to be aware of their own biases, values, and sociocultural framework, in actual practice, this kind of awareness is rare (García & Tehee, 2014). Skilful research is ethical research that recognizes and respects the cultural and ethical frames of all parties. Research that ignores cultural context will be deeply flawed and have very limited generalizability (Henrich, Heine, & Norenzayan, 2010).

In present-day United States, explicit bias is infrequent and exhibited at much lower frequency than fifty to seventy-five years ago. Implicit bias is pervasive: 75 percent of Americans display an implicit preference for White people relative to Black people (Banaji & Greenwald, 2013). There is a large body of evidence, both individual studies and meta-studies that report that automatic White preference, or hidden bias, predicts discriminatory behaviour, even among people who espouse egalitarian views (Banaji & Greenwald, 2013). This alarming and illuminating research indicates that self-reflection, one of the most frequently used methods by psychologists to analyze their own behaviour, is shockingly ineffective in helping the person to change behaviour. There is a profound need for change in the culture of American psychology in order for psychologists to "first, do no harm." SIP community members documented their experiences as a way to cut through abstract, academic ideas of what constitutes a competent psychologist or researcher. Effective psychological research is contextual and relational. Competent psychological research is honest. Honest research recognizes inherent biases and recognizes culture, and it is moral and ethically consistent with the individual or groups involved in the study.

According to Trimble and Mohatt (2006), compliance with and the enactment of moral and ethical principles begin with the researcher. They ask:

> What does it mean to be an ethical person when conducting research with ethnocultural communities? Does it imply that one must be a morally upstanding person who abides by a rigorous set of virtues that cannot be compromised? Does one approach ethical standards by viewing community-based dilemmas from a principled perspective guided by

> the fixed rules of objectivity, reason, and impartiality? Is that approach likely to be acceptable to the community's research partners? Is it possible that one's character and thus moral and ethical standards are incompatible with those likely to exist in the host research community? (p. 327)

In keeping with Juagquisho's (*Oren Lyons)* comments (1977) regarding respect, moral, and ethical human interactions, an interrelational view of harmony and balance in life, in health, and in communities, the SIP Commentary proposes that Respect (currently Principle E) be the very first Principle, as none of the other Principles can occur in an environment in which Respect on the part of both parties is missing. Two additional Principles are proposed and defined: cultural relevance and humility (p. 15).

Cultural relevance refers to services designed for and constructive to a particular community. It was first discussed in the education literature by Gloria Ladson-Billings (1995) as a service, "that empowers students to maintain cultural integrity, while succeeding academically" (p. 476). Essentially, it is the idea that good research should consider the culture in order to be related to the community on their terms. Sometimes a new approach must be designed in order to be relevant. Sometimes this might mean an adaptation of services or methods used with other populations. Most importantly, the community, not the researcher, is the final arbiter of cultural relevance. Researchers may not understand the importance of cultural relevance if they have not explored the notions of multicultural competence and cultural humility.

Multicultural competence is considered a first step *before* conducting community research. It is mandatory for a researcher to actively seek out the skills to become multiculturally competent rather than assuming that he or she already is (García & Tehee, 2014; Straits et al., 2012; Trimble, 2013; Trimble, Pedersen, & Rodela, 2009). Cultural humility, as first discussed by Tervalon and Murray-García (1998), suggests that cultural humility is the next logical step to move beyond cultural competence. They noted that cultural humility must be a lifelong practice of continued reflection and self-critique in which each individual researcher acknowledges the power of his or her position and the need for mutual benefit between the researcher and the communities and individuals with whom he or she works. Mutual benefit must be developed with the communities and individuals in a non-paternalistic way, where all parties understand how differences in understanding may influence assessment, diagnosis, treatment, and research outcomes and interpretations. Failure to obtain multicultural competence training and a lack of cultural humility is a set-up for the unintentional abuse of power. It is important to recognize that a lack of cultural competence is a natural consequence of living in this society and taking active steps to correct this lack of competence (Banaji & Greenwald, 2013; Tervalon & Murray-García, 1998).

Cultural humility encourages psychologists to generate creative and culturally appropriate ways of connecting with communities, thus increasing trust with their clients. For example, the psychologist who understands cultural humility will recognize that staying in the office and expecting clients to come to them is a culture-bound expectation of Western psychology. Indigenous communities often wait to see how a new psychologist will interact with the community at large before individuals from that community decide to trust her or him. The psychologist who understands cultural humility will not assume that laboratory research, specialized and compartmentalized research, and "objective" research constitute a "gold standard" to which everyone aspires. Table 14.1 from the SIP Commentary (García & Tehee, 2014, pp. 74–75) has been included in order to more clearly illustrate the Indigenous approach to research. It is heavily based upon the work of Manuel Ramirez (1998, pp. 18–20).

Community-Based Participatory Research

Community-based participatory research (CBPR) is defined as research where the community and researchers work together from the inception through design, implementation, and publication of the study (Minkler & Wallerstein, 2003; Santiago-Rivera et al., 1998; Watkins & Shulman, 2008). As Newbrough (1995) aptly noted, community can be defined by an emphasis on fraternity, liberty and equality centred on balance, justice, and fairness. The methodology of CBPR is not just how to do research in a community but rather a way of approaching research as a partnership in which all members are equal in a number of ways (Rivkin et al., 2011). It is important to note that CBPR describes the way that respectful research has been conducted with Indigenous people for years (Wallerstein & Duran, 2003). The guidelines for CBPR have similar themes of respect, equity, and empowerment.

To illustrate this point, it is useful to visit the *Basic Call to Consciousness* (Lyons, 1977), an address to the United Nations in Geneva delivered by Juagquisho (Oren Lyons), which describes the *Gayaneshakgowa*, the Great Law of Peace, of the Haudenosaunee Nation (Iroquois Confederacy). The nations of the Haudenosaunee gathered together in council in order to set down the principles of the Great Law of Peace. The Great Law of Peace was originally created to prevent the abuse of humans by other humans. It stipulated that all people were free and all had a right to protection under what the Peacemaker called the Great Tree of Peace. The basic principles of peace went further than the simple absence of conflict. It is related to the Kanienkehaka (Mohawk) words *Skennen* (peace), *Kariwiio* (good mind) and *Kasastensera* (strength), which are achieved by preventing abuse of the environment as well as people. The Great Law of Peace outlined an ordered society capable of protecting people against abuse and dedicated to a containment of hierarchy. Peace may seem like an unconventional word to use

Table 14.1 Major Differences Between European and Indigenous Approaches to Research in Psychology

Characteristics of Theories	
European	*Indigenous*
• Focus is specialized and compartmentalized. • There is separation of cognitive and affective development, of nature and nurture, and of effects of sociocultural and biological-genetic influences on personality development and adjustment.	• Focus is interdisciplinary. • Personality is viewed as holistic and interwoven with social, political, and spiritual environments.
• Isolation and separation are fostered by development of specialized terminology and methodology with little intercommunication and cooperation with researchers outside the discipline.	• Emphasis is on communication and cooperation not only with other social scientists and practitioners but also with representatives of other disciplines as well.
Characteristics of Researchers	
European	*Indigenous*
• Minimizes the importance of the roles of values, belief systems, and worldviews in personality and mental health.Minimizes the importance of understanding the relationship of own values and belief systems to preference for certain theories, systems of psychotherapy, and research methodologies.	• Aware of the relationship of own values and belief systems to personal interests in research and intervention. • Values ability to synthesize and to integrate different disciplines, approaches, and worldviews.
• Analytical thinking is emphasized. The ideal is the scientist who is totally objective and removed from the social, economic, and political realities of the people with whom s/he works.	• The ideal is the generalist who is knowledgeable about history, politics, economics, spirituality, and cultural traditions and is a skilled teacher. It is preferable that the psychologist has lived through some of the same life experiences as the client or participant.

(*Continued*)

Table 14.1 (Continued)

Role of Researchers	
European	*Indigenous*
• Allegedly objective and nonpolitical. • As an ideal, personal values and belief systems are kept separate from research and intervention. • The researcher or interventionist is the expert, and the participant or patient is viewed as being sick, uninformed, underdeveloped, unfortunate, or uncivilized and in need of education, enlightenment, and enculturation, as well as more sophisticated adjustment and development.	• Deep personal commitment to solving social problems. • The principal role is to create societal change that can promote fairness, justice, empowerment, and equality of opportunity. • Conceptualizer, participant, and change agent. Views self as a partner and equal to the client or participant.
• Primary responsibility in research is to self and to academic community.	• Primarily responsible to the community in which the research is conducted and to the participants. Places the needs of the participants, clients, and communities above those of academia and science.
• Being considered by peers to be a "true scientist and scholar" is a primary goal.	• Being considered a change agent for his or her people is the primary goal.
Approach to Research and Data Interpretation	
European	*Indigenous*
• Laboratory-setting research, which maximizes control and manipulation of variables, is the ideal. • The assumption that psychological reality is fixed in time. Instruments, research methods, and intervention approaches are considered to be valid for all peoples. • Data are interpreted using theories with no modifications or allowances made for differing views of patients or clients and participants. • Emphasis is on universalism (an etic perspective in cross-cultural research).	• Naturalist setting with non-obtrusive approaches for data collection is preferred. • Use of observational and life history approaches with person-environment and person-socio-historical-political interactions are given great importance. • Data are interpreted in the context of social, physical, and spiritual environments of participants with the use of theoretical orientations and concepts that are consonant with the worldviews of participants and clients. • Emphasis is placed on individual and cultural differences (an emic perspective in cross-cultural research).

when speaking of research methods, but in terms of CBPR, it is both parsimonious and elegant.

In his address, Juagquisho defined peace (*Skennen*) as,

> the active strivings of humans for the purpose of establishing universal justice . . . the ability to enact the principles of peace through education, public opinion and political and when necessary military unity. It is the product of a spiritually conscious society using it's abilities to reason.

When we work for peace (*Skennen*), we work towards developing our good mind (*Kariwiio*) and it is then that we can get the needed work done. It is then when humility can be the driving force and thoughts of superiority, prejudice, and privilege no longer drive community research (Lyons, 1977).

In Lakota culture, the idea that everything is connected and that we are all related can be captured in the phrase *mitakuye oyasin*, which is spoken during ceremony to greet all relatives and to thank all of life. This is a profound and complex concept that is shared by many Indigenous groups throughout the Americas. It is an integral part of the values statement in the SIP Commentary (García & Tehee, 2014, pp. 13–14). This concept is behind the position, held by many Indigenous psychologists, that isolating individual variables or individual participants is not appropriate if one wants research and knowledge to be generalizable. *Mitakuye oyasin* points to the imperative for considering the entire community in undertaking any research venture and involving them in all phases of the project. These concepts give us the basic principles under which honourable and ethical research can be conducted. As noted previously, the basic principles include respect, equity, and empowerment.

Before any work can be done, respect and trust must be established between the researcher and the community. The university researcher, or even an inside community researcher, must respect and trust the people of the local population as capable researchers and holders of the knowledge of their people and society. Reciprocally, the community must respect and trust the researcher as a holder of a particular knowledge that might be helpful for them. It is essential to let go of one's need for superiority and privilege and to be humble enough to learn from each other.

A research partnership also means that the development and fruits of research are shared with both the researcher and the community. Beginning with the conceptualization of the project and continuing through the development of the methodology, the implementation phase, and publication, the partnership is defined by the notion of equity. Equity is built during the conceptualization and development of the methodology through shared participation in the creative process. As the roles of individuals emerge in the partnership, it is expected that the work to prepare the study and implement the study will be shared. Financial equity is demonstrated by having paid university as well as community researchers. In non-partnership research, the researcher would draw a salary for the project as the experts, while the community members receive nothing except the goodwill of the researcher. In partnership research, it is expected that the funding stream will include community members as well as the researchers in the salary budget. Partnership research emphasizes equity that leads to empowerment.

The principle of empowerment suggests that the research process and outcomes should benefit a community in such a way that helps the community to make changes for the members (Santiago-Rivera et al., 1998). Following this, it is important for the university researcher to take the time to train local researchers rather than using their students or research technicians, who might not be familiar with the community culture. This helps the community to become more research independent and the researcher to gain greater buy-in from the community for the research project. As community members become involved in the research and the publications associated with the research, their contributions ensure that the inferences drawn from the research outcomes are culturally consistent and useful. In addition, the publication contributions help community researchers become more independent as researchers and are more likely to carry the information to the community. The university researcher gains by having publications of increased validity because the community vetted them.

In response to research abuses described previously and consistent with the philosophy of CBPR, several tribes in the United States and Canada have developed their own Institutional Review Boards (IRB) and research protocols. For example, the Akwsasne Task Force on the Environment Advisory Committee (ATFE, 1996), the Ho-Chunk Legislature (2005), and the Navajo Human Research Review Board, 2007a; Navajo Human Research Review Board, 2007b (2007) all outline CBPR guidelines for working within their respective communities.

Recommendations for the Training of Researchers

The areas in psychology found most wanting by the SIP in their Commentary were Competence (Standard 2), Training (Standard 7), and Research (Standard 8). Addressing each of these areas is essential to training researchers who are capable of engaging in partnership research with ethnocultural populations. There is an assumption in psychology that if the method is objective, then the people using the method are objective. This completely ignores the overwhelming evidence that implicit bias affects everyone in our society (Banaji & Greenwald, 2013).

> Implicit bias may operate outside of awareness, hidden from those who have it, but the discrimination that it produces can be clearly visible to researchers, and almost certainly also clearly visible to those who are disadvantaged by it.
>
> (Banaji & Greenwald, 2013, p. 209)

There is a strong tendency for psychologists in the fields of clinical and counselling psychology to exist in silos. For the most part, psychology training programs have ignored the research that social psychologists and community psychologists have been publishing for the past thirty years about the pervasive nature of bias (Kahneman, 2011), the unconscious ways that racism is perpetuated in our society, and the ways that racism is toxic to all of us (Banaji & Greenwald, 2013). Banaji and Greenwald (2013) go on to state that inherent bias must be identified and overtly addressed in order to be neutralized.

As made abundantly clear in the SIP Commentary, the skills necessary to learn about and address one's own bias and privilege are not taught in most psychology training programs. For the research relationship with ethnocultural groups to be based on respect, the researcher *must* have done significant homework on his or her own biases, prejudices, and stereotypes prior to contacting the community, rather than reading about how it manifests in others and doing "self-reflection." Work on one's own inherent biases is a prerequisite for learning appropriate social and communication skills in the ethnocultural context. Researchers who want to work with ethnocultural communities have to have the skills to assure the community that the colonization paradigm will not apply this time. As pointed out in the earlier quote, ethnocultural communities can tell if the researcher lacks multicultural competence.

It is common in psychology training programs for faculty to encourage self-reflection as a way of identifying bias. The stories in the SIP Commentary illustrate that self-reflection is a very poor method to gain true cultural competence (García & Tehee, 2014). If our perspective is narrow, then the mirror for self-reflection will be narrow. Gaining cultural competence is a matter of acknowledging the past thirty years of research, acknowledging that we all live in a racist society, stepping out of our comfort zones to learn how to address unconscious biases, widening our own circles, and *then* having a peer group that can help us to reflect rather than avoid (Irving, 2014).

Psychology programs have also encouraged students to be "good listeners" as a way of establishing empathy with others. Ultimately, "good listening" and "empathy" are culturally defined (García & Tehee, 2014). It is not possible to be a "good listener" without being aware of the inner filter of our inherent biases (Irving, 2014).

While CBPR was discussed in this chapter as an appropriate methodology for working with ethnocultural groups, other methods can also be appropriate. For many Indigenous cultures, it is essential to understand people within their context. Observational and life history approaches to determine person-environment and person-socio-historical-political interactions provide rich data in ethnocultural communities. This is consistent with Blume's (2014) proposal that psychological science consider Indigenous views, which can improve upon the current standards of research for everyone. Holistic perspectives supported by purposeful communal goals and a spiritual worldview may represent the best and most complete way to address critical community problems (Blume, 2014).

If you understand the basics then you can understand the possibilities.

I add my breath to your breath
That our days may be long on the Earth,
That the days of our people may be long,
That we may be one person,
That we may finish our roads together.
May our mother bless you with life.
May our Life Paths be fulfilled.
Keres song (Allen, 1986, p. 56)

References

Akwesasne Task Force on the Environment Advisory Committee. (1996). *Protocol for review of environmental and scientific research proposals*. Hogansburg, NY: ATFE.

Allen, P. G. (1986). *The sacred hoop: Recovering the feminine in American Indian traditions*. Boston: Beacon Press.

American Indian Law Center. (1999). *Model tribal research code: With materials for tribal regulation for research and checklist for Indian health boards*, 3rd ed. Albuquerque, NM: American Indian Law Center, Inc.

American Psychological Association. (2000). *Guidelines for research in ethnic minority communities*. Washington, DC: Council of National Psychhological Associations for the Advancement of Ethnic Minority Interests.

American Psychological Association (2002). *Guidelines on multicultural education, training, research, practice, and organizational change for psychologists*. Washington, DC: Author.

American Psychological Association (2010). *Ethical principles of psychologists and code of conduct* (2002, Amended June 1, 2010). Retrieved from http://www.apa.org/ethics/code/index.aspxBanaji, M. R., & Greenwald, A. G. (2013). *Blind spot: Hidden biases of good people*. New York: Delacorte Press.

Bengsten, V., Grigsby, E., Corry, E., & Hruby, M. (1977). Relating academic research to community concerns: A case in collaborative effort. *Journal of Social Issues, 33*(4), 75–92.

Blume, A. W. (2014). Sharing the light of the sacred fire: A proposal for a paradigm shift in psychology. *Journal of Indigenous Research*. Retrieved from http://digitalcommons.usu.edu/kicjir/vol3/iss1/4/

Burhansstipanov, L., Christopher, S., & Schumacher, A. (2005). Lessons learned from community-based participatory research in Indian Country. *Cancer Control, Cancer, Culture, and Literacy Supplement, 12*(Suppl 2), 70–76.

Canadian Institutes of Health Research. (2007). *CIHR guidelines for health research involving aboriginal people*. Retrieved from http://www.cihr-irsc.gc.ca/e/29134.html

Capriccioso, R. (2010, April 23). Havasupai blood case settled. *Indian Country Today*. Retrieved October, 21, 2010 from http://www.indiancountrytoday.com/archive/91728874.html

Casillas, D. M. (2006). *Evolving research approaches in tribal communities: A community empowerment training*. Unpublished master's thesis, University of South Dakota, Vermillion, SD.

Cassell, J., & Jacobs, S. (Eds.) (1987). *Handbook on ethical issues in anthropology*. Special publication of the American Anthropological Association. No. 23. Washington, DC: American Anthropological Association.

Castellano, M. B. (2004). Ethics of Aboriginal research. *Journal of Aboriginal Health, 1*, 98–114.

Childs, J. E., Ksiazek, T. G., Spiropoulou, C. F., Krebs, J. W., Morzunov, S., Maupin, G. O., Gage, K. L., Rollin, P. E., Sarisky, J., Enscore, R. E., Frey, J. K., Peters, C. J., & Nichol, S. T. (1994). Serologic and genetic identification of *Peromyscus maniculatus* as the primary rodent reservoir for a hantavirus in the southwestern United States. *Journal of Infectious Diseases, 169*, 1271–1280.

Corbie-Smith, G., Thomas, S. B., & St. George, D. M. M. 2002. Distrust, race and research. *Archives of Internal Medicine, 162*, 2458–2463.

Davis, J. D., Erickson, J. S., Johnson, S. R., Marshall, C. A., Running Wolf, P., & Santiago, R. L. (Eds.) (2002). *Work Group on American Indian Research and Program Evaluation Methodology (AIRPEM), Symposium on research and evaluation methodology: Lifespan issues related to American Indians/ Alaska Natives with disabilities*. Flagstaff: Northern Arizona University, Institute for Human Development, Arizona University Center on Disabilities, American Indian Rehabilitation Research and Training Center. Retrieved July 15, 2005 from http://www.nau.edu/ihd/airrtc/catalog.html

Davis, S. M., & Reid, R. (1999). Practicing participatory research in American Indian communities. *American Journal of Clinical Nutrition, 69*, 755S–759S.

Fisher, C. B., Hoagwood, K., Boyce, C., Duster, T., Frank, D. A., Grisso, T., Levine, R. J., Macklin, R., Spencer, M. B., Takanishi, R., Trimble, J. E., & Zayas, L. H. (2002). Research ethics for mental health science involving ethnic minority children and youths. *American Psychologist, 57*, 1024–1040.

Fisher, C. B., & Wallace, S. C. (2000). Through the community looking glass: Reevaluating the ethical and policy implications of research on adolescent risk and psychopathology. *Ethics and Behavior, 10*, 99–118.

Foulks, E. F. (1989). Misalliances in the barrow alcohol study. *American Indian and Alaskan Native Mental Health Research, 2*, 2–17.

García, M., & Tehee, M. (Eds.) (2014). *Society of Indian psychologists commentary on the American Psychological Association's (APA) ethical principles of psychologists and code of conduct*. Retrieved from http://www.aiansip.org

Goodenough, W. H. (1980). Ethnographic field techniques. In H. C. Triandis, & J. W. Berry (Eds.), *Handbook of cross-cultural psychology: Methodology* (Vol. 2, pp. 39–55). Boston: Allyn & Bacon.

Grosz, E. (1989). *Sexual subversions: Three French Feminists*. St. Leanads, NSW, Australia: Allen & Unwin.

Hendricks, L. (2004, February 28). Havasupai file $25M suit vs. ASU. *Arizona Daily Sun*, p. A1.

Henrich, J., Heine, S. J., & Norenzayan, A. (2010). The weirdest people in the world? *Behavioral and Brain Sciences, 33*, 61–135.

Hillabrant, W. (2002). *Research in Indian Country: Challenges and changes*. In J. D. Davis, J. S. Erickson, S. R. Johnson, C. A. Marshall, P. Running Wolf, & R. L. Santiago (Eds.) (2002). *Work group on American Indian Research and Program*

Evaluation Methodology (AIRPEM), symposium on research and evaluation methodology: Lifespan issues related to American Indians/ Alaska Natives with disabilities (pp. 19–31). Flagstaff: Northern Arizona University, Institute for Human Development, Arizona University Center on Disabilities, American Indian Rehabilitation Research and Training Center.

Ho-Chunk Legislature. (2005). Tribal Research Code, Ho-Chunk Nation 3 HCC § 3 (2005).

Ibrahim, F. A., & Cameron, S. C. (2005). Racial-cultural ethical issues in research. In R. T. Carter (Ed.), *Handbook of racial-cultural psychology and counseling: Theory and research* (Vol. 1, pp. 391–414). Hoboken, NJ: Wiley.

Irving, D. (2014). *Waking up white*. Cambridge, MA: Elephant Room Press.

Kahneman, D. (2011). *Thinking, fast and slow*. New York: Farrar, Straus & Giroux.

Ladson-Billings, G. (1995). Toward a theory of culturally relevant pedagogy. *American Research Journal, 32*(3), 465–491.

LaDuke, W. (2005). *Recovering the sacred: The power of naming and claiming*. Cambridge, MA: Southend Press.

Letiecq, B. L., & Bailey, S. J. (2004). Evaluating from outside the circle: Conducting cross-cultural evaluation research on a Native American reservation. *Evaluation Review, 28*, 342–357.

Lyons, O. (1977). *Public address: A basic call to consciousness: The haudenosaunee address to the western world*. Geneva, Switzerland: The United Nations.

Lyons, O. (1993). R.C.A.P. Public Hearings, Akwesasne. Retrieved from http://sisis.nativeweborg/mohawk/ovide.html

Malgady, R. G. (1996). The question of cultural bias in assessment and diagnosis of ethnic minority clients: Let's reject the null hypothesis. *Professional Psychology: Research and Practice, 27*, 73–77.

Minkler, M., & Wallerstein, N. (Eds.) (2003). *Community-based participatory research for health*. San Francisco: Jossey-Bass.

Navajo Human Research Review Board. (2007a). *IRB research protocol application guidelines*. Window Rock: Navajo Division of Health, Author.

Navajo Human Research Review Board. (2007b). *Procedural guidelines for principal investigators*. Window Rock: Navajo Division of Health, Author.

Newbrough, J. R. (1995). Toward community: A third position. *American Journal of Community Psychology, 23*, 9–36.

Nichol, S. T., Spiropoulou, D. F., Morzunov, S., Rollin, P. E., Ksiazek, T. G., Feldman, H. Sanchez, A., Childs, J., Zaki, S., & Peters, C. J. (1993). Genetic identification of a hantavirus associated with an outbreak of acute respiratory illness. *Science, 262*(832), 834–836.

Norton, I. M., & Manson, S. M. (1996). Research in American Indian and Alaska Native communities: Navigating the cultural universe of values and process. *Journal of Consulting and Clinical Psychology, 64*, 856–860.

Ramirez, M. (1998). *Multicultural/multiracial psychology: Mestizo perspectives in personality and mental health*. New Jersey: Jason Aronson.

Reverby, S. M. (2011). "Normal exposure" and inoculation syphilis: A PHS "Tuskegee" doctor in Guatemala, 1946–1948. *Journal of Policy History, 23*, 6–28.

Rivkin, I. D., Lopez, E. D. S., Quaintance, T. M., Trimble, J. E., Hopkins, S., Fleming, C., Orr, E., & Mohatt, G. V. (2011). Value of community partnership for understanding stress and coping in rural Yup'ik communities: The CANHR study. *Journal of Health Disparities Research and Practice, 4*(3), 1–17.

Rogler, L. H. (1999). Methodological sources of cultural insensitivity in mental health research. *American Psychologist, 54*(6), 424–433.

Santiago-Rivera, A., Morse, G., Haase, R., & McCaffrey, R. (2007). Exposure to environmental contamination, quality of life, and psychological distress in a Native American Community. *Environmental Psychology, 7*, 33–43.

Santiago-Rivera, A. L., Morse, G. S., Hunt, A., & Lickers, H. (1998). Building a community-based research partnership: Lessons from the Mohawk Nation of Akwesasne. *Journal of Community Psychology, 26*, 163–174.Smith, L. T. (1999). *Decolonizing methodologies: Research and indigenous peoples*. New York: Zed Books.

Straits, K. J. E., Bird, D. M., Tsinajinnie, E., Espinoza, J., Goodkind, J., Spencer, O., Tafoya, N., Willging, C., & the Guiding Principles Workgroup. (2012). *Guiding principles for engaging in research with Native American communities*, Version 1. UNM Center for Rural and Community Behavioral Health & Albuquerque Area Southwest Tribal Epidemiology Center. Retrieved from http://psychiatry.unm.edu/centers/crcbh/naprogram/guidingprinciples.html

Tervalon, M., & Murray-García, J. (1998). Cultural humility versus cultural competence: A critical distinction in defining physician training outcomes in multicultural education. *Journal of Health Care for the Poor and Underserved, 9*(2), 117–129.

Tierney, P. (2001). *Darkness in El Dorado: How scientists and journalists devastated the Amazon*. New York: Norton.

Trimble, J. E. (1977). Research in American Indian communities: Methodological issues and concerns. *Journal of Social Issues, 33*(4), 159–174.

Trimble, J. E. (2013). Advancing understanding of cultural competence, cultural sensitivity, and the effects of cultural incompetence. In M. Prinstein, & M. Patterson (Eds.), *The portable mentor: Expert guide to a successful career in psychology* (2nd ed., pp. 57–80). New York: Kluwer Academic/Plenum.

Trimble, J. E., & Fisher, C. (Eds.) (2006). *Handbook of ethical and responsible research with ethnocultural populations and communities*. Thousand Oaks, CA: Sage.

Trimble, J. E., & Mohatt, G. V. (2006). Coda: The virtuous and responsible researcher in another culture. In J. E. Trimble, & C. B. Fisher (Eds.), *Handbook of ethical and responsible research with ethnocultural populations and communities* (pp. 325–334). Thousand Oaks, CA: Sage.

Trimble, J. E., Pedersen, P., & Rodela, R. (2009). The real cost of multicultural incompetence: An epilogue. In D. K. Deardorff (Ed.), *Handbook of intercultural competence* (pp. 492–503). Thousand Oaks, CA: Sage.

Trimble, J. E., Scharron-del Rio, M., & Casillas, D. (2013). Ethical matters and contentions in the principled conduct of research with ethnocultural communities. In F. T. L. Leong, L. Comas- Dias, G. N. Hall, V. McLloyd, V., & J. E. Trimble (Eds.), *Handbook of multicultural psychology* (Vols. I and II, pp. 59–82). Washington, DC: American Psychological Association.

Universal Declaration of Ethical Principles for Psychologists. (2009). Retrieved October 14, 2009, from the International Union of Psychological Science Web site: http://www.am.org/iupsys

Wallerstein, N., & Duran, B. (2003). The conceptual, historical, and practice roots of community based participatory research and related participatory traditions. In M. Minkler, & N. Wallerstein (Eds.), *Community-based participatory research for health* (pp. 27–52). San Francisco: Jossey-Bass.

Washington, H. A. (2006). *Medical apartheid: The dark history of medical experimentation on Black Americans from colonial times to the present*. New York: Doubleday.
Watkins, M., & Shulman, H. (2008). *Toward psychologies of liberation*. Basingstoke, England: Palgrave Macmillan.
Whitt, L. (2009). *Science, colonialism, and Indigenous peoples: The cultural politics of law and knowledge*. Cambridge, UK: Cambridge University Press.

Biographies

Asma-na-hi Antoine, MEd., Toquaht, Nuu-chah-nulth. My name Asma-na-hi, which means "Caring for Precious Ones." It was given to me at a naming potlatch by my late grandfather's brother Archie Thompson. The name is derived from my mother's roots from Nuu-chah-nulth lands of Toquaht Nation. My last name, Antoine, comes from my father's roots of Carrier Sekani lands of Saik'uz Nation. I am a proud member of the "House of Happiness," along with my husband and children. I have earned a master's degree in Education Psychology and Leadership Studies from the Aboriginal Communities Counselling Program, now known as the Indigenous Communities Counselling Program at the University of Victoria. I am the Manager of Indigenous Education & Student Services at Royal Roads University. My foundation, responsibilities, and practices are rooted in a holistic perspective and are supported by positive relationships with local First Nations communities and relevant local, provincial, and national organizations. I believe practicing and sharing traditional knowledge will bring a brighter future for the next generation to have equal opportunities and support to succeed.

Beth Boyd, Ph.D. is an enrolled member of the Seneca Nation of Indians and a Full Professor in the Clinical Psychology doctoral program at the University of South Dakota. She directs the USD Clinical Psychology Program and is a member of the Disaster Mental Health Institute. Dr. Boyd has responded to numerous disasters, working with the American Red Cross, SAMHSA, the Indian Health Service, and the DMHI. Dr. Boyd is a Past President of the Society for the Psychological Study of Culture, Ethnicity and Race (Division 45), and the Society for the Clinical Psychology of Ethnic Minorities (Division 12, Section VI) of the American Psychological Association. Other APA service includes the Board for the Advancement of Psychology in the Public Interest; the Presidential Task Force on PTSD and Trauma in Children and Adolescents; the Commission on Ethnic Minority Recruitment, Retention & Training Implementation Task Force; and the Minority Fellowship Program Training Advisory Committee.

Dale Brotherton, Ph.D. is a Professor at Western Carolina University where he has served as a Faculty Member, Program Director, and Department Head. He received his doctorate in Family Therapy from Florida State University. His research interests include developmental tasks facing couples and family across the life span, models of family functioning, and the use of metaphor and nature as a way of better understanding the client and the developing culturally based therapeutic interventions.

Derek Burks, Ph.D. is an Assistant Professor at the University of Texas Southwestern Medical Center within the Department of Psychiatry. He also serves as a Psychologist and Clinical Director of telemental health at the Veterans Affairs North Texas Health Care System. He received his doctorate in Counselling Psychology from the University of Oklahoma. His research interests include empathy in health care, humanistic factors in psychotherapy, and developing multiculturally competent therapeutic interventions.

Denise M. Casillas, MA is an enrolled member of the Cheyenne River Sioux Tribe. She is in the process of completing her Ph.D. in Clinical Psychology through the University of South Dakota. Her research interest focuses on the ethical research in Native American communities.

Michael Chandler is a Developmental Psychologist and Professor Emeritus working at the University of British Columbia. His ongoing program of research explores the role that culture plays in setting the course of identity development. In particular, his work has made it clear that both individual youth and entire Indigenous communities that lose a sense of their own personal and cultural continuity are at special risk of suicide and a host of other negative outcomes. These efforts have earned Dr. Chandler the Killam Memorial Senior Research Prize and the Killam Teaching Prize. He has also been named Canada's only Distinguished Investigator of both the Canadian Institutes of Health Research and the Michael Smith Foundation for Health Research, which resulted in his being chosen as a member of the Advisory Board of CIHR's Institute of Aboriginal Health. Professor Chandler's program of research dealing with identity development and suicide in Indigenous communities lead to his twice being named a Distinguished Fellow of the Peter Wall Institute for Advanced Studies—work singled out for publication as a book and an invited SRCD Monograph—the only program of Canadian research featured in WHO's recently released report on the social determinants of health.

Stephen Colmant is a Prescribing Psychologist and Faculty Member at the Southern New Mexico Residency Program in Las Cruces, NM. He completed a Ph.D. in Counselling Psychology at Oklahoma State University in 2005 and a post-doctorate Masters in Clinical Psychopharmacology in 2015. His two main areas of research have been understanding trauma in

Indian boarding schools and incorporating traditional healing practices (sweat therapy) into counselling and psychotherapy.

Eduardo Duran has been working in Indian Country for thirty years. He has been instrumental in developing clinical theory and methods that integrate ancient traditional approaches with modern Western strategies in an effort to make healing relevant to Native peoples. Duran has published several books and articles that are bringing much-needed dialogue to the discipline of psychology and is inspiring new interpretations to issues that afflict all human beings. In his latest book *Healing the Soul Wound* Duran takes traditional thought and metaphor and applies these towards the development of a hybrid epistemological approach that inspires a new vision for healing of our collective soul wounds.

Evan Allen Eason, Ph.D., ABPP, is a Counseling Psychologist and graduate of the Arkansas School for Mathematics and Sciences, Hendrix College, and Oklahoma State University. He is currently a Supervisory Psychologist for the PTSD Clinical Team at the Veterans Healthcare System of the Ozarks and an Adjunct Assistant Professor of Clinical Psychology at the University of Arkansas. He has worked in collaboration with the National Center for PTSD on the facilitation and implementation of evidence-based psychotherapies. Dr. Eason is proficient in CBCT-PTSD, CBT-I, CPT, DBT, MI, and PE evidence-based psychotherapies. He was formerly an Assistant Professor in Ethnic Studies and Multicultural Psychology at Kansas State University and has more than twenty refereed publications and regional, national, and international presentations. Multicultural areas of interest include dominant-minority relations, postcolonialism, microagressions, American Indians, Indigenous and non-Western healing, cross-cultural group sweating practices, religion/spirituality, and diversity in-group psychotherapy. Representative publications of possible interest to the current audience include "Diversity and Group Theory, Practice, and Research"; "Sweat Therapy Theory, Practice, and Efficacy"; and "Walking in Beauty: An American Indian Perspective on Social Justice."

Larry W. Emerson is Tsénahabiłnii, Tó'aheidlíiní. His cheis (paternal grandparents) are Hoghanłání and his maternal grandparents are Kiiyaa'áanii. He is a Community Activist, Farmer, Artist, and Scholar living in Tsédaak'áán, Diné Nation, east of Shiprock, New Mexico, Diné Nation. His 2003 Ph.D. is from the Joint Doctoral Program of San Diego State University and Claremont Graduate University in California. His dissertation was entitled *Hozhonahazdlii: Towards a Practice of Diné Decolonization*. His interest are in Indigenous studies and scholarship, social justice, decolonizing research methodologies, Diné peacemaking, education, and health.

Judith Firehammer is a Clinical Psychologist of Irish and Swiss ancestry who was born and raised in Montana. She completed a bachelor's degree in Photography at Montana State University and another in Psychology at the University of Montana before pursuing a career as a psychologist. She studied clinical psychology at the California School of Professional Psychology in the San Francisco Bay Area and completed her postdoctoral work with Indian Health Service in New Mexico. Over the past fifteen years, her work has been devoted to providing direct services to multicultural and underserved populations in community, educational, and medical settings. Her interests include resilience after trauma, issues affecting women, social justice, Jungian psychotherapy, creativity, and integrating spirituality in healing. She currently lives and works in Bozeman, Montana, with her husband and their two young daughters.

Melinda A. García is a Clinical, Community, and Organizational Psychologist of Meso-American Indigenous, European, and African descent. She has over forty years of experience in a variety of settings, including inpatient, outpatient, communities, organizations, and academia. She has many specialties because she is very curious and is always trying to puzzle out how everything relates to everything else. She enjoys sharing what she has learned with others in ways that are immediately applicable. Her approach integrates Indigenous, Western, and Eastern approaches to health. To honor her Elders and ancestors, she is a mentor, a musician, a seamstress, a beader, a writer, a storyteller, an activist, and a frustrated gardener. She is in independent practice in Albuquerque, New Mexico.

J. T. Garrett (Eastern Band of the Cherokee Nation) is Director of Public Health and Human Services for the Eastern Band of Cherokee Indians. He earned his Doctorate of Education in Public Health at the University of Tennessee at Knoxville. He has served for over forty years with organizations that include the Carteret County Health Department, the Indian Health Service/U.S. Public Health Service, the National Institute of Environmental Health Science, the Administration on Aging, and the Governor's Office for the North Carolina Commission on Indian Affairs. Dr. Garrett has authored *The Cherokee Herbal* (2003), *Cherokee Full Circle: A Practical Guide to Ceremonies and Traditions* (2002), *Meditations with the Cherokee: Prayers, Songs, and Stories of Healing and Harmony* (2001), and *Medicine of the Cherokee: The Way of Right Relationship* (1996), all published through Inner Traditions/Bear & Company.

Michael Tlanusta Garrett, Ph.D. (Eastern Band of the Cherokee Nation) is a Guidance Director and Certified School Counsellor with Broward County Public Schools in Fort Lauderdale, Florida. He received his doctorate in Counseling and Counsellor Education from UNC-Greensboro. His major research interests include exploring the relationship between cultural values, acculturation, and wellness with implications for developmental, culturally based therapeutic interventions; strength-based work to improve wellness and resilience of children, adolescents, and adults in families, schools, and communities; better understanding bicultural competence;

prevention of school dropouts and enhancing school persistence among at-risk youth; counselling Indigenous and other diverse populations; and spiritual issues in counselling.

Lisa Grayshield, Ph.D. (Washoe Nation) is Associate Professor of Counseling & Educational Psychology at New Mexico State University. She received her doctorate in Counsellor Education and Supervision from the University of Nevada—Reno. Her major research interests include Indigenous Ways of Knowing in counseling and psychology, with specific focus on the incorporation of Indigenous knowledge forms as viable options for the way counselling and psychology are conceptualized, taught, practiced, and researched.

Gawehogeh Wendy Hill, Cayuga Nation, Bear Clan. I work as a Traditional Healer in numerous Indigenous communities. I do one-on-one spiritual sessions to help people to come to a better place in their life situations and provide hands-on healing for physical problems. The other work I do is a variety of workshops on "Understanding the Spirit and Our Health," "Using the Good Mind," "Helping Young People with Their Self-Esteem," "Empowerment," "Colonization Effects on Parenting," "Spiritual Gifts." Other communities have utilized my skills to help with their relationship issues with band members, councillors, and conflicts in their communities. I was trained in Conflict Resolution twenty years ago while I worked in a women's prison in Kitchener. The training has stayed with me throughout my work in this field, and I have fine-tuned it for Native peoples' issues. The other training I provide is Effective/Compassionate Communication. I have been working in the relationship-building field for over twenty years, as I worked as a Cultural Resource Worker at the Pine Tree Native Centre. Being in this position, I was instrumental in teaching various non-Native and Native organizations/schools/police/governmental people history and cultural understandings to improve relationships. I have worked extensively with the local communities to help them to heal. Today I travel to many Native communities throughout North America bringing awareness and healing. I speak on prophecies and awareness of the needs of our spirit. My most important goal is to help others to learn to have a peaceful relationship with themselves and others.

Ashley Hyatt is a doctoral student in Clinical and Counselling Psychology at the Ontario Institute for Studies in Education at the University of Toronto. Ashley has been active in community-based Indigenous research and programming since beginning her undergraduate degree at University of Waterloo. Her area of research is life transitions for Aboriginal youth, especially in the areas of education and employment. She is deeply interested in creating and nurturing respectful relationships with the Aboriginal community both as an aspiring counsellor and as a researcher.

Gloria K. King, Navajo Nation, Rainbow Star Healing.

Jeff King is a Professor at Western Washington University's Department of Psychology, where he is also Director for the Center for Cross-Cultural Research. He is a licensed clinical psychologist and has provided clinical services to primarily American Indian populations for the past twenty-five years. He is also currently the President of the First Nations Behavioral Health Association, a non-profit organization that provides advocacy at the national level for cultural competence and the reduction in disparity in mental health care for Native Americans and other ethnic minority populations. Dr. King has published a number of chapters/articles regarding cultural competency, Western European culture/science and Indigenous knowledge, and cross-cultural assessment. He has also provided expert witness testimony regarding Indian child welfare, child custody, and abuse cases. Dr. King is a tribally enrolled member of the Muscogee (Creek) Nation of Oklahoma.

Colleen MacDougall was born in Virden, Manitoba, in 1981. She lived predominantly in Winnipeg until 2008. She has Scottish, Irish, and English ancestry. In 2008, she moved to Victoria, British Columbia, which lies on Coast Salish Territory, to pursue her master's in Counselling for Indigenous Communities. Colleen chose the specialized training after working in Winnipeg within Indigenous communities where she had transformative experiences with the families she had the honour to work with, which included traditional healing modalities and ceremony. Since graduating with her master's program in 2011, she has been working at Hulitan Family and Community Services Society in Victoria. She is currently working as a Child and Youth Mental Health Therapist in the L, KI, L Program. L, KI, L refers to "Confidence and the positive feeling arising from an appreciation of one's own ability" and originates from the SENĆOŦEN language of the W_SÁNEĆ people.

Anne Marshall is a Professor of Counselling Psychology in the Department of Educational Psychology and Leadership Studies (Faculty of Education) and Director of the Centre for Youth & Society at the University of Victoria, Canada. She is the co-developer of the Indigenous Communities Counselling Psychology (ICCP) graduate program, the first of its kind in Canada. Dr. Marshall's community-engaged research focuses on youth well-being, transitions, and mental health in cultural and community contexts. Much of her work involves Indigenous communities and marginalized youth. She is the co-author of *Knowledge Translation in Context: Indigenous, Policy, and Community Settings*, published in 2011 by University of Toronto Press.

Glen McCabe is a Métis man born and raised in Winnipeg's "inner city." He spent much time in the company of his Aboriginal relatives on the outskirts of Winnipeg learning the ways of community and healing. As a teenager and young adult, staff and members of Robertson United Church in Winnipeg's "inner city" mentored him. He earned his Ph.D. in Clinical Psychology from the University of Manitoba and was one of the first Canadian Aboriginal people to receive a doctorate in Clinical Psychology. He is currently a professor in Counselling Psychology at the University of Manitoba and is very involved in Indigenous advisory work there and in the community at large. He has been highly engaged in community development programs and is an invited guest at many conferences as a keynote speaker on the topic of Indigenous human rights and healing. He was the Regional Mental Health Consultant with First Nations and Inuit Health in Manitoba. He is one of the founding members of the Aboriginal Health and Wellness Centre in downtown Winnipeg and has been designated as a Fire Keeper and Knowledge Keeper in the Aboriginal community of Manitoba. He also provides consultative and therapeutic psychological healing services at the community level. One of his articles, "Mind, Body, Emotions and Spirit: Reaching to the Ancestors for Healing," is one of the most sought out and read articles of its type anywhere. Dr. McCabe is also an accomplished musician and songwriter, often using Indigenous themes in his creative work.

Brenda McDaniel is Assistant Professor in the Department of Psychology at Oklahoma State University.

Terry Mitchell is an associate professor of Community Psychology at Wilfrid Laurier University and the Balsillie School of International Affairs. She is also a registered Clinical Psychologist with a private practice. She is the Director of the Laurier Indigenous Rights and Social Justice Research Group and past Director, and current Board Member of the Laurier Centre for Community Research Learning and Action. She was a Visiting Scholar at the Institute of Indigenous Studies at the Universidad de La Frontera in Chile. Her research focuses on colonial trauma, Indigenous rights, and resource governance.

Roy Moodley, Ph.D., is Associate Professor of Counselling Psychology at the Ontario Institute for Studies in Education, University of Toronto, Canada, and Director of the Centre for Diversity in Counselling and Psychotherapy. His research interests include critical multicultural counseling/psychotherapy; race and culture in psychotherapy; traditional healing practices; gender and identity. He is the author/editor or co-editor of several books, including *Integrating Traditional Healing Practices into Counseling and Psychotherapy* (Sage, 2005) and *Caribbean Healing Traditions: Implications for Health and Mental Health* (Routledge, 2013).

Gayle S. Morse (Gayle Skawen:nio Morse) is the current Director of the Community Counseling Program at the Sage Colleges. She has also conducted research examining the effects of polychlorinated biphenyls and other toxic chemicals on human health. Currently she is looking at the neurological effects of toxic chemicals and disability as well as treatments for toxic exposure. Dr. Morse is a Member of the American Psychological Association (APA) and is the current Chair of the Board for the Advancement of Psychology in the Public Interest and the President-Elect of the Society of Indian Psychologists. Finally, she is an enrolled member of the Mohawk Tribe, and draws from the tribe the principles of respect, trust, and empowerment that have guided her both professionally and personally.

Linda O'Neill is an Associate Professor in Counselling at the University of Northern British Columbia in Prince George, British Columbia, and a Community Trauma Counsellor. Before moving into academia, she lived for twenty-five years in a small northern community in British Columbia where she became a passionate supporter for Aboriginal youth in the education system. In this northern setting, she also became an ally through mentorship from Elders and other community members. Linda and her research teams have worked to develop trauma-informed training for all helping practitioners in her efforts to ensure that survivors of adverse events are supported to live life fully with less trauma symptoms and to assist helping practitioners in sustaining their work with survivors.

Olga Oulanova is a registered Clinical and Rehabilitation Psychologist working in private practice in Toronto, Ontario. She completed her Ph.D. in Clinical/Counselling Psychology at the University of Toronto. Dr. Oulanova's research and publications have focused on the exploration of the healing process following suicide bereavement, the integration of alternative and complementary healing practices with psychotherapy, and medical education. Dr. Oulanova teaches part-time at OISE/University of Toronto.

Ruby Peterson (Pankwa'las), MEd was raised by her mother and grandparents in Alert Bay, British Columbia, and she is a proud 'N*a*mgis First Nations member. She has traveled extensively and has worked for over twenty years in the social service and counselling sectors of practice, working with children, youth, and families and developing community wellness initiatives. She completed a Bachelor of Social Work degree in 2000 and a Masters of Education in Aboriginal Community Counselling in 2011. She is passionate about voicing the need to include the history of colonial policy and its impacts in context Aboriginal community wellness needs, which is also a part of her own healing story. Her counselling focus is largely on trauma, grief, and abuse, with special interest in the legacy of intergenerational trauma, abuse suicides, and addiction. She enjoys volunteering and giving back to community where she can and is grateful to her Elders and teachers for the lessons she has learned about traditional Indigenous knowledge wellness teachings. Her family is her pride and joy, and she takes great joy in the gift of being a mom and an auntie. Her family recently moved to West Kelowna, British Columbia, where she now works with Okanagan Nation Alliance as the Syilx Residential School Support Lead.

Tarrell Awe Agahe Portman, Ph.D. (White River Cherokee) is Professor and Dean of the College of Education at Winona State University. She received her doctorate in Counsellor Education from the University of Arkansas-Fayetteville. Her major research interests include translation of theory to practice in counselling as it interacts with three specific areas of counsellor development: supervision and consultation, multiculturalism (particularly American Indians and giftedness), and education reform (action research in education).

Allison Reeves earned her Ph.D. in Clinical and Counselling Psychology at the University of Toronto (Ontario Institute for Studies in Education), where her research focused on recovery from colonial and intergenerational traumas among Indigenous peoples. Specifically, she studied recovery from sexual abuse and complex trauma using principles and methods of Indigenous healing. Her CIHR-funded postdoctoral fellowship looked at unique considerations for healing among Indigenous men. She is currently the Staff Psychologist at Anishnawbe Health Toronto where she continues to carry out community-based research. She also teaches health courses at two Canadian universities.

Rockey Robbins, Ph.D. (Cherokee/Choctaw) is an Associate Professor at the University of Oklahoma, where he teaches multicultural counselling, behaviour disorders, and personality assessment. He has published over fifty articles in psychology and education journals during his twelve-year experience as a professor. His research areas include re-norming psychological instruments for use with American Indians, means of coping for Indian students in boarding schools, needs of therapists who work with Indian clients, and studies that focus on American Indian family resiliency. The area in which he is currently doing most of his research is in American Indian spirituality. He is currently working on articles related to traditional American Indian spirituality as it is related to psychological health, an American Indian spirituality development model, and Christian colonialization. He has also published five programs: Through the Diamond Threshold, Leadership Skills Building with Indian adolescents, an Indian Women's Identity group, Family Therapy with American Indians, and a Prevention Program for Cherokees. He has conducted hundreds of workshops and speaking engagements across the United States and Europe related to American Indian topics.

Mary Lou Smoke, LL.D. (Hon). Mary Lou Smoke's spirit name is *Asayenes Kwe* (Shooting Star Woman). She is of the Bear Clan and is from Batchawana Bay First Nation. Mary Lou is also an accomplished singer and makes use of traditional Anishnabec forms of music within her healing practice and service to Indigenous communities. She is an Adjunct Professor at Western University. She is a media activist and cohosts the Smoke Signals CHRW Radio Program from London, Ontario.

Dan Smoke, LL. D. (Hon). Dan Smoke is the life partner of Mary Lou, and Dan's spirit name is also *Asayenes* (Star Falling in Flight). He is from the Snipe Clan, from the Six Nations Grand River Territory. Both he and Mary Lou travel widely across North America, offering their traditional teachings and traditional healing practices to anyone seeking assistance. He is an Adjunct Professor at Western University. He is a media activist and cohosts the Smoke Signals CHRW Radio Program from London, Ontario.

Suzanne L. Stewart, Ph.D. is a leading scholar in the field of counselling psychology, whose work was among the first to address Aboriginal social problems within the field of psychology using an *Aboriginal knowledges* perspective. Dr. Stewart is a member of the Yellowknife Dene First Nation of Canada. She is a registered Psychologist and Associate Professor in Counselling Psychology at the Ontario Institute for Studies in Education, University of Toronto, where she is also Special Advisor to the Dean on Aboriginal Education. Dr. Stewart's research and teaching interest include Indigenous mental health and healing in psychology (homelessness, youth mental health, identity, and work-life development) and Indigenous pedagogies in teacher education, higher education, and psychotherapy practice/training. She currently holds the Canada Research Chair in Aboriginal Homelessness and Life Transitions and is committed to advancing Indigenous healing through the discipline of psychology and through influencing policy change at all levels.

Edil Torres-Rivera, has a Ph.D. in Counselling Psychology with a concentration in multicultural counseling from the University of Connecticut, Storrs. He is a Professor at the Chicago School of Professional Psychology, Chicago Campus. Edil Torres-Rivera is a native Puerto Rican with a career of over twenty years in counseling. This includes twelve years in the U.S. Army. Dr. Torres-Rivera's research interests are in multicultural counseling, group work, chaos theory, liberation psychology, Indigenous counselling, Puerto Rican studies, identity development, and gang/prison-related behaviour. Specifically, his primary research focuses on complexity and how Indigenous healing techniques are a necessary ingredient when working with ethnic minority populations in the United States. Dr. Torres-Rivera has additional interests in studying the implications of social injustice and oppression in counselling and psychotherapy with ethnic minorities in the United States. His community work includes consultation services to the Pyramid Lake Paiute Tribe Council in Nevada, Visiting Professor to the Universidad del Valle, Guatemala, and former Director of the Graduate School of Education's School Counseling Program in Singapore.

Joseph E. Trimble, Ph.D., is a Distinguished University Professor and Professor of Psychology at Western Washington University, also he is a President's

Professor at the Center for Alaska Native Health Research at the University of Alaska Fairbanks. He was a former Senior Scholar at the Tri-Ethnic Center for Prevention Research at Colorado State University and a Research Associate for the National Center for American Indian and Alaska Native Mental Health Research at the University of Colorado Health Sciences Center. From 2000 to 2001, he was a Fellow and Visiting Professor at the Radcliffe Institute for Advanced Studies at Harvard University Throughout his long career, he has focused his efforts on promoting psychological and sociocultural mental health research with Indigenous populations, especially American Indians and Alaska Natives. Since 1972, he has continuously served as a member of numerous scientific review committees and research panels for several federal agencies. He is the editor or author of 20 books and over 140 journal articles and chapters and the recipient of 20 fellowships, awards, and honors.

Barbara Waterfall, B.A., RSW, M.S.W., Ph.D. Barbara Waterfall is of Métis-Anishnabec background. She carries two spirit names, *Waabshki Mshkode Bzhiki Kwe* (White Buffalo Woman) and *Zaawaa Nimkii Aankwad Kwe* (Yellow Thundercloud Woman). She is a member of the Crane Clan. She is an accomplished singer and songwriter and employs traditional Anishnabec music within her healing practice. She is currently the Coordinator and a Professor in the Indigenous Wellness & Addictions Prevention Program at Canadore College in North Bay, Ontario. She has thirty years of experience in the human services field and has taught for eighteen years in both the university and community college systems. Her areas of specialization are in addictions recovery, trauma, Indigenous-centred teaching and practice, and the inclusion of spirituality in teaching and practice.

Lorna Williams (Lorna Wanosts'a7 Williams), OBC is Lil'wat. Her life has been devoted to promoting and restoring Indigenous culture and language. She worked as an Indigenous educator and language specialist for more than fifty years in diverse settings, including Indigenous communities, public schools, and adult education settings. Dr. Williams recently retired from the University of Victoria as Associate Professor and Canada Research Chair in Indigenous Knowledge and Learning (co-appointment with Faculty of Education and Department of Linguistics).

Index

For Product Safety Concerns and Information please contact our EU representative GPSR@taylorandfrancis.com
Taylor & Francis Verlag GmbH, Kaufingerstraße 24, 80331 München, Germany

www.ingramcontent.com/pod-product-compliance
Ingram Content Group UK Ltd.
Pitfield, Milton Keynes, MK11 3LW, UK
UKHW021429080625
459435UK00011B/208

* 9 7 8 0 3 6 7 1 9 6 1 5 8 *